# Novel food ingredients for weight control

**Related titles:**

*Food, diet and obesity*
(ISBN 978-1-85573-958-1)
Obesity is a global epidemic, with large proportions of adults and children overweight or obese in many developed and developing countries. As a result, there is an unprecedented level of interest and research on the complex interactions between our genetic susceptibility, diet and lifestyle in determining individual risk of obesity. With its distinguished editor and international team of contributors, this collection sums up the key themes in weight control research, focusing on their implications and applications for food product development and consumers.

*Improving the fat content of foods*
(ISBN 978-1-85573-965-9)
Dietary fats have long been recognised as having a major impact on health, negative in the case of consumers' excessive intake of saturated fatty acids, positive in the case of increasing consumers' intake of long chain n-3 polyunsaturated fatty acids. However, progress in ensuring that consumers achieve a nutritionally optimal fat intake has been slow. This important collection reviews the range of steps needed to improve the fat content of foods whilst maintaining sensory quality.

*Benders' dictionary of nutrition and food technology (8th edition)*
(ISBN 978-1-84569-051-9)
A new edition of this classic reference work. Updated to reflect recent advances in food science (for example an increased number of entries on genetics) and with broader coverage of food technology, this dictionary will remain an essential tool for all those who work in nutrition and food sciences.

Details of these books and a complete list of Woodhead's titles can be obtained by:

- visiting our web site at www.woodheadpublishing.com
- contacting Customer Services (e-mail: sales@woodhead-publishing.com; fax: +44 (0) 1223 893694; tel.: +44 (0) 1223 891358 ext. 130; address: Woodhead Publishing Ltd, Abington Hall, Abington, Cambridge CB21 6AH, England)

# Novel food ingredients for weight control

Edited by
C. J. K. Henry

CRC Press
Boca Raton Boston New York Washington, DC

WOODHEAD PUBLISHING LIMITED
Cambridge England

Published by Woodhead Publishing Limited, Abington Hall, Abington, Cambridge CB21 6AH, England
www.woodheadpublishing.com

Published in North America by CRC Press LLC, 6000 Broken Sound Parkway, NW, Suite 300, Boca Raton, FL 33487, USA

First published 2007, Woodhead Publishing Limited and CRC Press LLC


British Library Cataloguing in Publication Data
A catalogue record for this book is available from the British Library.

Library of Congress Cataloging in Publication Data
A catalog record for this book is available from the Library of Congress.

Woodhead Publishing ISBN 978-1-84569-030-4 (book)
Woodhead Publishing ISBN 978-1-84569-311-4 (e-book)
CRC Press ISBN 978-0-8493-9147-7
CRC Press order number WP9147

The publishers' policy is to use permanent paper from mills that operate a sustainable forestry policy, and which has been manufactured from pulp which is processed using acid-free and elementary chlorine-free practices. Furthermore, the publishers ensure that the text paper and cover board used have met acceptable environmental accreditation standards.

Typeset by SNP Best-set Typesetter Ltd., Hong Kong
Printed by TJ International Limited, Padstow, Cornwall, England

# Contents

# Contributor contact details

(* = main contact)

**Editor**
C. J. K. Henry
Oxford Brookes University
Headington Campus
Gipsy Lane
Oxford
OX3 0BP
UK

email: jhenry@brookes.ac.uk

## Chapter 1

Monika Leonhardt* and Wolfgang Langhans
Institute of Animal Sciences
ETH Zürich
Schorenstrasse 16
8603 Schwerzenbach
Switzerland

email: monika-leonhardt@ethz.ch

## Chapter 2

Henk F. J. Hendriks*, Gertruud C. M. Bakker, Wilrike J. Pasman, Annette Stafleu and Wendy A. M. Blom
TNO Quality of Life
P.O. Box 360
3700 AJ Zeist
The Netherlands

email: henk.hendriks@tno.nl

## Chapter 3

Isabelle Aeberli* and Michael B. Zimmermann
Institute of Food Science and Nutrition
Human Nutrition, LFV D11
ETH Zürich
8092 Zürich
Switzerland

email: isabelle.aeberli@ilw.agrl.ethz.ch

## Chapter 4

Andreu Palou* and M. Luisa Bonet
Departament de Biologia Fonamental i Cienciès de la Salut
Universitat de les Illes Balears
Crta. Valldemossa Km 7.5
07122 Palma de Mallorca
Baleares
Spain

email: andreu.palou@uib.es

## Chapter 5

G. Harvey Anderson*, Tina Akhavan and Rena Mendelson*
Department of Nutritional Sciences
Faculty of Medicine
University of Toronto
150 College Street
M5S 3E2
Toronto
ON, Canada

email: harvey.anderson@utoronto.ca
mendelso@ryerson.ca

## Chapter 6

Julie-Anne Nazare*, Martine Laville*, Costas G. Biliaderis, Athina Lazaridou, Gunilla Önning, Marjatta Salmenkallio-Marttila and Angeliki Triantafyllou
Centre de Recherche en Nutrition Humaine Rhône-Alpes*
Faculté de Médecine RTH Laennec
8, rue Guillaume Paradin
69372 Lyon cedex 08
France

email: julie-anne.nazare@recherche.univ-lyon1.fr
martine.laville@chu-lyon.fr

## Chapter 7

Nathalie M. Delzenne*, Patrice D. Cani, Evelyne Delmée and Audrey M. Neyrinck
Unit of Pharmacokinetics, Metabolism, Nutrition and Toxicology
Université catholique de Louvain
Avenue Mounier 73
PMNT 7369 1200 Brussels
Belgium

email: delzenne@pmnt.ucl.ac.be

## Chapter 8

Anne M. Birkett*
National Starch Food Innovation
10 Finderne Avenue
Bridgewater
New Jersey 08807
USA

email: anne.birkett@nstarch.com

and

Ian L. Brown
University of Colorado
Health Sciences Center, Denver
Colorado 80262
USA

email: ian.brown@clovercorp.com.au

## Chapter 9

Bruce R. Hamaker*, Genyi Zhang and Mahesh Venkatachalam
Whistler Center for Carbohydrate Research
Department of Food Science
Purdue University
West Lafayette
Indiana 47907-2009
USA

email: hamakerb@purdue.edu

## Chapter 10

Julian D. Stowell
Danisco Sweeteners
41–51 Brighton Road
Redhill
Surrey
RH1 6YS
UK

email: julian.stowell@danisco.com

## Chapter 11

Gerhard Gerstner*
Jungbunzlauer Ladenburg GmbH
Dr.-Albert-Reimann-Str. 18
DE-68526 Ladenburg
Germany

email: gerhard.gerstner@jungbunzlauer.com

and

Michael de Vrese
Federal Research Center for Nutrition and Food
Kiel
Germany

## Chapter 12

J. L. Sebedio
UMR, 1019 INRA-Université d'Auvergne
Unité de Nutrition Humaine
58 rue Montalembert
63122 St Genès Champanelle
France

email: jls@clermont.inra.fr

## Chapter 13

Maria Sörhede Winzell and Bo Ahrén*
Department of Clinical Sciences, Medicine
Lund University
BMC, B11
SE-221 84 Lund
Sweden

email: Bo.Ahren@med.lu.se

## Chapter 14

Iwona Rudkowska and Peter J. H. Jones*
Richardson Centre for Functional Foods and Nutraceuticals
196 Innovation Drive
University of Manitoba, Smartpark
Winnipeg
MB
R3T 2N2
Canada

email: peter.jones@mcgill.ca

## Chapter 15

Eckhard Flöter and Gerrit van Duijn*
Unilever Research & Development
Room A6411
P.O. Box 114
3130 AC Vlaardingen
The Netherlands

email: Gerrit-van.Duijn@unilever.com

# Preface

Obesity and type 2 diabetes have become major public health concerns worldwide with an exponential increase in numbers over recent years. Currently (2007) there are more than a billion overweight adults, surpassing the number of under nourished adults for the first time in human history. Obesity is not merely a problem of the developed world, but also of the developing world – notably China, India and South America. As obesity and diabetes are intimately interlinked, their management and treatment may need to be considered together. It is now well recognised that the etiology of obesity is multi-factorial, and that foods we consume may have a contributory role. It is with this in mind that the current book has been developed.

The book is largely organised into the following themes:

- Part I discusses ingredients implicated in the body's response to appetite and satiety;
- Part II concentrates on ingredients derived from cereals, fruits and vegetables that can assist in weight control;
- Part III details ingredients such as calcium, CLA and *trans*-free oils and fats that may contribute to regulate body weight.

This unique book has brought together many key researchers on new product development for weight management and should serve as a ready reference for those interested and involved in the development of foods for weight management.

I am privileged to have collaborated with some of the most gifted international scientists working on the development of specific products and ingredients that may help control body weight. I unreservedly thank all the contributors for their unbridled support in sharing their expertise. We hope that readers will find the book a useful resource to combat the global pandemic of obesity.

*C. J. K. Henry*
*Oxford*

# Part I

# Food and obesity

# 1

# Lipid metabolism: its role in energy regulation and obesity

**M. Leonhardt and W. Langhans, ETH Zürich, Switzerland**

## 1.1 Introduction

Fat is an important macronutrient. It provides substrates for energy turnover, is an integral part of biological membranes and regulates gene expression (Jump *et al.* 2005). In the Western world dietary fats constitute about 40% of human energy intake (Mu and Hoy 2004), and several studies have revealed a positive relationship between the level of fat intake and body weight in humans (Bray and Popkin 1998; Astrup *et al.* 2000; Saris *et al.* 2000; Satia-Abouta *et al.* 2002; Huot *et al.* 2004; Mosca *et al.* 2004). High-fat diets may increase the obesity risk because of: (a) the usually high energy density of such diets (Rolls 2000; Westerterp-Plantenga 2001), (b) the often high palatability of fat-rich foods (Drewnowski 1998) and (c) the finding that fats seem to have a lower short-term satiating capacity than carbohydrates [for review see Blundell and Stubbs (1999)].

Obesity is now a global health problem of epidemic proportions. Worldwide more than 1.1 billion adults and 10% of all children are currently classified as overweight or obese (Haslam and James 2005). Although the important contribution of high fat intake to the development of obesity is widely accepted, it is also clear that fat cannot be the only culprit [for review see Willett (1998)]. The tremendous increase in obesity is – in addition to a high fat intake – related to genetic susceptibility and decreased physical activity (Kopelman 2000). Obesity is a major risk for chronic diseases including type 2 diabetes, coronary heart disease and different forms of cancer (Kopelman 2000; Haslam and James 2005).

This review focuses on lipid metabolism including *de novo* lipogenesis (DNL), and on the role of adipose tissue as an endocrine organ.

Pharmacological and dietary substances that inhibit fatty acid synthesis are presented and their potential for the treatment of obesity is discussed.

## 1.2 Lipid metabolism: from digestion and synthesis to storage

The most important lipid components of our diet are triacylglycerols (TAG, about 100 g/day), followed by phospholipids (about 5 g/day) and small amounts of glycerolipids, sterols and fat-soluble vitamins (Mu and Hoy 2004). The efficiency of the organism in digesting and absorbing TAG is very high (about 95%). TAG consist of a glycerol molecule acylated with three fatty acids. The positions are numbered by the stereochemical numbering system, i.e. fatty acids may be designated sn1-, sn2- and sn3-. In human diets the fatty acids vary in chain length from C2 to C24, and from saturated to unsaturated fatty acids with up to six double bonds (Mu and Porsgaard 2005). Quantitatively relevant fat sources in the diet are oils – such as olive oil, soybean oil and fish oil – milk fat and adipose tissue of certain animals including marine species (Mu and Hoy 2004).

Fat digestion occurs in the stomach and intestine. After chewing, a food bolus is formed and transported to the stomach, where a partial hydrolysis of TAG into diacylglycerols and free fatty acids (FFA) takes place (Mu and Hoy 2004). In humans the lipases in the stomach, are derived from the tongue (lingual lipase) or from the stomach, with gastric lipase being the predominant enzyme (Denigris *et al.* 1988; Hamosh 1990). Gastric predigestion accounts for about 15% of fat digestion and facilitates the digestion process in the small intestine. Pancreatic lipase is the major contributor to TAG hydrolysis (Lowe 1997). The appearance of TAG degradation products in the proximal intestine causes gall bladder emptying, pancreatic lipase secretion and cholecystokinin release (Meyer and Jones 1974; Watanabe *et al.* 1988). TAG are emulsified by bile acids, which are strong detergents, markedly increasing the available surface for pancreatic lipase binding, hence promoting TAG digestion. The degradation process is region-specific and ideally results in the formation of sn2-monoacylglycerols and FFA, which are then absorbed by enterocytes (Mu and Hoy 2004). In the smooth endoplasmic reticulum of the enterocytes, new TAG are synthesized and lipoproteins are formed, which are subsequently secreted into the lymph. Two major lipoproteins are secreted by the intestine: chylomicrons (CM) and very low density lipoproteins (VLDL). CMs are TAG-rich lipoproteins synthesized in the small intestine after a meal to transport lipids, whereas VLDL are formed during fasting when the level of exogenous lipids is too low to drive CM formation. Intestinal lipoproteins are secreted into tiny lymph vessels inside each of the intestinal villi, and then enter the circulation in the subclavian vein via the thoracic duct (Mu and Hoy 2004; Williams *et al.* 2004). Nevertheless, not all lipids are transported via lymphatics, and some can also be transported directly to the liver via the hepatic portal vein. The most important factor affecting the portal–lymph distribution is the chain length of fatty acids: short- and medium-chain fatty acids are mainly transported via the portal vein, whereas long-chain fatty acids are transported via the lymphatic system (St Onge and Jones 2002). Lipoprotein lipase located at or close to the capillary endothelial wall in extra-hepatic tissues, such as heart, skeletal muscle and adipose tissue, rapidly hydrolyzes circulating CM TAG. The resulting CM remnants are recognized and removed by the liver. The action of lipoprotein lipase provides FFA and 2-monoacylglycerols for tissue utilization. In white adipose tissue, FFA are re-esterified with glucose-derived glycerol-3-phosphate for the storage of energy as TAG, whereas in other tissues FFA are mainly oxidized to drive cell metabolism or thermogenesis (Mead *et al.* 2002).

## 1.3 Adipose tissue

White adipose tissue was long seen as a passive reservoir for the storage of fat derived from the diet or from endogenous synthesis. Meanwhile it is clear that white adipose tissue is also an important endocrine organ [for review see Kershaw and Flier (2004)]. The proteins that are produced and released by adipose tissue are called adipokines. It is important to note that white adipose tissue is not a homogeneous organ. The two best-described adipose tissue depots are subcutaneous and visceral adipose tissues. FFA, glycerol and hormones from visceral adipose tissue are directly released into the hepatic portal vein and thus have direct access to the liver, whereas the subcutaneous fat depots release their adipokines and metabolites into the systemic circulation. Therefore it is clear that visceral adipose tissue has a greater effect on hepatic metabolism than subcutaneous adipose tissue. Finally, the two adipose tissues have different adipokine secretion patterns, with visceral adipose tissue secreting mainly interleukin-6 (IL-6) and plasminogen activator inhibitor (PAI), whereas the secretion of leptin and adiponectin is relatively greater from subcutaneous than from visceral adipose tissue. Furthermore, visceral and subcutaneous adipocytes also carry different receptors on their surfaces and, hence, respond differently to signals. For example, expression of β3-adrenergic, glucocorticoid, and androgen receptors is greater in visceral than in subcutaneous adipose tissue. All these differences might contribute to the fact that enlarged visceral but not subcutaneous adipose tissue is associated with increased risk for several diseases and in particular the metabolic syndrome (Kershaw and Flier 2004). In the following section we will discuss the most important proteins secreted by white adipose tissue.

### 1.3.1 Adipose tissue-derived proteins

*Leptin*

Leptin was first characterized in 1994 (Zhang *et al.* 1994) and is one of the most important adipose tissue-derived hormones (Stanley *et al.* 2005). Leptin is the product of the *ob* gene which is predominantly expressed in adipocytes (Zhang *et al.* 1994), but also in gastric epithelium (Bado *et al.* 1998) and placenta (Masuzaki *et al.* 1997). The name 'leptin' has its roots in the Greek word 'leptos', meaning thin, and leptin was initially viewed as an adipocyte-derived signal that functions primarily to prevent obesity (Flier 2004). Indeed, the effects of leptin on energy homeostasis are well documented: exogenous leptin administration, both centrally and peripherally reduces food intake and increases energy expenditure (Friedman and Halaas 1998; Rosenbaum and Leibel 1998; Kershaw and Flier 2004). Adipocytes secrete leptin, however, in direct proportion to adipocyte size, and the majority of obese animals and humans have increased plasma leptin instead of an absolute or relative leptin deficiency (Kershaw and Flier 2004). Furthermore, short-term fasting results in a larger suppression of circulating leptin than would be expected from the loss of fat mass alone (Dubuc *et al.* 1998; Mars *et al.* 2005, 2006). A more recent concept proposes that a decrease in plasma leptin concentration might serve as an important signal from fat to brain informing the brain that the body is starving. Consequently, in the absence of leptin, the brain senses energy deficiency despite massive obesity and thus leptin's primary role may be as a hormone of starvation rather than one of plenty (Flier 2004).

Leptin signals via a single-transmembrane-domain receptor. Alternative mRNA splicing and post-translational processing results in multiple isoforms of the receptor (Ob-R), such as the long, short and secreted form of the Ob-R (Stanley *et al.* 2005). Many effects of leptin on food intake and energy expenditure are mediated primarily via hypothalamic pathways. It is therefore hardly surprising that the long form of the Ob-R is expressed widely within the hypothalamus, in particular in the arcuate nucleus (ARC), but also in areas of the brain stem that are involved in the control of food intake. Two major types of ARC neurons carry the long form of the Ob-R: (1) neurons expressing the orexigenic neuropeptides neuropeptide Y (NPY) and agouti-related peptide (AgRP), and (2) neurons expressing proopiomelanocortin (POMC) and cocaine- and amphetamine-regulated transcript (CART). Through the Ob-R, leptin inhibits the activity of orexigenic NPY/AgRP neurons and activates anorectic POMC/CART neurons. The absence of leptin action has profound effects on body weight. Lack of circulating leptin or of functional leptin receptors due to mutations in the pertinent genes leads to hyperphagia, obesity and neuroendocrine disturbances. This holds for the leptin- or leptin receptor-deficient *ob/ob* or *db/db* mouse, but also for genetic leptin deficiency in humans. The lack of leptin phenotype can be ameliorated by administration of exogenous leptin (Stanley *et al.* 2005). Finally, leptin has many functions besides control of energy homeostasis: it regulates the onset of puberty, promotes proliferation and differentiation of hematopoic cells, alters cytokine production by immune cells, stimulates endothelial cell growth and angiogenesis, and accelerates wound healing (Kershaw and Flier 2004).

*Adiponectin*

Adiponectin, also called adipocyte complement-related protein (Acrp30) or adipose most abundant gene transcript (apM1), is a protein hormone with circulating blood levels that are up to 1000-fold higher than those of other hormones such as leptin and insulin (Stanley *et al.* 2005).

The exact function of adiponectin is largely unknown, but it is postulated to regulate energy homeostasis (Stanley *et al.* 2005): peripheral administration of adiponectin to rodents has been shown to attenuate body weight gain by increasing oxygen consumption without affecting food intake (Berg *et al.* 2001; Fruebis *et al.* 2001; Yamauchi *et al.* 2001; Yang *et al.* 2001). The plasma concentration of adiponectin is inversely correlated with adiposity in primates (Hotta *et al.* 2001) including humans (Yang *et al.* 2001; Faraj *et al.* 2003). Furthermore, plasma adiponectin increases during food restriction in rodents (Berg *et al.* 2001) including after weight loss induced by a calorie-restricted diet (Hotta *et al.* 2000) or gastric partition surgery in obese humans (Yang *et al.* 2001).

Plasma adiponectin levels correlate negatively with insulin resistance (Hotta *et al.* 2001), and adiponectin knock-out mice demonstrate severe diet-induced insulin resistance (Stanley *et al.* 2005), suggesting that adiponectin improves insulin sensitivity. Recently, two distinct adiponectin receptors have been cloned: adipoR1, which is highly expressed in skeletal muscle, and adipoR2, which is highly expressed in the liver. Adiponectin receptors have also been detected in the hypothalamus (Qi *et al.* 2004). All in all, adiponectin or potent adipoR agonists might have potential for the treatment of diabetes and obesity.

*Resistin*

Resistin was identified in 2001 (Steppan *et al.* 2001), and rodent studies confirmed its adipose tissue-specific expression. Circulating resistin is increased in obese rodents (Rajala *et al.* 2004) and it appears to increase insulin resistance (Steppan *et al.* 2001; Banerjee and Lazar 2003). Mice lacking resistin have similar body weight as wild-type mice, but they exhibit lower blood glucose levels after fasting, due to reduced hepatic glucose production (Banerjee *et al.* 2004). Recently, Graveleau *et al.* (2005) demonstrated that resistin directly impaired glucose transport in primary mouse cardiomyocytes. All these findings suggest that resistin contributes to the development of insulin resistance in obese rodents. Nevertheless, whether resistin also plays a role in human obesity and diabetes is still unclear (Banerjee and Lazar 2003).

*Acylation-stimulating protein*

Acylation-stimulating protein (ASP) is produced in white adipose tissue and its synthesis requires three proteins: C3, adipsin and factor B (Faraj *et al.* 2004). ASP promotes fatty acid uptake and TAG synthesis, and it decreases lipolysis and FFA release from adipocytes (Cianflone *et al.* 2003). ASP-deficient mice are hyperphagic, but their energy expenditure is increased resulting in reduced body fat compared with wild-type mice (Xia *et al.* 2004). Also, these mice are resistant to diet-induced weight gain (Rajala and Scherer 2003). Several human studies indicate that ASP positively correlates with adiposity and insulin resistance (Cianflone *et al.* 2003). Consistent with this finding, plasma ASP levels decrease with body weight loss (Faraj *et al.* 2003).

*Tumor necrosis factor-α*

Adipocytes are a predominant source of tumor necrosis factor α (TNF-α) and express both types of TNF-α receptors (Faraj *et al.* 2004). The association of TNF-α with type 2 diabetes and insulin resistance is well documented (Hotamisligil *et al.* 1993; Ruan and Lodish 2003), and mice lacking TNF-α function are protected from obesity-induced insulin resistance (Uysal *et al.* 1997). TNF-α reduces insulin signaling in many peripheral tissues such as liver, muscles and white adipose tissue (Faraj *et al.* 2004). In adipose tissue, TNF-α represses genes involved in the uptake and storage of FFA and lipogenesis, whereas it increases expression of genes favoring FFA and cytokine release (Ruan *et al.* 2002). In humans, weight loss decreased circulating TNF-α, but plasma levels of TNF-α did not correlate with measures of insulin resistance (Bruun *et al.* 2003), and systemic administration of a TNF-α antibody failed to improve insulin sensitivity in obese subjects with established type 2 diabetes (Ofei *et al.* 1996). Therefore, in contrast to rodents, it is not so clear that TNF-α contributes to obesity-induced insulin resistance in humans (Faraj *et al.* 2004).

*Interleukin-6*

Interleukin-6 (Il-6) is produced by a number of cells, including monocytes, endothelial cells, smooth muscle cells and adipocytes (Faraj *et al.* 2004). Up to 35% of the basal supply of Il-6 is derived from white adipose tissue (Mohamed-Ali *et al.* 1997). In obese male subjects, plasma levels of Il-6 were increased and correlated with measures of insulin resistance (Bruun *et al.* 2003). These findings appear to suggest a causal role for Il-6 in obesity and insulin resistance (Kershaw and Flier 2004). In contrast to this assumption, however, mice with targeted deletion of Il-6 develop mature-onset obesity and display impaired glucose clearance (Wallenius *et al.* 2002), whereas over-expression of Il-6 in pancreatic cells of non-obese diabetic mice resulted in delayed onset of diabetes mellitus and prolonged survival (Dicosmo *et al.* 1994). Therefore, increased Il-6 plasma levels may be a consequence rather than a cause of obesity and may be an attempt to prevent metabolic perturbations (Faraj *et al.* 2004). At the moment it is unclear whether IL-6 mimetic or antagonizing strategies may achieve a role in treating metabolic diseases.

This brief summary of some important factors produced and secreted by adipose tissue highlights the importance of adipose tissue as an endocrine organ playing a major role in energy homeostasis. It can be expected that even more genes expressed in adipose tissue will be identified and characterized in the future, and that these discoveries will promote our understanding of the role of adipose tissue at the crossroads of energy balance regulation, obesity and inflammation.

## 1.4 *De novo* lipogenesis

In situations where carbohydrates, proteins and fats are ingested in high amounts, excess dietary fat can easily be stored as TAG in adipose tissue. The storage capacity for carbohydrates in the form of glycogen is limited, however, and in humans no protein has been identified whose sole function is to serve as an amino acid reservoir. Therefore, the body must be capable of transforming surplus non-fat energy into fat. This process is called *de novo* lipogenesis (DNL). In humans, DNL occurs in the liver and, possibly to a lesser extent, in adipose tissue (Hellerstein *et al.* 1996). Obviously, the key component of DNL is the biosynthesis of FFA – mainly palmitate – which is a complex process that starts from acetyl-coenzyme A (CoA) and takes place in the cytosol (Fig. 1.1). Acetyl-CoA is generated in the mitochondria, but citrate and not acetyl-CoA is transported into the cytosol. There, the citrate is cleaved to acetyl-CoA and oxaloacetate by the enzyme ATP-citrate lyase (CL). The enzyme acetyl-CoA carboxylase (ACC) catalyzes the production of malonyl-CoA. This is the controlling step in fatty acid synthesis. The fatty acid synthase (FAS) is responsible for the overall synthesis of fatty acids. It is a single polypeptide containing seven distinct enzymatic activities. FAS catalyzes a series of condensation reactions each accompanied by decarboxylation and two reductions with the reduced form of nicotinamide adenine dinucleotide phosphate (NADPH) as a hydrogen donor, and this reaction is repeated until formation of a palmitate molecule is achieved (Hellerstein *et al.* 1996). DNL is stimulated by a low-fat, high-carbohydrate diet in weight-stable human subjects (Hudgins *et al.* 1996), but it is generally assumed that fatty acid biosynthesis is an unimportant metabolic pathway in humans. Schwarz *et al.* (1995) quantified that even humans receiving a diet with 50% energy surplus as carbohydrate synthesize less than 5 g fatty acids in the liver per day. Yet, we have to keep in mind that: (a) it is difficult to assess DNL in humans (Schutz 2004) and that (b) it is unknown how longer-term overfeeding with a high-carbohydrate diet affects DNL in lean and obese subjects (Schutz 2000). Furthermore,

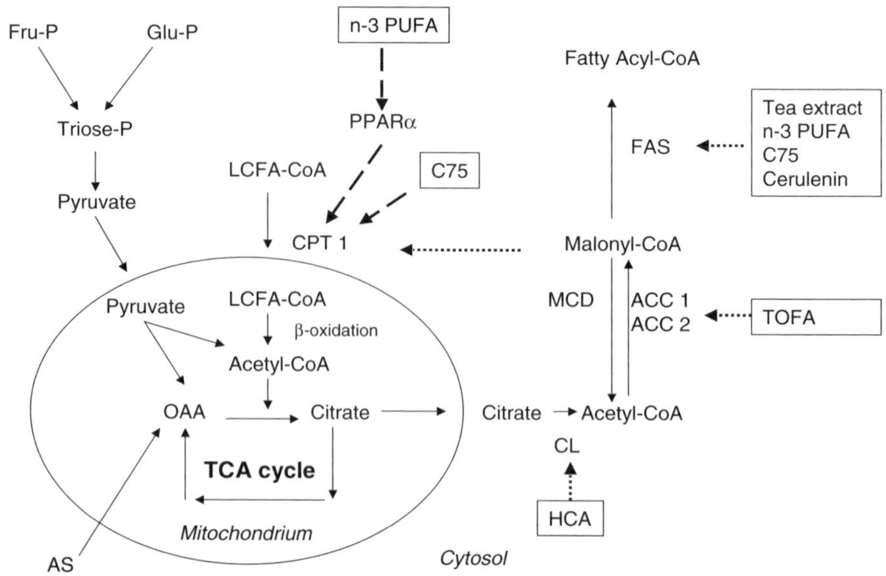


**Fig. 1.1** Diagram depicting the effects of several substances on DNL and CPT 1 activity: dashed arrow, activation; dotted arrow, inhibition. Abbreviations: ACC, acetyl-CoA carboxylase; AS, amino acids; CL, ATP-citrate lyase; CPT 1, carnitine palmitoyl transferase 1; FAS, fatty acid synthase; Fru, fructose; Glu, glucose; HCA, hydroxycitric acid; MCD, malonyl-CoA decarboxylase; OAA, oxaloacetate; PPAR-α, peroxisome proliferator-activated receptor-α; TCA, tricarboxylic acid; LCFA-CoA, long-chain fatty acid-CoA; P, phosphate; n-3 PUFA, n-3 polyunsaturated fatty acid.

DNL also contributes to multiple cellular processes. McGarry and Foster (1980) found that malonyl-CoA, the first intermediate product of DNL, is a potent inhibitor of the carnitine palmitoyl transferase 1 (CPT 1), the enzyme that catalyses the rate-controlling step in mitochondrial fatty acid oxidation (Foster 2004) (Fig. 1.1). This finding might explain why so many non-lipogenic tissues, such as heart and brain, also express enzymes of DNL; the ability to generate malonyl-CoA allows cells to block mitochondrial fatty acid oxidation quickly by switching to carbohydrate utilization. The finding that certain neurons in the brain, notably in the hypothalamus, express enzymes involved in DNL and fatty acid oxidation is surprising because under normal conditions the brain almost exclusively metabolizes glucose (Seeley and York 2005). Presumably, intermediates in the DNL pathway, such as malonyl-CoA, serve as energy sensors that signal higher brain centers to produce appropriate responses, i.e. changes in food intake and energy expenditure (Dowell *et al.* 2005). Therefore, DNL in specialized neurons of the brain appears to play a crucial role in the control of energy balance (Ronnett *et al.* 2005).

### 1.4.1 Importance of *de novo* lipogenesis assessed by transgenic animal technology

The general importance of DNL is emphasized by the finding that the generation of homozygous knock-out mice lacking important enzymes of DNL – such as CL (Beigneux *et al.* 2004), ACC 1 (Abu-Elheiga *et al.* 2005) and also FAS (Chirala *et al.* 2003) – is impossible because these mice have lethal development defects, suggesting an important role for DNL in embryonic development (Beigneux *et al.* 2004).

As already mentioned, one important step of DNL is the carboxylation of acetyl-CoA to form malonyl-CoA that is catalyzed by ACC (Fig. 1.1). Malonyl-CoA is an important metabolic intermediate that signals to the cell that surplus energy is available (Ruderman *et al.* 2003). Furthermore, besides being an intermediate in DNL, malonyl-CoA also plays a pivotal role in the control of fatty acid oxidation (Abu-Elheiga *et al.* 2000). Two isoforms of ACC (ACC 1 and ACC 2) have been identified in animals and humans. ACC 1 is a cytosolic protein that is highly expressed in lipogenic tissues, such as liver and adipose tissue. ACC 2 is associated with mitochondria suggesting that it is mainly involved in the control of mitochondrial fatty acid oxidation. In line with this assumption, ACC 2 is expressed in tissues such as muscle and brain, in which little or no DNL takes place (Abu-Elheiga *et al.* 2000). Whereas the genetic lack of ACC 1 is lethal (Abu-Elheiga *et al.* 2005), mice lacking ACC 2 have a normal life span, a higher fatty acid oxidation rate and less adipose tissue weight (Abu-Elheiga *et al.* 2001). Furthermore, ACC 2-deficient mice turned out to be protected against obesity and diabetes induced by a high-fat, high-carbohydrate diet (Abu-Elheiga *et al.* 2003). Therefore, ACC 2 seems to be an interesting therapeutic target in the fight against obesity and related disorders.

All these findings support the important role of DNL in energy homeostasis, but also in embryonic development. With respect to the latter aspect it is very important to consider possible teratogenic consequences of anti-obesity drugs aimed at inhibiting DNL.

### 1.4.2 Substances reducing the rate of *de novo* lipogenesis and their possible therapeutic potential for the control of obesity

*Pharmacological substances*

C75

C75, an inhibitor of the enzyme FAS, was initially developed for the treatment of certain cancers (Kuhajda *et al.* 2000) because many common human cancers express high levels of FAS. Subsequent tests revealed that systemic and intracerebroventricular (i.c.v.) administration of C75 in mice reduced food intake and body weight (Loftus *et al.* 2000), making FAS also an interesting target in the therapy of obesity. C75 blocks the conversion of malonyl-CoA into fatty acids and, hence, increases tissue levels of malonyl-CoA

(Loftus *et al.* 2000). A C75-induced increase in hypothalamic malonyl-CoA and a decrease in AMP-activated kinase activity and subsequent changes in the expression of hypothalamic orexigenic (NPY, AgRP) and anorectic (POMC, CART) neuropeptides are presumably involved in the feeding-inhibitory effect of C75 (Kumar *et al.* 2002; Ronnett *et al.* 2005). Yet, not all findings support the assumption that hypothalamic malonyl-CoA levels are involved in the feeding-inhibitory effect of i.c.v. C75 (Wortman *et al.* 2003). In addition, some results (Clegg *et al.* 2002; Takahashi *et al.* 2004; Rohrbach *et al.* 2005) indicate that intraperitoneally (i.p.) injected C75 has unspecific aversive effects in rodents.

Although C75 clearly increases malonyl-CoA, which should inhibit CPT 1 and, hence, mitochondrial fatty acid oxidation (McGarry and Foster 1980) (Fig. 1.1), the published results on the effect of C75 on CPT 1 activity and fatty acid oxidation are controversial. Bentebibel *et al.* (2006) demonstrated that the CoA derivative of C75 is a potent inhibitor of CPT 1 and fatty acid oxidation, whereas Thupari *et al.* (2002) showed that i.p. injected C75 increased CPT 1 and fatty acid oxidation in adipose tissue and liver despite a high tissue level of malonyl-CoA. C75 stimulated CPT 1 and increased intracellular ATP levels also in primary cortical neuronal cultures, similar to its effects in peripheral tissues (Kim *et al.* 2004; Landree *et al.* 2004). C75 also increased whole-body and in particular skeletal-muscle fatty acid oxidation when injected i.c.v. in mice. Phentolamine, an α-adrenergic blocking agent, prevented the C75-induced increases in whole-body fatty acid oxidation, implicating the sympathetic nervous system in this effect (Cha *et al.* 2005). One consequence of an increase in whole-body fatty acid oxidation is that energy expenditure is also increased, and this effect in response to C75 was more pronounced in mice with diet-induced obesity compared with lean mice (Tu *et al.* 2005). Finally, FAS seems to generate signals that may be essential for the differentiation of preadipocyte, because inhibition of FAS by C75 prevented preadipocyte differentiation (Schmid *et al.* 2005).

All in all, C75 [for review see also Ronnett *et al.* (2005)] is presumably not a drug that can be used for the treatment of human obesity, but it is an interesting substance that allows researchers to study the roles of FAS and CPT 1 in the control of food intake, body weight and adipose tissue mass (Kuhajda *et al.* 2005).

#### Cerulenin and 5-(tetradecyloxy)-2-furoic acid

Cerulenin is another inhibitor of FAS that reduced food intake when injected i.p. in mice, albeit not as potently as C75 (Loftus *et al.* 2000). Another difference between cerulenin and C75 is that cerulenin does not activate CPT 1 (Jin *et al.* 2004). *In vitro* cerulenin decreased fatty acid oxidation by increasing cytosolic malonyl-CoA levels (Thupari *et al.* 2001). When cerulenin was injected i.c.v., however, it increased energy expenditure and CPT 1 activity in soleus muscle, possibly via sympathetic nervous system activation (Jin *et al.* 2004). 5-(Tetradecyloxy)-2-furoic acid (TOFA) is an inhibitor of the enzyme acetyl-CoA carboxylase; it increases ATP levels in neuronal cells *in vitro* (Landree *et al.* 2004), but does not affect food intake *in vivo*. Pretreatment with TOFA actually reversed the anorectic effect of C75 (Loftus *et al.* 2000), suggesting that the absolute energy status of hypothalamic neurons is not crucial for the control of food intake. As is the case for C75, cerulenin and TOFA can presumably not directly be used for the treatment of obesity. Yet again, all these substances are interesting tools with which to study the role of DNL in the control of food intake and body weight.

*Food ingredients*

Hydroxycitric acid

Hydroxycitric acid (HCA) is a compound found in fruit rinds of *Garcina cambogia*, *Garcina indica* and *Garcina atroviridis*. These plants are cultivated on the Indian subcontinent and in western Sri Lanka (Jena *et al.* 2002). HCA has been shown to potently inhibit the extramitochondrial enzyme CL (Fig. 1.1), which catalyses the cleavage of citrate to acetyl-CoA and oxalacetate, another key step in DNL (Sullivan *et al.* 1972). Sullivan *et al.* (1974b) demonstrated that oral administration of HCA dose-dependently reduced *in vivo* lipogenesis in liver, adipose tissue and small intestine. Furthermore, HCA caused a significant reduction in food consumption and body weight in rodent studies when animals had access to a high-glucose diet that contained only 1% fat (Sullivan *et al.* 1974a). Recently, we demonstrated that HCA also reduced food intake and body weight in adult rats after substantial body weight loss, when HCA was given with a high-glucose (Leonhardt *et al.* 2001, 2004c; Leonhardt and Langhans 2002) or a high-fructose diet (Brandt *et al.* 2006) that contained 120 g/kg of fat.

The mechanism involved in the feeding-inhibitory effect of HCA is poorly understood. HCA reduces the availability of cytosolic acetyl-CoA level (Michno *et al.* 2004) and thereby prevents the formation of malonyl-CoA (Fig. 1.1). HCA should therefore stimulate fatty acid oxidation. Changes in peripheral, in particular, hepatic fatty acid oxidation are supposed to be involved in the control of food intake [for review see Leonhardt and Langhans (2004)]. In cell culture experiments HCA reduced cytosolic malonyl-CoA levels (Saha *et al.* 1997) and increased fatty acid oxidation (Chen *et al.* 1994). However, whether this also occurs *in vivo* is unclear. In one of our studies (Leonhardt *et al.* 2004a) HCA reduced the respiratory quotient (RQ); this has also been shown in other animal (Ishihara *et al.* 2000) and human (Lim *et al.* 2002; Tomita *et al.* 2003) studies. A reduction in RQ could be related to an increase in fatty acid oxidation and/or a reduction in DNL. DNL is an energy-consuming process, and the conversion of carbohydrate to fat costs about 0.25 MJ per MJ of ingested carbohydrates (Acheson and Flatt 2002). As a result, inhibition of DNL should decrease energy expenditure. Indeed, HCA reduced energy expenditure in addition to the RQ (Leonhardt *et al.* 2004a), suggesting that the reduced RQ was mainly related to the suppression of DNL. HCA also reduced DNL, RQ and energy expenditure in humans (Kovacs and Westerterp-Plantenga, 2006). Another argument against the assumption that an increase in hepatic fatty acid oxidation causes the feeding-inhibitory effect of HCA is that this effect was shown to be independent of vagal afferents (Leonhardt *et al.* 2004b), whereas several findings strongly suggest that the feeding-stimulatory effect caused by an inhibition of peripheral fatty acid oxidation is signaled to the brain by vagal afferents [for review see Leonhardt and Langhans (2004)].

Wielinga *et al.* (2005) recently demonstrated that HCA delayed glucose absorption, but it is unclear whether this effect is involved in the feeding-inhibitory effect of HCA. Finally, HCA inhibited serotonin reuptake, thereby increasing serotonin availability in isolated rat brain cortical slices (Ohia *et al.* 2002) and HCA reduced the synthesis and release of acetylcholine in experiments on slices of rat caudate nuclei (Ricny and Tucek 1982). However, so far it is unknown whether HCA can cross the blood–brain barrier, which would be a precondition for a direct effect of HCA on brain areas involved in food intake control.

Therefore, whereas a reduction in food intake and body weight by HCA was shown in many rodent studies, the efficacy of HCA in humans appears to be inconsistent and variable: effects of HCA on food intake, body weight, visceral fat accumulation or fatty acid oxidation have been reported in some (Lim *et al.* 2002, 2003; Westerterp-Plantenga and Kovacs 2002; Hayamizu *et al.* 2003; Tomita *et al.* 2003; Preuss *et al.* 2004), but not all (Kriketos *et al.* 1999; Mattes and Bormann 2000; van Loon *et al.* 2000; Kovacs *et al.* 2001a,b), studies. Different experimental designs or differences in the HCA preparations employed might explain the discrepant findings. For example, the bioavailability of various HCA preparations differs (Lim *et al.* 2005).

Finally, so far it is unclear whether long-term HCA treatment may have adverse effects. Most animal studies indicate that HCA is a safe, natural supplement that does not cause any changes in major organs or in hematology, clinical chemistry and histopathology (Ohia *et al.* 2002; Shara *et al.* 2004; Soni *et al.* 2004; Oikawa *et al.* 2005). However, in one study a high dose of HCA caused potent testicular atrophy and toxicity (Saito *et al.* 2005), and we recently observed that long-term application of HCA increased liver lipid content and plasma cholesterol levels in rats (Brandt *et al.* 2006). One explanation for the unexpected effects of HCA on lipid metabolism might be that HCA stimulates the enzyme ACC (Hackenschmidt *et al.* 1972). Thus, HCA acts as an inhibitor of DNL only if cytoplasmatic acetyl-CoA is produced by the citrate cleavage enzyme reaction, whereas HCA will not affect (Zambell *et al.* 2003) or even activate fatty acid synthesis whenever an alternative source of cytoplasmatic acetyl-CoA, e.g. acetate, is available (Hackenschmidt *et al.* 1972). It is still unclear whether HCA also enhances lipid synthesis and hepatic lipid accumulation in humans under certain circumstances. Consequently, long-term treatment with HCA may only be recommended with caution.

### Green and black tea extracts

Green and black teas are popular drinks consumed all over the world. Epidemiological studies suggest that green tea in particular has preventive effects on chronic inflammatory diseases, cardiovascular diseases and cancer (Sueoka *et al.* 2001). Green tea or green tea extracts contain large amounts of polyphenolic components such as epicatechin, epicatechin gallate, epigallocatechin and epigallocatechin gallate (EGCG) (Dulloo *et al.* 1999). EGCG is the most abundant of these substances, constituting more than 50% of the total amount of polyphenolic components in green tea, and is believed to be the most pharmacologically active tea catechin (Dulloo *et al.* 1999). Dulloo *et al.* (1999) demonstrated in humans that treatment with green tea extracts resulted in a significant increase in 24-h energy expenditure and a stimulation of fat oxidation. In rats, orally and i.p. administered EGCG reduced food intake and body weight (Kao *et al.* 2000). Recently Wolfram *et al.* (2005) confirmed that EGCG prevents body weight gain in mice, although in their study EGCG had no effect on food intake. Further, FAS and ACC 1 mRNA levels were decreased in adipose tissue of EGCG-supplemented mice (Wolfram *et al.* 2005) suggesting that EGCG might inhibit DNL (Fig. 1.1). Indeed Wang and Tian (2001) demonstrated that EGCG is an inhibitor of FAS and that the inhibition is related to β-ketoacyl reductase activity of FAS. *In vitro*, EGCG inhibits FAS as effectively as C75 (Wang *et al.* 2003), but the inhibition kinetics of the two substances differ considerably: the inhibition of FAS by EGCG is mainly a reversible fast-binding inhibition, whereas C75 causes an irreversible, slow-binding inactivation (Wang and Tian 2001). In a recent study (Zhang *et al.* 2006), the ability of green tea extracts to inhibit FAS was even more potent than that of EGCG, suggesting that other components of green tea can also inhibit FAS. The same group also identified catechin gallate in green tea extracts as a very potent inhibitor of FAS (Zhang *et al.* 2006). Finally, it is not only green tea extracts that can inhibit FAS; keemun black tea extracts also contain potent FAS inhibitors (Du *et al.* 2005), and these components are possibly theaflavins. Unfortunately, only 10–23% of the inhibitory activity of black tea is extracted by the general method of boiling with water (Du *et al.* 2005).

All in all, green and black tea extracts seem to have anti-obesity effects, i.e. they decrease in body weight and adipose tissue mass, in particular by increasing energy expenditure and by reducing DNL through inhibition of FAS.

### Polyunsaturated fatty acids

Polyunsaturated fatty acids (PUFAs), in particular those of the n-3 family, seem to act as fuel partitioners in that they direct glucose away from glycolysis towards glycogen storage and shift fatty acids away from TAG synthesis and storage in adipose tissue towards fatty acid oxidation (Clarke 2000, 2001). These effects appear to be mainly related to the fact that PUFAs activate PPARs (Fig 1.1), induce genes encoding proteins involved in fatty acid oxidation (Clarke 2000) and inhibit genes involved in DNL such as FAS, presumably by suppressing the abundance of the sterol regulatory element-binding protein (Sekiya *et al.* 2003; Jump *et al.* 2005). Recently, Dentin *et al.* (2005) demonstrated that some of the n-3 PUFAs suppressive effects on glycolysis and lipogenesis are also mediated through the inhibition of carbohydrate responsive element-binding protein. Most of the n-3 PUFAs-induced changes in fatty acid metabolism have been shown for the liver. As the liver plays a central role in whole-body lipid meta-bolism, effects on whole-body lipid metabolism can be expected (Jump *et al.* 2005).

Another feature of n-3 PUFAs is that they also increase brown adipose tissue uncoupling protein 1 mRNA level in rats (Takahashi and Ide 2000) and induce a marked stimulation of brown fat thermogenesis (Oudart *et al.* 1997). In both studies, n-3 PUFAs had no major effect on food intake, but epididymal white fat mass was reduced, suggesting that n-3 PUFA indeed increased energy expenditure (Oudart *et al.* 1997; Takahashi and Ide 2000). Whether PUFAs also increase thermogenesis in humans is unknown.

n-3 PUFAs may be interesting as a nutrient supplement in the therapy of obesity, but it has to be mentioned that n-3 PUFAs had adverse effects on glycemic control in obese individuals (Mori *et al.* 2000; Woodman *et al.* 2002). The mechanism of this negative effect is unknown, but an increase in hepatic gluconeogenesis caused by an increase in hepatic fatty acid oxidation might contribute (Woodman *et al.* 2002). Nevertheless, in another study with overweight patients, n-3 PUFAs (as fish oil) combined with a weight-loss regimen were more effective at improving glucose–insulin metabolism than either weight loss or fish oil supplementation alone (Mori *et al.* 1999). Therefore, further studies should examine whether n-3 PUFAs have adverse effects on insulin sensitivity in obese people under certain circumstances.

## 1.5 Future trends

The process of DNL has gained more and more attention over the last few years, and it seems that the enzymatic pathways involved are not only interesting targets for obesity therapy (Abu-Elheiga *et al.* 2001, 2003; Kuhajda *et al.* 2005) but also for the treatment of other diseases such as cancer (Kuhajda *et al.* 2000). Modern transgenic animal technology allowing inducible gain-of-function and loss-of-function manipulations of a target gene in a specific organ will help to better understand the role of DNL in energy homeostasis. Organ-specific interference with enzymes of the DNL pathway for the treatment of obesity is presumably necessary because DNL seems to be important for normal embryonic development, especially of the brain (Beigneux *et al.* 2004).

Currently, several different food ingredients are being screened that inhibit DNL, or more precisely FAS, such as protein concentrates from *Amaranthus cruentus* seeds (Escudero *et al.* 2006) and whey protein (Morifuji *et al.* 2005). However, only animal studies are available so far, and whether these substances are useful supplements for humans is not clear yet. In general, it has to be considered that inhibition of FAS entails an increase in cytosolic malonyl-CoA levels, causing inhibition of CPT 1 and consequently of mitochondrial fatty acid oxidation. Short-term inhibition of fatty acid oxidation improves hyperglycemia (Deems *et al.* 1998), but long-term inhibition causes accumulation of TAG in liver and muscle and reduces insulin sensitivity (Dobbins *et al.* 2001).

In summary, all substances discussed in this review have been shown to suppress DNL, but their efficacy to cause weight loss is less clear and also the safety of long-term therapeutic use of some of these substances appears questionable. Consequently, the use of these substances can only be recommended with caution. Further screening of food ingredients that interfere with the enzymes of DNL might lead to the discovery of supplements that have a high efficacy and are safe.

## 1.6 References

ABU-ELHEIGA L, BRINKLEY W R, ZHONG L, CHIRALA S S, WOLDEGIORGIS G and WAKIL S J (2000), The subcellular localization of acetyl-CoA carboxylase 2. *Proceedings of the National Academy of Sciences of the United States of America*, **97**, 1444–1449.

ABU-ELHEIGA L, MATZUK M M, ABO-HASHEMA K A and WAKIL S J (2001), Continuous fatty acid oxidation and reduced fat storage in mice lacking acetyl-CoA carboxylase 2. *Science*, **291**, 2613–2616.

ABU-ELHEIGA L, MATZUK M M, KORDARI P, OH W, SHAIKENOV T, GU Z W and WAKIL S J (2005), Mutant mice lacking acetyl-CoA carboxylase 1 are embryonically lethal. *Proceedings of the National Academy of Sciences of the United States of America*, **102**, 12011–12016.

ABU-ELHEIGA L, OH W K, KORDARI P and WAKIL S J (2003), Acetyl-CoA carboxylase 2 mutant mice are protected against obesity and diabetes induced by high-fat/high-carbohydrate diets. *Proceedings of the National Academy of Sciences of the United States of America*, **100**, 10207–10212.

ACHESON K J and FLATT J P (2002), Minor importance of de novo lipogenesis on energy expenditure in human. *British Journal of Nutrition*, **87**, 189.

ASTRUP A, GRUNWALD G K, MELANSON E L, SARIS W H M and HILL J O (2000), The role of low-fat diets in body weight control: a meta-analysis of ad libitum dietary intervention studies. *International Journal of Obesity*, **24**, 1545–1552.

BADO A, LEVASSEUR S, ATTOUB S, KERMORGANT S, LAIGNEAU J P, BORTOLUZZI M N, MOIZO L, LEHY T, GUERRE-MILLO M, MARCHAND-BRUSTEL Y and LEWIN M J M (1998), The stomach is a source of leptin. *Nature*, **394**, 790–793.

BANERJEE R R and LAZAR M A (2003), Resistin: molecular history and prognosis. *Journal of Molecular Medicine*, **81**, 218–226.

BANERJEE R R, RANGWALA S M, SHAPIRO J S, RICH A S, RHOADES B, QI Y, WANG J, RAJALA M W, POCAI A, SCHERER P E, STEPPAN C M, AHIMA R S, OBICI S, ROSSETTI L and LAZAR M A (2004), Regulation of fasted blood glucose by resistin. *Science*, **303**, 1195–1198.

BEIGNEUX A P, KOSINSKI C, GAVINO B, HORTON J D, SKARNES W C and YOUNG S G (2004), ATP-citrate lyase deficiency in the mouse. *Journal of Biological Chemistry*, **279**, 9557–9564.

BENTEBIBEL A, SEBASTIÁN D, HERRERO L, LÓPEZ-VIÑAS E, SERRA D, ASINS G, GÓMEZ-PUERTAS P and HEGARD F G (2006), Novel effect of C75 on carnitine palmitoyltransferase I activity and palmitate oxidation. *Biochemistry*, **45**, 4339–4350.

BERG A H, COMBS T P, DU X L, BROWNLEE M and SCHERER P (2001), The adipocyte-secreted protein Acrp30 enhances hepatic insulin action. *Nature Medicine*, **7**, 947–953.

BLUNDELL J E and STUBBS R J (1999), High and low carbohydrate and fat intakes: limits imposed by appetite and palatability and their implications for energy balance. *European Journal of Clinical Nutrition*, **53**, S148–S165.

BRANDT K, LANGHANS W, GEARY N and LEONHARDT M (2006), Beneficial and deleterious effects of hydroxycitrate in rats fed a high-fructose diet. *Nutrition*, **22**, 905–912.

BRAY G A and POPKIN B M (1998), Dietary fat intake does affect obesity! *American Journal of Clinical Nutrition*, **68**, 1157–1173.

BRUUN J M, VERDICH C, TOUBRO S, ASTRUP A and RICHELSEN B (2003), Association between measures of insulin sensitivity and circulating levels of interleukin-8, interleukin-6 and tumor necrosis factor-alpha. Effect of weight loss in obese men. *European Journal of Endocrinology*, **148**, 535–542.

CHA S H, HU Z, CHOHNAN S and LANE M D (2005), Inhibition of hypothalamic fatty acid synthase triggers rapid activation of fatty acid oxidation in skeletal muscle. *Proceedings of the National Academy of Sciences of the United States of America*, **102**, 14557–14562.

CHEN S, OGAWA A, OHNEDA M, UNGER R H, FOSTER D W and MCGARRY J D (1994), More direct evidence for a malonyl-CoA-carnitine palmitoyltrans-ferase I interaction as a key event in pancreatic beta-cell signaling. *Diabetes*, **43**, 878–883.

CHIRALA S S, CHANG H, MATZUK M, ABU-ELHEIGA L, MAO J Q, MAHON K, FINEGOLD M and WAKIL S J (2003), Fatty acid synthesis is essential in embryonic development: Fatty acid synthase null mutants and most of the heterozygotes die in utero. *Proceedings of the National Academy of Sciences of the United States of America*, **100**, 6358–6363.

CIANFLONE K, XIA Z N and CHEN L Y (2003), Critical review of acylation-stimulating protein physiology in humans and rodents. *Biochimica et Biophysica Acta*, **1609**, 127–143.

CLARKE S D (2000), Polyunsaturated fatty acid regulation of gene transcription: a mechanism to improve energy balance and insulin resistance. *British Journal of Nutrition*, **83**, S59–S66.

CLARKE S D (2001), Polyunsaturated fatty acid regulation of gene transcription: A molecular mechanism to improve the metabolic syndrome. *Journal of Nutrition*, **131**, 1129–1132.

CLEGG D J, WORTMAN M D, BENOIT S C, MCOSKER C C and SEELEY R J (2002), Comparison of central and peripheral administration of C75 on food intake, body weight, and conditioned taste aversion. *Diabetes*, **51**, 3196–3201.

DEEMS R O, ANDERSON R C and FOLEY J E (1998), Hypoglycemic effects of a novel fatty acid oxidation inhibitor in rats and monkeys. *American Journal of Physiology*, **43**, R524–R528.

DENIGRIS S J, HAMOSH M, KASBEKAR D K, LEE T C and HAMOSH P (1988), Lingual and gastric lipases – species-differences in the origin of prepancreatic digestive lipases and in the localization of gastric lipase. *Biochimica et Biophysica Acta*, **959**, 38–45.

DENTIN R, BENHAMED F, PEGORIER J P, FOUFELLE F, VIOLLET B, VAULONT S, GIRARD J and POSTIC C (2005), Polyunsaturated fatty acids suppress glycolytic and lipogenic genes through the inhibition of ChREBP nuclear protein translocation. *Journal of Clinical Investigation*, **115**, 2843–2854.

DICOSMO B F, PICARELLA D and FLAVELL R A (1994), Local production of human Il-6 promotes insulitis but retards the onset of insulin-dependent diabetes-mellitus in nonobese diabetic mice. *International Immunology*, **6**, 1829–1837.

DOBBINS R L, SZCZEPANIAK L S, BENTLEY B, ESSER V, MYHILL J and MCGARRY J D (2001), Prolonged inhibition of muscle carnitine palmitoyltransferase-1 promotes intramyocellular lipid accumulation and insulin resistance in rats. *Diabetes*, **50**, 123–130.

DOWELL P, HU Z Y and LANE M D (2005), Monitoring energy balance: Metabolites of fatty acid synthesis as hypothalamic sensors. *Annual Review of Biochemistry*, **74**, 515–534.

DREWNOWSKI A (1998), Energy density, palatability, and satiety: implications for weight control. *Nutrition Review*, **56**, 347–353.

DU Y T, WANG X, WU X D and TIAN W X (2005), Keemun black tea extract contains potent fatty acid synthase inhibitors and reduces food intake and body weight of rats via oral administration. *Journal of Enzyme Inhibition and Medicinal Chemistry*, **20**, 349–356.

DUBUC G R, PHINNEY S D, STERN J S and HAVEL P J (1998), Changes of serum leptin and endocrine and metabolic parameters after 7 days of energy restriction in men and women. *Metabolism*, **47**, 429–434.

DULLOO A G, DURET C, ROHRER D, GIRARDIER L, MENSI N, FATHI M, CHANTRE P and VAN-DERMANDER J (1999), Efficacy of a green tea extract rich in catechin polyphenols and caffeine in increasing 24-h energy expenditure and fat oxidation in humans. *American Journal of Clinical Nutrition*, **70**, 1040–1045.

ESCUDERO N L, ZIRULNIK F, GOMEZ N N, MUCCIARELLI S I and GIMENEZ M S (2006), Influence of a protein concentrate from *Amaranthus cruentus* seeds on lipid metabolism. *Experimental Biology and Medicine*, **231**, 50–59.

FARAJ M, HAVEL P J, PHELIS S, BLANK D, SNIDERMAN A D and CIANFLONE K (2003), Plasma acylation-stimulating protein, adiponectin, leptin, and ghrelin before and after weight loss induced by gastric bypass surgery in morbidly obese subjects. *Journal of Clinical Endocrinology and Metabolism*, **88**, 1594–1602.

FARAJ M, LU H L and CIANFLONE K (2004), Diabetes, lipids, and adipocyte secretagogues. *Biochemistry and Cell Biology*, **82**, 170–190.

FLIER J S (2004), Obesity wars: Molecular progress confronts an expanding epidemic. *Cell*, **116**, 337–350.

FOSTER D W (2004), The role of the carnitine system in human metabolism. *Annals of the New York Academy of Sciences*, **1033**, 1–16.

FRIEDMAN J M and HALAAS J L (1998), Leptin and the regulation of body weight in mammals. *Nature*, **395**, 763–770.

FRUEBIS J, TSAO T S, JAVORSCHI S, EBBETS-REED D, ERICKSON M R S, YEN F T, BIHAIN B E and LODISH H F (2001), Proteolytic cleavage product of 30-kDa adipocyte complement-related protein increases fatty acid oxidation in muscle and causes weight loss in mice. *Proceedings of the National Academy of Sciences of the United States of America*, **98**, 2005–2010.

GRAVELEAU C, ZAHA V G, MOHAJER A, BANERJEE R R, DUDLEY-RUCKER N, STEPPAN C M, RAJALA M W, SCHERER P E, AHIMA R S, LAZAR M A and ABEL E D (2005), Mouse and human resistins impair glucose transport in primary mouse cardiomyocytes, and oligomerization is required for this biological action. *Journal of Biological Chemistry*, **280**, 31679–31685.

HACKENSCHMIDT J, BARTH C and DECKER K (1972), Stimulation of acetyl-CoA carboxylase by (–)-hydroxycitrate. *FEBS Letters*, **27**, 131–133.

HAMOSH M (1990), Lingual and gastric lipases. *Nutrition*, **6**, 421–428.

HASLAM D W and JAMES W P T (2005), Obesity. *Lancet*, **366**, 1197–1209.

HAYAMIZU K, ISHII Y, KANEKO I, SHEN M Z, OKUHARA Y, SHIGEMATSU N, TOMI H, FURUSE M, YOSHINO G and SHIMASAKI H (2003), Effects of *Garcinia cambogia* (hydroxycitric acid) on visceral fat accumulation: A double-blind, randomized, placebo-controlled trial. *Current Therapeutic Research*, **64**, 551–567.

HELLERSTEIN M K, SCHWARZ J M and NEESE R A (1996), Regulation of hepatic de novo lipogenesis in humans. *Annual Review of Nutrition*, **16**, 523–557.

HOTAMISLIGIL G S, SHARGILL N S and SPIEGELMAN B M (1993), Adipose expression of tumor-necrosis-factor-alpha – direct role in obesity-linked insulin resistance. *Science*, **259**, 87–91.

HOTTA K, FUNAHASHI T, ARITA Y, TAKAHASHI M, MATSUDA M, OKAMOTO Y, IWAHASHI H, KURIYAMA H, OUCHI N, MAEDA K, NISHIDA M, KIHARA S, SAKAI N, NAKAJIMA T, HASEGAWA K, MURAGUCHI M, OHMOTO Y, NAKAMURA T, YAMASHITA S, HANAFUSA T and MATSUZAWA Y (2000), Plasma concentrations of a novel, adipose-specific protein, adiponectin, in type 2 diabetic patients. *Arteriosclerosis Thrombosis and Vascular Biology*, **20**, 1595–1599.

HOTTA K, FUNAHASHI T, BODKIN N L, ORTMEYER H K, ARITA Y, HANSEN B C and MATSUZAWA Y (2001), Circulating concentrations of the adipocyte protein adiponectin are decreased in parallel with reduced insulin sensitivity during the progression to type 2 diabetes in rhesus monkeys. *Diabetes*, **50**, 1126–1133.

HUDGINS L C, HELLERSTEIN M, SEIDMAN C, NEESE R, DIAKUN J and HIRSCH J (1996), Human fatty acid synthesis is stimulated by a eucaloric low fat, high carbohydrate diet. *Journal of Clinical Investigation*, **97**, 2081–2091.

HUOT I, PARADIS G and LEDOUX M (2004), Factors associated with overweight and obesity in Quebec adults. *International Journal of Obesity*, **28**, 766–774.

ISHIHARA K, OYAIZU S, ONUKI K, LIM K and FUSHIKI T (2000), Chronic (–)-hydroxycitrate administration spares carbohydrate utilization and promotes lipid oxidation during exercise in mice. *Journal of Nutrition*, **130**, 2990–2995.

JENA B S, JAYAPRAKASHA G K, SINGH R P and SAKARIAH K K (2002), Chemistry and biochemistry of (–)-hydroxycitric acid from Garcinia. *Journal of Agricultural and Food Chemistry*, **50**, 10–22.

JIN Y J, LI S Z, ZHAO Z S, AN J J, KIM R Y, KIM Y M, BAIK J H and LIM S K (2004), Carnitine palmitoyltransferase-1 (CPT-1) activity stimulation by cerulenin via sympathetic nervous system activation overrides cerulenin's peripheral effect. *Endocrinology*, **145**, 3197–3204.

JUMP D B, BOTOLIN D, WANG Y, XU J H, CHRISTIAN B and DEMEURE O (2005), Fatty acid regulation of hepatic gene transcription. *Journal of Nutrition*, **135**, 2503–2506.

KAO Y H, HIIPAKKA R A and LIAO S S (2000), Modulation of endocrine systems and food intake by green tea epigallocatechin gallate. *Endocrinology*, **141**, 980–987.

KERSHAW E E and FLIER J S (2004), Adipose tissue as an endocrine organ. *Journal of Clinical Endocrinology and Metabolism*, **89**, 2548–2556.

KIM E K, MILLER I, AJA S, LANDREE L E, PINN M, MCFADDEN J, KUHAJDA F P, MORAN T H and RONNETT G V (2004), C75, a fatty acid synthase inhibitor, reduces food intake via hypothalamic AMP-activated protein kinase. *Journal of Biological Chemistry*, **279**, 19970–19976.

KOPELMAN P G (2000), Obesity as a medical problem. *Nature*, **404**, 635–643.

KOVACS E M R and WESTERTERP-PLANTENGA M S (2006), Effects of (–)-hydroxycitrate on net fat synthesis as de novo lipogenesis. *Physiology & Behavior*, **88**, 371–381.

KOVACS E M, WESTERTERP-PLANTENGA M S, DE VRIES M, BROUNS F and SARIS W H (2001a), Effects of 2-week ingestion of (–)-hydroxycitrate and (–)-hydroxycitrate combined with medium-chain triglycerides on satiety and food intake. *Physiology & Behavior*, **74**, 543–549.

KOVACS E M R, WESTERTERP-PLANTENGA M S and SARIS W H M (2001b), The effects of 2-week ingestion of (–)-hydroxycitrate and (–)-hydroxycitrate combined with medium-chain triglycerides on satiety, fat oxidation, energy expenditure and body weight. *International Journal of Obesity*, **25**, 1087–1094.

KRIKETOS A D, THOMPSON H R, GREENE H and HILL J O (1999), (–)-Hydroxycitric acid does not affect energy expenditure and substrate oxidation in adult males in a post-absorptive state. *International Journal of Obesity*, **23**, 867–873.

KUHAJDA F P, LANDREE L E and RONNETT G V (2005), The connections between C75 and obesity drug-target pathways. *Trends in Pharmacological Sciences*, **26**, 541–544.

KUHAJDA F P, PIZER E S, LI J N, MANI N S, FREHYWOT G L and TOWNSEND C A (2000), Synthesis and antitumor activity of an inhibitor of fatty acid synthase. *Proceedings of the National Academy of Sciences of the United States of America*, **97**, 3450–3454.

KUMAR M V, SHIMOKAWA T, NAGY T R and LANE M D (2002), Differential effects of a centrally acting fatty acid synthase inhibitor in lean and obese mice. *Proceedings of the National Academy of Sciences of the United States of America*, **99**, 1921–1925; erratum. **99**, 7809.

LANDREE L E, HANLON A L, STRONG D W, RUMBAUGH G, MILLER I M, THUPARI J N, CONNOLLY E C, HUGANIR R L, RICHARDSON C, WITTERS L A, KUHAJDA F P and RONNETT G V (2004), C75, a fatty acid synthase inhibitor, modulates AMP-activated protein kinase to alter neuronal energy metabolism. *Journal of Biological Chemistry*, **279**, 3817–3827.

LEONHARDT M and LANGHANS W (2002), Hydroxycitrate has long-term effects on feeding behavior, body weight regain and metabolism after body weight loss in male rats. *Journal of Nutrition*, **132**, 1977–1982.

LEONHARDT M and LANGHANS W (2004), Fatty acid oxidation and control of food intake. *Physiology & Behavior*, **83**, 645–651.

LEONHARDT M, BALKAN B and LANGHANS W (2004a), Effect of hydroxycitrate on respiratory quotient, energy expenditure, and glucose tolerance in male rats after a period of restrictive feeding. *Nutrition*, **20**, 911–915.

LEONHARDT M, HRUPKA B and LANGHANS W (2001), Effect of hydroxycitrate on food intake and body weight regain after a period of restrictive feeding in male rats. *Physiology & Behavior*, **74**, 191–196.

LEONHARDT M, HRUPKA B J and LANGHANS W (2004b), Subdiaphragmatic vagal deafferentation fails to block the anorectic effect of hydroxycitrate. *Physiology & Behavior*, **82**, 263–268.

LEONHARDT M, MUNCH S, WESTERTERP-PLANTENGA M and LANGHANS W (2004c), Effects of hydroxycitrate, conjugated linoleic acid, and guar gum on food intake, body weight regain, and metabolism after body weight loss in male rats. *Nutrition Research*, **24**, 659–669.

LIM K, RYU S, NHO H S, CHOI S K, KWON T, SUH H, SO J, TOMITA K, OKUHARA Y and SHIGEMATSU N (2003), (–)-Hydroxycitric acid ingestion increases fat utilization during exercise in untrained women. *Journal of Nutritional Science and Vitaminology*, **49**, 163–167.

LIM K, RYU S, OHISHI Y, WATANABE I, TOMI H, SUH H, LEE W K and KWON T (2002), Short-term (–)-hydroxycitrate ingestion increases fat oxidation during exercise in athletes. *Journal of Nutritional Science and Vitaminology*, **48**, 128–133.

LIM K, RYU S, SUH H, ISHIHARA K and FUSHIKI T (2005), (–)-Hydroxycitrate ingestion and endurance exercise performance. *Journal of Nutritional Science and Vitaminology*, **51**, 1–7.

LOFTUS T M, JAWORSKY D E, FREHYWOT G L, TOWNSEND C A, RONNETT G V, LANE M D and KUHAJDA F P (2000), Reduced food intake and body weight in mice treated with fatty acid synthase inhibitors. *Science*, **288**, 2379–2381.

LOWE M E (1997), Structure and function of pancreatic lipase and colipase. *Annual Review of Nutrition*, **17**, 141–158.

MARS M, DE GRAAF C, DE GROOT C P G M, VAN ROSSUM C T M and KOK F J (2006), Fasting leptin and appetite responses induced by a 4-day 65%-energy-restricted diet. *International Journal of Obesity*, **30**, 122–128.

MARS M, DE GRAAF C, DE GROOT L C P G and KOK F J (2005), Decreases in fasting leptin and insulin concentrations after acute energy restriction and subsequent compensation in food intake. *American Journal of Clinical Nutrition*, **81**, 570–577.

MASUZAKI H, OGAWA Y, SAGAWA N, HOSODA K, MATSUMOTO T, MISE H, NISHIMURA H, YOSHIMASA Y, TANAKA I, MORI T and NAKAO K (1997), Nonadipose tissue production of leptin: Leptin as a novel placenta-derived hormone in humans. *Nature Medicine*, **3**, 1029–1033.

MATTES R D and BORMANN L (2000), Effects of (–)-hydroxycitric acid on appetitive variables. *Physiology & Behavior*, **71**, 87–94.

MCGARRY J D and FOSTER D W (1980), Regulation of hepatic fatty-acid oxidation and ketone-body production. *Annual Review of Biochemistry*, **49**, 395–420.

MEAD J R, IRVINE S A and RAMJI D P (2002), Lipoprotein lipase: structure, function, regulation, and role in disease. *Journal of Molecular Medicine*, **80**, 753–769.

MEYER J H and JONES R S (1974), Canine pancreatic responses to intestinally perfused fat and products of fat digestion. *American Journal of Physiology*, **226**, 1178–1187.

MICHNO A, SKIBOWSKA A, RASZEJA-SPECHT A, CWIKOWSKA J and SZUTOWICZ A (2004), The role of adenosine triphosphate-citrate lyase in the metabolism of acetyl-coenzyme A and function of blood platelets in diabetes mellitus. *Metabolism*, **53**, 66–72.

MOHAMED-ALI V, GOODRICK S, RAWESH A, KATZ D R, MILES J M, YUDKIN J S, KLEIN S and COPPACK S W (1997), Subcutaneous adipose tissue releases interleukin-6, but not tumor necrosis factor-alpha, in vivo. *Journal of Clinical Endocrinology and Metabolism*, **82**, 4196–4200.

MORI T A, BAO D Q, BURKE V, PUDDEY I B, WATTS G F and BEILIN L J (1999), Dietary fish as a major component of a weight-loss diet: effect on serum lipids, glucose, and insulin metabolism in overweight hypertensive subjects. *American Journal of Clinical Nutrition*, **70**, 817–825.

MORI T A, BURKE V, PUDDEY I B, WATTS G F, O'NEIL D N, BEST J D and BEILIN L J (2000), Purified eicosapentaenoic and docosahexaenoic acids have differential effects on serum lipids and lipoproteins, LDL particle size, glucose, and insulin in mildly hyperlipidemic men. *American Journal of Clinical Nutrition*, **71**, 1085–1094.

MORIFUJI M, SAKAI K, SANBONGI C and SUGIURA K (2005), Dietary whey protein downregulates fatty acid synthesis in the liver, but upregulates it in skeletal muscle of exercise-trained rats. *Nutrition*, **21**, 1052–1058.

MOSCA C L, MARSHALL J A, GRUNWALD G K, CORNIER M A and BAXTER J (2004), Insulin resistance as a modifier of the relationship between dietary fat intake and weight gain. *International Journal of Obesity*, **28**, 803–812.

MU H L and HOY C E (2004), The digestion of dietary triacylglycerols. *Progress in Lipid Research*, **43**, 105–133.

MU H L and PORSGAARD T (2005), The metabolism of structured triacylglycerols. *Progress in Lipid Research*, **44**, 430–448.

OFEI F, HUREL S, NEWKIRK J, SOPWITH M and TAYLOR R (1996), Effects of an engineered human anti-TNF-alpha antibody (CDP571) on insulin sensitivity and glycemic control in patients with NIDDM. *Diabetes*, **45**, 881–885.

OHIA S E, OPERE C A, LEDAY A M, BAGCHI M, BAGCHI D and STOHS S J (2002), Safety and mechanism of appetite suppression by a novel hydroxycitric acid extract (HCA-SX). *Molecular and Cellular Biochemistry*, **238**, 89–103.

OIKAWA D, HIRAKAWA H, HAYAMIZU K, NAKAMURA Y, SHIBA N, NAKANISHI T, IWAMOTO H, TACHIBANA T and FURUSE M (2005), Dietary Garcinia cambogia does not modify skin properties of mice with or without excessive sucrose intake. *Phytotherapy Research*, **19**, 294–297.

OUDART H, GROSCOLAS R, CALGARI C, NIBBELINK M, LERAY C, LEMAHO Y and MALAN A (1997), Brown fat thermogenesis in rats fed high-fat diets enriched with n-3 polyunsaturated fatty acids. *International Journal of Obesity*, **21**, 955–962.

PREUSS H G, BAGCHI D, BAGCHI M, RAO C V S, SATYANARAYANA S and DEY D K (2004), Efficacy of a novel, natural extract of (–)-hydroxycitric acid (HCA-SX) and a combination of HCA-SX, niacin-bound chromium and Gymnema sylvestre extract in weight management in human volunteers: A pilot study. *Nutrition Research*, **24**, 45–58.

QI Y, TAKAHASHI N, HILEMAN S M, PATEL H R, BERG A H, PAJVANI U B, SCHERER P E and AHIMA R S (2004), Adiponectin acts in the brain to decrease body weight. *Nature Medicine*, **10**, 524–529.

RAJALA M W and SCHERER P E (2003), Minireview: The adipocyte – at the crossroads of energy homeostasis, inflammation, and atherosclerosis. *Endocrinology*, **144**, 3765–3773.

RAJALA M W, QI Y, PATEL H R, TAKAHASHI N, BANERJEE R, PAJVANI U B, SINHA M K, GINGERICH R L, SCHERER P E and AHIMA R S (2004), Regulation of resistin expression and circulating levels in obesity, diabetes, and fasting. *Diabetes*, **53**, 1671–1679.

RICNY J and TUCEK S (1982), Acetyl-coenzyme A and acetylcholine in slices of rat caudate nuclei incubated with (–)-hydroxycitrate, citrate, and EGTA. *Journal of Neurochemistry*, **39**, 668–673.

ROHRBACH K W, HAN S P, GAN J P, O'TANYI E J, ZHANG H W, CHI C L, TAUB R, LARGENT B L and CHENG D (2005), Disconnection between the early onset anorectic effects by C75 and hypothalamic fatty acid synthase inhibition in rodents. *European Journal of Pharmacology*, **511**, 31–41.

ROLLS B J (2000), The role of energy density in the overconsumption of fat. *Journal of Nutrition*, **130**, 268S–271S.

RONNETT G V, KIM E K, LANDREE L E and TU Y J (2005), Fatty acid metabolism as a target for obesity treatment. *Physiology & Behavior*, **85**, 25–35.

ROSENBAUM M and LEIBEL R L (1998), The physiology of body weight regulation: Relevance to the etiology of obesity in children. *Pediatrics*, **101**, 525–539.

RUAN H and LODISH H F (2003), Insulin resistance in adipose tissue: direct and indirect effects of tumor necrosis factor-alpha. *Cytokine & Growth Factor Reviews*, **14**, 447–455.

RUAN H, MILES P D G, LADD C M, ROSS K, GOLUB T R, OLEFSKY J M and LODISH H F (2002), Profiling gene transcription in vivo reveals adipose tissue as an immediate target of tumor necrosis factor-alpha – Implications for insulin resistance. *Diabetes*, **51**, 3176–3188.

RUDERMAN N B, SAHA A K and KRAEGEN E W (2003), Minireview: malonyl CoA, AMP-activated protein kinase, and adiposity. *Endocrinology*, **144**, 5166–5171.

SAHA A K, VAVVAS D, KUROWSKI T G, APAZIDIS A, WITTERS L A, SHAFRIR E and RUDERMAN N B (1997), Malonyl-CoA regulation in skeletal muscle: its link to cell citrate and the glucose-fatty acid cycle. *American Journal of Physiology*, **272**, E641–E648.

SAITO M, UENO M, OGINO S, KUBO K, NAGATA J and TAKEUCHI M (2005), High dose of Garcinia cambogia is effective in suppressing fat accumulation in developing male Zucker obese rats, but highly toxic to the testis. *Food and Chemical Toxicology*, **43**, 411–419.

SARIS W H M, ASTRUP A, PRENTICE A M, ZUNFT H J F, FORMIGUERA X, VERBOEKET-VAN DE VENNE W P H G, RABEN A, POPPITT S D, SEPPELT B, JOHNSTON S, VASILARAS T H and KEOGH G F (2000), Randomized controlled trial of changes in dietary carbohydrate/fat ratio and simple vs complex carbohydrates on body weight and blood lipids: the CARMEN study. *International Journal of Obesity*, **24**, 1310–1318.

SATIA-ABOUTA J, PATTERSON R E, SCHILLER R N and KRISTAL A R (2002), Energy from fat is associated with obesity in US men: results from the prostate cancer prevention trial. *Preventive Medicine*, **34**, 493–501.

SCHMID B, RIPPMANN J F, TADAYYON M and HAMILTON B S (2005), Inhibition of fatty acid synthase prevents preadipocyte differentiation. *Biochemical and Biophysical Research Communications*, **328**, 1073–1082.

SCHUTZ Y (2000), Human overfeeding experiments: potentials and limitations in obesity research. *British Journal of Nutrition*, **84**, 135–137.

SCHUTZ Y (2004), Dietary fat, lipogenesis and energy balance. *Physiology & Behavior*, **83**, 557–564.

SCHWARZ J M, NEESE R A, TURNER S, DARE D and HELLERSTEIN M K (1995), Short-term alterations in carbohydrate energy intake in humans. Striking effects on hepatic glucose production, de novo lipogenesis, lipolysis, and whole-body fuel selection. *Journal of Clinical Investigation*, **96**, 2735–2743.

SEELEY R J and YORK D A (2005), Fuel sensing and the central nervous system (CNS): implications for the regulation of energy balance and the treatment for obesity. *Obesity Reviews*, **6**, 259–265.

SEKIYA M, YAHAGI N, MATSUZAKA T, NAJIMA Y, NAKAKUKI M, NAGAI R, ISHIBASHI S, OSUGA J, YAMADA N and SHIMANO H (2003), Polyunsaturated fatty acids ameliorate hepatic steatosis in obese mice by SREBP-1 suppression. *Hepatology*, **38**, 1529–1539.

SHARA M, OHIA S E, SCHMIDT R E, YASMIN T, ZARDETTO-SMITH A, KINCAID A, BAGCHI M, CHATTERJEE A, BAGCHI D and STOHS S J (2004), Physico-chemical properties of a novel (–)-hydroxycitric acid extract and its effect on body weight, selected organ weights, hepatic lipid peroxidation and DNA fragmentation, hematology and clinical chemistry, and histopathological changes over a period of 90 days. *Molecular and Cellular Biochemistry*, **260**, 171–186.

SONI M G, BURDOCK G A, PREUSS H G, STOHS S J, OHIA S E and BAGCHI D (2004), Safety assessment of (–)-hydroxycitric acid and Super CitriMax (R), a novel calcium/potassium salt. *Food and Chemical Toxicology*, **42**, 1513–1529.

ST ONGE M P and JONES P J (2002), Physiological effects of medium-chain triglycerides: potential agents in the prevention of obesity. *Journal of Nutrition*, **132**, 329–332.

STANLEY S, WYNNE K, MCGOWAN B and BLOOM S (2005), Hormonal regulation of food intake. *Physiological Reviews*, **85**, 1131–1158.

STEPPAN C M, BAILEY S T, BHAT S, BROWN E J, BANERJEE R R, WRIGHT C M, PATEL H R, AHIMA R S and LAZAR M A (2001), The hormone resistin links obesity to diabetes. *Nature*, **409**, 307–312.

SUEOKA N, SUGANUMA M, SUEOKA E, OKABE S, MATSUYAMA S, IMAI K, NAKACHI K and FUJIKI H (2001), A new function of Green Tea: prevention of lifestyle-related diseases. *Annals of the New York Academy of Sciences*, **928**, 274–280.

SULLIVAN A C, HAMILTON J G, MILLER O N and WHEATLEY V R (1972), Inhibition of lipogenesis in rat liver by (–)-hydroxycitrate. *Archives of Biochemistry and Biophysics*, **150**, 183–190.

SULLIVAN A C, TRISCARI J, HAMILTON J G and MILLER O N (1974a), Effect of (–)-hydroxycitrate upon the accumulation of lipid in the rat. II. Appetite. *Lipids*, **9**, 129–134.

SULLIVAN A C, TRISCARI J, HAMILTON J G, MILLER O N and WHEATLEY V R (1974b), Effect of (–)-hydroxycitrate upon the accumulation of lipid in the rat. I. Lipogenesis. *Lipids*, **9**, 121–128.

TAKAHASHI K A, SMART J L, LIU H Y and CONE R D (2004), The anorexigenic fatty acid synthase inhibitor, C75, is a nonspecific neuronal activator. *Endocrinology*, **145**, 184–193.

TAKAHASHI Y and IDE T (2000), Dietary n-3 fatty acids affect mRNA level of brown adipose tissue uncoupling protein 1, and white adipose tissue leptin and glucose transporter 4 in the rat. *British Journal of Nutrition*, **84**, 175–184.

THUPARI J N, LANDREE L E, RONNETT G V and KUHAJDA F P (2002), C75 increases peripheral energy utilization and fatty acid oxidation in diet-induced obesity. *Proceedings of the National Academy of Sciences of the United States of America*, **99**, 9498–9502.

THUPARI J N, PINN M L and KUHAJDA F P (2001), Fatty acid synthase inhibition in human breast cancer cells leads to malonyl-CoA-induced inhibition of fatty acid oxidation and cytotoxicity. *Biochemical and Biophysical Research Communications*, **285**, 217–223.

TOMITA K, OKUHARA Y, SHIGEMATSU N, SUH H and LIM K (2003), (–)-Hydroxycitrate ingestion increases fat oxidation during moderate intensity exercise in untrained men. *Bioscience Biotechnology and Biochemistry*, **67**, 1999–2001.

TU Y J, THUPARI J N, KIM E K, PINN M L, MORAN T H, RONNETT G V and KUHAJDA F P (2005), C75 alters central and peripheral gene expression to reduce food intake and increase energy expenditure. *Endocrinology*, **146**, 486–493.

UYSAL K T, WIESBROCK S M, MARINO M W and HOTAMISLIGIL G S (1997), Protection from obesity-induced insulin resistance in mice lacking TNF-alpha function. *Nature*, **389**, 610–614.

VAN LOON L J, VAN ROOIJEN J J, NIESEN B, VERHAGEN H, SARIS W H and WAGENMAKERS A J (2000), Effects of acute (–)-hydroxycitrate supplementation on substrate metabolism at rest and during exercise in humans. *American Journal of Clinical Nutrition*, **72**, 1445–1450.

WALLENIUS V, WALLENIUS K, AHREN B, RUDLING M, CARLSTEN H, DICKSON S L, OHLSSON C and JANSSON J O (2002), Interleukin-6-deficient mice develop mature-onset obesity. *Nature Medicine*, **8**, 75–79.

WANG X and TIAN W X (2001), Green tea epigallocatechin gallate: a natural inhibitor of fatty-acid synthase. *Biochemical and Biophysical Research Communications*, **288**, 1200–1206.

WANG X, SONG K S, GUO Q X and TIAN W X (2003), The galloyl moiety of green tea catechins is the critical structural feature to inhibit fatty-acid synthase. *Biochemical Pharmacology*, **66**, 2039–2047.

WATANABE S, LEE K Y, CHANG T M, BERGERORNSTEIN L and CHEY W Y (1988), Role of pancreatic-enzymes on release of cholecystokinin-pancreozymin in response to fat. *American Journal of Physiology*, **254**, G837–G842.

WESTERTERP-PLANTENGA M S (2001), Analysis of energy density of food in relation to energy intake regulation in human subjects. *British Journal of Nutrition*, **85**, 351–361.

WESTERTERP-PLANTENGA M and KOVACS E M R (2002), The effect of (–)-hydroxycitrate on energy intake and satiety in overweight humans. *International Journal of Obesity*, **26**, 870–872.

WIELINGA P Y, WACHTERS-HAGEDOORN R E, BOUTER B, VAN DIJK T H, STELLAARD F, NIEUWENHUIZEN A G, VERKADE H J and SCHEURINK A J W (2005), Hydroxycitric acid delays intestinal glucose absorption in rats. *American Journal of Physiology*, **288**, G1144–G1149.

WILLETT W C (1998), Is dietary fat a major determinant of body fat? *American Journal of Clinical Nutrition*, **67**, 556S–562S.

WILLIAMS C M, BATEMAN P A, JACKSON K G and YAQOOB P (2004), Dietary fatty acids and chylomicron synthesis and secretion. *Biochemical Society Transactions*, **32**, 55–58.

WOLFRAM S, RAEDERSTORFF D, WANG Y, TEIXEIRA S R, ELSTE V and WEBER P (2005), TEAVIGO (TM) (epigallocatechin gallate) supplementation prevents obesity in rodents by reducing adipose tissue mass. *Annals of Nutrition and Metabolism*, **49**, 54–63.

WOODMAN R J, MORI T A, BURKE V, PUDDEY I B, WATTS G F and BEILIN L J (2002), Effects of purified eicosapentaenoic and docosahexaenoic acids on glycemic control, blood pressure, and serum lipids in type 2 diabetic patients with treated hypertension. *American Journal of Clinical Nutrition*, **76**, 1007–1015.

WORTMAN M D, CLEGG D J, D'ALESSIO D, WOODS S C and SEELEY R J (2003), C75 inhibits food intake by increasing CNS glucose metabolism. *Nature Medicine*, **9**, 483–485.

XIA Z N, STANHOPE K L, DIGITALE E, SIMION O M, CHEN L Y, HAVEL P and CIANFLONE K (2004), Acylation-stimulating protein (ASP)/complement C3adesArg deficiency results in increased energy expenditure in mice. *Journal of Biological Chemistry*, **279**, 4051–4057.

YAMAUCHI T, KAMON J, WAKI H, TERAUCHI Y, KUBOTA N, HARA K, MORI Y, IDE T, MURAKAMI K, TSUBOYAMA-KASAOKA N, EZAKI O, AKANUMA Y, GAVRILOVA O, VINSON C, REITMAN M L, KAGECHIKA H, SHUDO K, YODA M, NAKANO Y, TOBE K, NAGAI R, KIMURA S, TOMITA M, FROGUEL P and KADOWAKI T (2001), The fat-derived hormone adiponectin reverses insulin resistance associated with both lipoatrophy and obesity. *Nature Medicine*, **7**, 941–946.

YANG W S, LEE W J, FUNAHASHI T, TANAKA S, MATSUZAWA Y, CHAO C L, CHEN C L, TAI T Y and CHUANG L M (2001), Weight reduction increases plasma levels of an adipose-derived anti-inflammatory protein, adiponectin. *Journal of Clinical Endocrinology and Metabolism*, **86**, 3815–3819.

ZAMBELL K L, FITCH M D and FLEMING S E (2003), Acetate and butyrate are the major substrates for de novo lipogenesis in rat colonic epithelial cells. *Journal of Nutrition*, **133**, 3509–3515.

ZHANG R, XIAO W P, WANG X, WU X D and TIAN W X (2006), Novel inhibitors of fatty-acid synthase from green tea (Camellia sinensis Xihu Longjing) with high activity and a new reacting site. *Biotechnology and Applied Biochemistry*, **43**, 1–7.

ZHANG Y Y, PROENCA R, MAFFEI M, BARONE M, LEOPOLD L and FRIEDMAN J M (1994), Positional cloning of the mouse obese gene and its human homolog. *Nature*, **372**, 425–432.

# 2

# Hunger and satiety: relation to body weight control

**H. F. J. Hendriks, G. C. M. Bakker, W. J. Pasman, A. Stafleu and W. A. M. Blom, TNO Quality of Life, Zeist, The Netherlands**

## 2.1 Introduction

Currently more than 1 billion adults are overweight – and at least 300 million of them are clinically obese. Obesity levels range from below 5% in China, Japan and certain African nations, to over 75% in urban Samoa. But even in relatively low prevalence countries like China, rates are almost 20% in some cities. Childhood obesity is already epidemic in some areas and is on the rise in others. An estimated 22 million children under five are estimated to be overweight worldwide. According to the US Surgeon General, in the USA the number of overweight children has doubled and the number of overweight adolescents has trebled since 1980. The principal causes of the epidemic of overweight and obesity are sedentary lifestyles and high-fat, energy-dense diets, resulting in increased energy intake and decreased energy expenditure. Body weight may be managed by increasing physical activity to increase energy expenditure and by lowering food intake to decrease in energy intake. Energy intake is predominately determined by two processes: satiety and satiation. We start eating when we get hungry (= absence of satiety) and stop when we feel full (satiation).

Thus, there is an urgent need for food products that help to maintain body weight at the present low level of physical activity. Substances that speed up the process of satiation (feeling full) and/or induce longer-term feelings of satiety (absence of hunger) may help to control weight. The development of suitable biomarkers is very important for efficacy and safety studies of newly developed foods or ingredients aimed at long-term weight management.

## 2.2 Factors influencing satiety and satiation

Research on the regulation of food intake has been carried out for many years, but the mechanism of the human regulation of food intake has not been elucidated yet. Three main levels of food intake regulation may be distinguished. These include the level of the gastrointestinal tract and the level of the hypothalamus in the brain. These first two levels will provide input to the cortex resulting in behavior after further integration with cognitive processes (third level).

The gastrointestinal tract and nervous system, both central and enteric, are involved in two-way extrinsic communication by parasympathetic and sympathetic nerves, each comprising efferent fibers and afferent sensory fibers required for gut–brain signaling. Afferent nerves are equipped with numerous sensors at their terminals in the gut related to visceral mechano-, chemo- and noci-receptors, whose excitations may trigger a variety of visceral reflexes regulating gastrointestinal functions and appetitive behavior. Food intake depends upon various influences from the central nervous system as well as from the body energy stores.

The complexity and the central level of integration of food intake regulatory signals are the reason for the lack of full understanding of food intake regulation in humans. Animal research has unraveled part of this central regulation which takes place mainly in the hypothalamus. However, the regulation of food intake in humans may be different from animals but investigating these central mechanisms is extremely difficult in humans. Apart from the complexity and limited technological possibilities, new hormonal factors involved in food intake regulation are still being identified (e.g. ghrelin and obestatin). Lastly, humans do not eat solely in response to a metabolic need for nutrients, but also in response to non-physiological factors that are hard to control in a research setting.

### 2.2.1 Non-physiological factors influencing food intake

External non-physiological factors modulate physiologically derived hunger and satiety signals. Non-physiological factors such as hedonic (palatability, taste, texture, odour), social (culture, religion), psychological (preferences, aversions, emotions, dieting behaviour), environmental (temperature, time of day, other people), economic (cost, availability) and pharmacological (anorectants) factors influence food intake. The extent to which different individuals respond to these various factors may vary markedly. This may explain some discrepancies among human food intake studies, and some reports of high between-subject variability.

### 2.2.2 Physiological factors influencing food intake

The regulation of food intake is a complex interaction between numerous signals acting both peripherally and centrally, each varying over time.

Consuming a meal may be divided into three phases: a pre-prandial, a prandial and a postprandial (pre-absorptive and post-absorptive) phase. In addition, food intake is usually divided into two phases: satiation (meal termination) and satiety (absence of satiety leads to meal initiation). Roughly speaking, factors important during the prandial phase are involved in satiation, and factors important during the postprandial phase are involved in satiety. However, in practice this distinction is less clear.

*Satiation (meal termination)*

During the pre-prandial phase, visual, olfactory, gustatory and tactile inputs stimulate processes at multiple sites (i.e. salivary glands, gastrointestinal tract, pancreas, and cardiovascular and renal systems). These processes result in a cascade of physiological processes, termed the 'cephalic phase response', which occurs within seconds to minutes after exposure to foods. The taste and smell of foods stimulate, for example, gastrin and gastric acid release (Mattes, 1997). The cephalic phase responses improve or optimize the efficiency of the digestion, absorption and utilization of nutrients (Halford and Blundell, 2000).

During the prandial phase the central nervous system receives sensory afferent inputs reflecting the amount of food eaten and initial estimations of its nutrient content. Mechanoreceptors in the gut detect the distension of the gut caused by the presence of food. This helps to estimate the volume of food consumed. Fullness is directly correlated to gastric content, and hunger and desire to eat are inversely correlated. Oral ingestion of a physiological amount of nutrients leads to the greatest suppression of appetite. Orosensory stimulation (taste and smell perception) enhances the appetite-suppressing effects produced by gastric distension, probably partly caused by slower gastric emptying (Cecil *et al.*, 1998).

Chemoreceptors in the gastrointestinal tract detect the chemical presence of nutrients, and provide information on the composition of the foods consumed. Factors such as cholecystokinine (CCK) and glucagon-like peptide 1 (GLP-1) are released in response to the chemical presence of food in the gastrointestinal tract. CCK is a hormone released in the duodenum in response to consumption of fat (i.e. long-chain fatty acids) or protein (i.e. amino acids). GLP-1 is a hormone released in the blood by mucosal cells of the gut in response to the presence of carbohydrates and fat (MacIntosh *et al.*, 2001). CCK and GLP-1 suppress appetite by decreasing gastric emptying – by affecting the pyloric pressure, stomach motility and stomach muscle relaxation. By decreasing stomach emptying, the stomach distension increases, leading to sensations of fullness (Geliebter *et al.*, 1988; Rolls *et al.*, 1998). GLP-1 stimulates the islet B-cells in the pancreas to secrete insulin, thereby lowering blood glucose levels in response to carbohydrate consumption.

The effect of nutrients on satiety and satiation depends on the position of the nutrients in the digestive tract. The presence of physiological amounts of nutrients in the intestine provides a weak stimulus for the regulation of appetite. The same physiological amount of nutrients in the stomach leads to an increased suppression of appetite.

*Satiety (meal initiation)*

Owing to its central role in the regulation of energy metabolism, the role of glucose in meal initiation has been extensively investigated. Although absolute concentrations of glucose do not seem to be very important in the regulation of food intake (Chapman, 1998; Gielkens *et al.*, 1998), transient and dynamic declines in blood glucose concentration seem to be strongly related to meal initiation (Campfield and Smith, 1990; Kovacs *et al.*, 2002). In addition, intraduodenal glucose influences appetite, possibly through glucoreceptors or osmoreceptors in the intestine, which may induce satiety through direct vagal stimulation or via the release of insulin and/or incretin hormones such as GLP-1 (Lavin *et al.*, 1996). Unlike glucose, the role of insulin in the regulation of food intake is not clear, since studies examining exogenous insulin as well as studies investigating endogenous insulin give mixed results (Campfield *et al.*, 1996; Chapman, 1998).

Ghrelin is abundantly synthesized in the fundus of the human stomach (Ariyasu *et al.*, 2001), and is suggested to be involved in meal initiation. Plasma ghrelin concentrations rise before each meal and they decrease between meals (Cummings *et al.*, 2002). Moreover, an intravenous infusion of ghrelin in humans has been shown to increase food intake potently and enhance appetite by approximately 28% (Wren *et al.*, 2001). In response to oral and intravenous administration of glucose, plasma ghrelin concentrations decrease. Intake of an equivalent volume of water, however, does not influence ghrelin concentrations (Shiiya *et al.*, 2002), suggesting that secretion of ghrelin is not affected by stomach expansion. Moreover, ghrelin responses are dependent on energy dose and on type and composition of the macronutrients (Blom *et al.*, 2005, 2006). Ghrelin concentrations appear to be positively associated with appetite scores and inversely associated with intermeal interval. Such associations suggest that suppression of ghrelin concentrations may postpone initiation of the next meal. These are interesting results that need to be investigated further.

Peptide YY (PYY), which is also a gut hormone, is postprandially released in response to medium- and long-chain fatty acids but not after sucrose polyester ingestion (Maas *et al.*, 1998). PYY suppresses 24-h food intake in humans (Batterham *et al.*, 2002) and is correlated with measures of appetite (MacIntosh *et al.*, 1999).

*Long-term regulation of food intake*

Long-term food intake regulation is essential in food-weight management. The hormone leptin appears to be involved in long-term food intake regulation. Leptin is synthesized mainly by adipose tissue; it acts through receptors present in afferent visceral nerves and the hypothalamic arcuate nucleus, whose neurons are capable of expressing and releasing neuropeptide Y and agouti-related protein which activate ingestive behavior through the paraventricular nucleus.

Plasma leptin concentrations correlate positively with total body fat stores (Sinha *et al.*, 1996). An energy deficit of more than 24 h leads to decreases of plasma leptin concentration (Boden *et al.*, 1996), whereas an energy surplus of more than 24 h results in increased leptin concentrations (Kolaczynski *et al.*, 1996). Plasma leptin is negatively correlated with appetite and food intake when the energy balance is severely disturbed (Keim *et al.*, 1998; Chin-Chance *et al.*, 2000).

When subjects are in energy balance, the relation between leptin concentrations and food intake and appetite is less clear (Karhunen *et al.*, 1997; Joannic *et al.*, 1998; Romon *et al.*, 1999). Therefore, leptin seems to have a role in the regulation of food intake when energy stores are depleted or increased, rather than during energy balance.

The balance and interaction between anorexigenic (e.g. CCK, PYY) and orexigenic (ghrelin) factors originating from the gastrointestinal tract appear to play an important role in short-term regulation of food intake. An impairment of this balance may result in disorders of feeding behavior and weight gain (obesity) or weight loss (cachexia). Understanding this balance is essential in developing foods that help people maintain a healthy body weight.

## 2.3 The impact of different food components on satiety

In the past 20 years, numerous studies have been carried out to investigate the impact of different food components on satiety. Research has been done on three levels:

1 Effects of food components on subjective ratings of hunger and satiety.
2 Effects of food components on energy intake.
3 Effects of food components on body weight and long-term energy balance.

Much work has been done using a paradigm developed 20 years ago (Kissileff *et al.*, 1984) consisting of a preload or a test meal, after which subjects are followed up for several hours. In this paradigm subjects ingest preloads that differ in one particular property of food, whereas other properties are held constant, e.g. the fat content of a certain food is varied, while an attempt is made to hold the other properties (e.g. weight, volume, taste) constant. After the preloads, subjects record their feelings of hunger and satiety, and/or get a test meal from which they can eat *ad libitum*. The degree to which a particular property suppresses subsequent energy intake, and/or ratings of hunger and satiety, is then a measure of the satiating efficiency.

Many of the longer-term studies use a somewhat different approach to investigate the impact of properties of food on satiety. In many of these studies, subjects are offered diets that differ in one or more properties, from which they eat *ad libitum* for a certain amount of time. For example, in one study on the longer-term effects of the fat content of the diet on energy intake and energy balance, one group of subjects was offered a diet with foods of regular fat content, and another group of subjects was provided with the same foods but with a reduced fat content (de Graaf *et al.*, 1997). The time span of these studies varies from a few days to a few years, with many more short-term studies than longer-term studies. The effects of the various food components on satiety are described below.

### 2.3.1 Macronutrient content

The results of a number of studies suggest that the order of satiating efficiency of macronutrients is protein > carbohydrate > fat > alcohol, although this conclusion was not confirmed in one study (Raben *et al.*, 2003). The weak effect of fat on satiety is well documented. In many studies that covertly manipulated the fat content of foods, subjects did not respond to higher fat levels in preloads with subsequent lower hunger ratings and/or lower food and energy intakes. This is a consistent finding across studies with various foods (e.g. foods with fat replacers, regular foods with high/low fat levels) (de Graaf *et al.*, 1996) and with different groups of subjects (Rolls *et al.*, 1994).

The low satiating efficiency of fat is confirmed in short- and long-term studies on the *ad libitum* energy intake and energy balance from diets with various levels of fat. These studies show that *ad libitum* energy intake is lower on low-fat diets than on high-fat diets (e.g. Lissner *et al.*, 1987). Astrup *et al.* (2002) summarized the data from 13 clinical trials on low-fat diet and concluded that 'The evidence strongly supports the low-fat diet as the optimal choice for the prevention of weight gain and obesity.'

The results of a number of studies suggest that, per calorie, protein is the most satiating macronutrient (Raben *et al.*, 2003). This hypothesis was confirmed in a long-term trial (Haulrik *et al.*, 2002) in which it was shown that a high-protein diet led to a lower body weight. The results of some studies suggest that carbohydrates are more satiating than fats (Rolls and Hammer, 1995). In general, high-carbohydrate/low-fat diets lead to a lower energy intake than high-fat/low-carbohydrate diets. However, it is not clear whether this effect is related to the lower energy density of carbohydrates compared with fat. Complex carbohydrates may be more satiating than simple carbohydrates. Initial studies using complex carbohydrates, such as the exopolysaccharide Reuteran® in low quantities, did not show a clear effect on subjective measures of hunger and satiety nor on hunger-related hormones (Blom *et al.*, 2005). In a small additional clinical study, several tens of grams

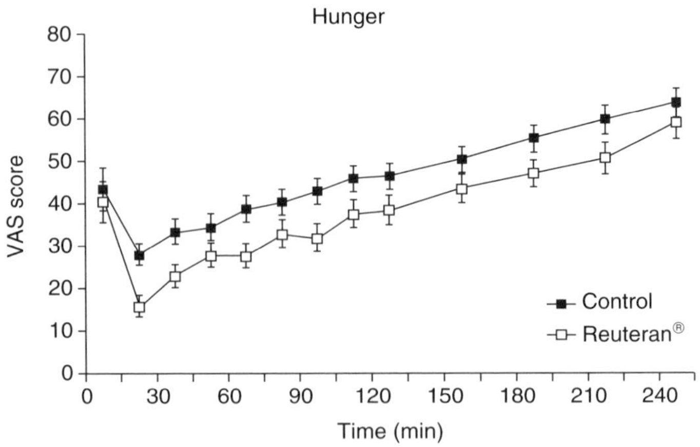


**Fig. 2.1** Effect of Reuteran® on hunger (VAS score is the score on a visual analog scale).

of Reuteran® appeared to postpone feelings of hunger (see Fig. 2.1) and stimulate satiety, but also appeared to suppress blood glucose and insulin levels.

The effect of alcohol on satiety is difficult to investigate because alcohol has strong behavioural effects. Results of studies of de Castro and Orozco (1990) indicated that the energy intakes from meals with alcohol are on average higher than the energy intakes from meals without alcohol.

### 2.3.2 Fiber

Fiber contributes to post-ingestive satiety. This result is clear from many studies (Holt *et al.*, 1995; Delargy *et al.*, 1997; Marlett *et al.*, 2002). The mechanisms through which fiber exerts these effects are, however, less clear. These mechanisms may include slower gastric emptying, increasing bulk, and/or increased transient time and nutrient exposure in the gut. The fiber content of foods also contributes to a lower glycemic index, which may facilitate the control of food intake (Jenkins *et al.*, 2002; Rizkalla *et al.*, 2002).

### 2.3.3 Weight and energy density

The weight and energy density of foods play a crucial role with respect to the impact of food components on satiety. From a large number of short-term studies it is clear that humans primarily regulate their food intake on the basis of the weight of foods, and not the energy content (Poppitt and Prentice, 1996). For example, when subjects have *ad libitum* access to foods (e.g. yoghurts) with varying energy densities (e.g. by manipulating the fat content), these subjects will generally ingest equal weights of the different foods. The energy intake is then positively related to the energy density. The constant weight intake can be conceived of as a learned response, based on the association between the sensory properties of foods and their post-ingestive hunger and satiety consequences. For example, after a number of exposures we learn that we need to eat a certain amount of certain foods for breakfast (e.g. two sandwiches with cheese) in order to stay satiated until lunch. This learning must be based on the association between the sensory properties of bread and cheese, and the associated post-ingestive consequences.

The idea that we gradually learn this association between sensory properties and post-ingestive consequences, explains why in many short-term studies, subjects do not respond very sensitively to covert manipulations of the energy content of foods (Stubbs *et al.*, 2000). These learned associations enable us to know how much to eat of various foods, e.g. for breakfast or other meals. The regulation on the basis of weight may also explain the weak satiating efficiency of fat that is found in many studies. Foods/diets with a high fat content generally have a high energy density, and consequently a low satiating efficiency.

### 2.3.4 Physical state: solid versus liquid

Solid foods have a larger effect on satiety than liquid foods with an equivalent composition (Hulshof *et al.*, 1993). Some studies found that sugar-containing drinks have little impact on satiety, implying that the energy content of these drinks is simply added to the energy intake from other foods (Tordoff and Alleva, 1990; Raben *et al.*, 2002).

## 2.4 The need for biomarkers of satiety

At present, there are no validated biomarkers of satiety and satiation. Information on satiation and satiety can only be assessed by means of subjective introspection, such as by measuring the intervals between spontaneous requests for meals (satiety) or by measuring the energy intake from the meal (satiation). There is a need for more objective measures (biomarkers) of satiety and satiation, for example for efficacy testing of bioactive functional food (food with claimed health benefits based or scientific evidence) ingredients. Biomarkers will give more insight into the processes and mechanisms involved in satiety than subjective reports. Therefore biomarkers are more suitable for claim support. Another advantage of objective measures of satiety is that the number of subjects needed in an efficacy study could be diminished, because in general there is less variation in objective parameters compared with subjective reports.

## 2.5 Developing new biomarkers

Biomarkers of satiety and satiation could be defined as physiological measures that relate to subjectively rated appetite and/or actual food intake. Markers can be either indicators of appetite, or they can be proven to be causal factors of appetite (Diplock *et al.*, 1999). Biomarkers should be:

- able to give relatively immediate outcomes to enable interventions on a reasonable time scale;
- validated and of high quality;
- clearly linked to the phenomenon rather than accurately measured;
- sensitive and specific, and reproduced by many centers;
- measurable in easily accessible biological materials (like urine and blood) according to ethical standards and minimally invasive;
- developed on the understanding that dynamic measurements are as useful as, or more useful than, static ones.

### 2.5.1 Biomarkers in blood

Recently developed techniques and acquired knowledge on the regulation of blood parameters known to be involved in signaling satiety and satiation – such as cholecystokinin, glucose, insulin, leptin, GLP-1 and others – enable the measurement of physiological correlates of satiation and satiety. In addition to these 'classic' parameters, new techniques can be used to find biomarkers of satiety. Nuclear magnetic resonance (NMR) spectroscopy combined with pattern recognition is a promising technique to identify potential biomarkers in blood and urine. With NMR techniques, a broad range of compounds with different physico-chemical properties can be detected simultaneously. Sophisticated statistical software is needed to explore patterns in NMR data. From these patterns it is possible to nominate potential biomarkers. Fractionation of the samples and subsequent NMR liquid chromatographic and mass-spectrometric analysis on the fractions will elucidate the structure of the biomarkers. In addition, proteomics, metabolomics and transcriptomics are promising techniques that can be used for identifying biomarkers of satiety (Werf *et al.*, 2001). Transcriptomics and proteomics can be employed to determine changes in gene expression and proteome relevant to the state of hunger or satiety. One such example has recently been published: consuming a breakfast relatively high in protein resulted in higher concentrations of ghrelin, glucagon, gastric inhibitory peptide (GIP), CCK and GLP-1 compared with consuming a breakfast relatively high in carbohydrates (Blom *et al.*, 2005). These conditions also differentially affected lymphocyte gene expression. Consumption of the high-carbohydrate breakfast resulted in expression of glycogen metabolism genes, whereas consumption of the high-protein breakfast resulted in expression of genes involved in protein biosynthesis (Van Erk *et al.*, 2006).

### 2.5.2 Central biomarkers

There is limited knowledge of how the brain contributes to the regulation of food intake in humans. After eating, the human brain senses a biochemical change and then signals satiation, but precisely when this occurs is unknown. With respect to central nervous system biomarkers of satiety and satiation, there have been a number of recent studies in the literature using imaging techniques. The two most important techniques used to study appetite are positron emission tomography (PET) and functional magnetic resonance imaging (fMRI) (Berns, 1999). These studies have identified various regions in the brain that can distinguish between fasted state and that after food ingestion (for example, Liu *et al.*, 2000; Smeets *et al.*, 2005a, 2005b). Some studies suggest that the responses of the brain to a meal differ between obese and lean individuals (Matsuda *et al.*, 1999; Gautier *et al.*, 2000). The rapid development of brain imaging techniques during the past decade, however, provides non-invasive methods enabling the investigation of brain function in response to various stimuli. The applicability of these techniques is limited, because specific and expensive technology is required and only specific brain areas may be investigated.

## 2.6 Future trends

Many components of foods have an effect on satiety and satiation, as they have an effect on energy metabolism and on hormones related to hunger and satiety. For example, protein-rich and solid foods have a higher satiating effect, whereas high-fat and liquid foods have a low satiating efficiency. This knowledge can be used to develop new foods with a higher satiating efficiency.

Another issue is the identification of new components/substances that have an effect on satiety and satiation. New developments in molecular biology, pharmacology and nutrigenomics enhance our insight in the complex pathways involved in energy balance. From these insights new substances will become available that will affect mechanisms involved in hunger and satiety, like *Hoodia gordonii* and Rimonabant®. New substances with a plausible mechanism should first be tested in animal studies with respect to toxicological aspects, and their potential to influence short- and long-term energy balance. This may be followed by short-term safety and efficacy tests in humans. Eventually, the substances may be used in more-long-term trials with humans. Relevant biomarkers of satiety need to be identified. Specific focus is needed for the identification of those short-term biomarkers that will predict long-term body weight changes.

Several reviews (Egger *et al.*, 1999; Allison *et al.*, 2001; Zemel, 2005) have been published on the effect of supplements on weight loss, such as chromium, conjugated linoleic acid (CLA), hydroxycitric acid (HCA), chitosan and Ma Huang (ephedra). In general there is no convincing evidence for the efficacy of the substances reviewed.

Apart from influencing feelings of hunger and satiety, two other potential mechanisms are involved in products aimed at weight loss or weight maintenance:

1 Reduction of energy intake. Examples are substances purported to block the absorption of fat; fat replacers, like Olestra (sucrose polyester); low-calorie products, such as light products and meal replacers.
2 Increasing energy expenditure. Examples are substances with an effect on fat burning, changes in basal metabolism and thermogenesis increase energy expenditure, like caffeine and ephedra.

For the design of new products that influence feelings of hunger and satiety it is necessary to identify food components with a satiating effect. Products could either speed up satiation (so that one stops eating sooner) or induce long-term satiety (so that one is not feeling hungry for a prolonged period after eating the product). These could be products or substances with an effect on noradrenalin and serotonin, such as St John's Wort and capsaicin, or products or substances that influence stomach filling, such as fiber, resistant starch or pectin. Products may need to be combined with interventions on other lifestyle factors such as physical activity to obtain optimal weight management.

To evaluate whether new or existing weight management products are effective in influencing satiety and satiation, biomarkers of both satiety and satiation should be used in controlled human intervention studies. Upon intervention, the marker should change in a statistically significant as well as physiological relevant way.

## 2.7 References

ALLISON D B, FONTAINE K R, HESHKA S, MENTORE J L and HEYMSFIELD S B (2001), 'Alternative treatments for weight loss: a critical review', *Crit Rev Food Sci Nutr*, **41** (1), 1–28.

ARIYASU H, TAKAYA K, TAGAMI T, OGAWA Y, HOSODA K, AKAMIZU T, SUDA M, KOH T, NATSUI K, TOYOOKA S, SHIRAKAMI G, USUI T, SHIMATSU A, DOI K, HOSODA H, KOJIMA M, KANGAWA K and NAKAO K (2001), 'Stomach is a major source of circulating ghrelin, and feeding state determines plasma ghrelin-like immunoreactivity levels in humans', *J Clin Endocrinol Metab*, **86** (10), 4753–4758.

ASTRUP A, BUEMANN B, FLINT A and RABEN A (2002), 'Low-fat diets and energy balance: how does the evidence stand in 2002?', *Proc Nutr Soc*, **61** (2), 299–309.

BATTERHAM R L, COWLEY M A, SMALL C J, HERZOG H, COHEN M A, DAKIN C L, WREN A M, BRYNES A E, LOW M J, GHATEI M A, CONE R D and BLOOM S R (2002), 'Gut hormone PYY (3–36) physiologically inhibits food intake', *Nature*, **418** (6898), 650–654.

BERNS G S (1999), 'Functional neuroimaging', *Life Sci*, **65** (24), 2531–2540.

BLOM W A M, STAFLEU A, DE GRAAF C, KOK F J, SCHAAFSMA G and HENDRIKS H F J (2005), 'Ghrelin response to carbohydrate-enriched breakfast is related to insulin', *Am J Clin Nutr*, **81** (2), 367–375.

BLOM W A M, LLUCH A, STAFLEU A, VINOY S, HOLST J J, SCHAAFSMA G J and HENDRIKS H F J (2006), 'Effect of a high protein breakfast on the postprandial ghrelin response', *Am J Clin Nutr*, **83** (2), 211–220.

BODEN G, CHEN X, MOZZOLI M and RYAN I (1996), 'Effect of fasting on serum leptin in normal human subjects', *J Clin Endocrinol Metab*, **81** (9), 3419–3423.

CAMPFIELD L A and SMITH F J (1990), 'Transient declines in blood glucose signal meal initiation', *Int J Obesity*, **14** (Suppl 3), 15–31.

CAMPFIELD L, SMITH F, ROSENBAUM M and HIRSCH J (1996), 'Human eating: evidence for a physiological basis using a modified paradigm', *Neurosci Biobehav Rev*, **20** (1), 133–137.

CECIL J, FRANCIS J and READ N (1998), 'Relative contributions of intestinal, gastric, oro-sensory influences and information to changes in appetite induced by the same liquid meal', *Appetite*, **31** (3), 377–390.

CHAPMAN I M (1998), 'Effect of intravenous glucose and euglycemic insulin infusions on short-term appetite and food intake', *Am J Physiol*, **274** (43), R596–R603.

CHIN-CHANCE C, POLONSKY K S and SCHOELLER D A (2000), 'Twenty-four-hour leptin levels respond to cumulative short-term energy imbalance and predict subsequent intake', *J Clin Endocrinol Metab*, **85** (8), 2685–2691.

CUMMINGS D E, WEIGLE D S, FRAYO R S, BREEN P A, MA M K, DELLINGER E P and PURNELL J Q (2002), 'Plasma ghrelin levels after diet-induced weight loss or gastric bypass surgery', *N Engl J Med*, **346** (21), 1623–1630.

DE CASTRO J M and OROZCO S (1990), 'Moderate alcohol intake and spontaneous eating patterns of humans: evidence of unregulated supplementation', *Am J Clin Nutr*, **52** (2), 246–253.

DE GRAAF C, HULSHOF T, WESTSTRATE J A and HAUTVAST J G (1996), 'Nonabsorbable fat (sucrose polyester) and the regulation of energy intake and body weight', *Am J Physiol*, **270** (6 Pt 2), R1386–R1393.

DE GRAAF C, DRIJVERS J J, ZIMMERMANNS N J, VAN HET H K, WESTSTRATE J A, VAN DEN B H, VELTHUIS-TE WIERIK E J, WESTERTERP K R, VERBOEKET-VAN DE VENNE W P and WESTERTERP-PLANTENGA M S (1997), 'Energy and fat compensation during long-term consumption of reduced fat products', *Appetite*, **29** (3), 305–323.

DELARGY H J, O'SULLIVAN K R, FLETCHER R J and BLUNDELL J E (1997), 'Effects of amount and type of dietary fiber (soluble and insoluble) on short-term control of appetite', *Int J Food Sci Nutr*, **48** (1), 67–77.

DIPLOCK A T, AGGETT P J, ASHWELL M, BORNET F, FERN E B and ROBERTFROID M B (1999), 'Scientific concepts of functional foods in Europe: Consensus Document', *Br J Nutr*, **81**, S1–S27.

EGGER G, CAMERON-SMITH D and STANTON R (1999), 'The effectiveness of popular, non-prescription weight loss supplements, *Med J Aus*, **171** (11–12), 599–600.

GAUTIER J F, CHEN K, SALBE A D, BANDY D, PRATLEY R E, HEIMAN M, RAVUSSIN E, REIMAN E M and TATARANNI P A (2000), 'Differential brain responses to satiation in obese and lean men', *Diabetes*, **49** (5), 838–846.

GELIEBTER A, WESTREICH S and GAGE D (1988), 'Gastric distention by balloon and test-meal intake in obese and lean subjects', *Am J Clin Nutr*, **48** (3), 592–594.

GIELKENS H A, VERKIJK M, LAM W F, LAMERS C B and MASCLEE A A (1998), 'Effects of hyperglycemia and hyperinsulinemia on satiety in humans', *Metabolism*, **47** (3), 321–324.

HALFORD J and BLUNDELL J (2000), 'Pharmacology of appetite suppression', *Prog Drug Res*, **54**, 25–58.

HAULRIK N, TOUBRO S, DYERBERG J, STENDER S, SKOV A R and ASTRUP A (2002), 'Effect of protein and methionine intakes on plasma homocysteine concentrations: a 6-mo randomized controlled trial in overweight subjects', *Am J Clin Nutr*, **76** (6), 1202–1206.

HOLT S H, MILLER J C, PETOCZ P and FARMAKALIDIS E (1995), 'A satiety index of common foods', *Eur J Clin Nutr*, **49** (9), 675–690.

HULSHOF T, DE GRAAF C and WESTSTRATE J A (1993), 'The effects of preloads varying in physical state and fat content on satiety and energy intake', *Appetite*, **21** (3), 273–286.

JENKINS D J, KENDALL C W, AUGUSTIN L S, FRANCESCHI S, HAMIDI M, MARCHIE A, JENKINS A L and AXELSEN M (2002), 'Glycemic index: overview of implications in health and disease', *Am J Clin Nutr*, **76** (1), 266S–273S.

JOANNIC J L, OPPERT J M, LAHLOU N, BASDEVANT A, AUBOIRON S, RAISON J, BORNET F and GUY-GRAND B (1998), 'Plasma leptin and hunger ratings in healthy humans', *Appetite*, **30** (2), 129–138.

KARHUNEN L, HAFFNER S, LAPPALAINEN R, TURPEINEN A, MIETTINEN H and UUSITUPA M (1997), 'Serum leptin and short-term regulation of eating in obese women', *Clin Sci (Lond)*, **92** (6), 573–578.

KEIM N, STERN J and HAVEL P (1998), 'Relation between circulating leptin concentrations and appetite during a prolonged, moderate energy deficit in women', *Am J Clin Nutr*, **68** (4), 794–801.

KISSILEFF H R, GRUSS L P, THORNTON J and JORDAN H A (1984), 'The satiating efficiency of foods', *Physiol Behav*, **32** (2), 319–332.

KOLACZYNSKI J W, OHANNESIAN J P, CONSIDINE R V, MARCO C C and CARO J F (1996), 'Response of leptin to short-term and prolonged overfeeding in humans', *J Clin Endocrinol Metab*, **81** (11), 4162–4165.

KOVACS E M, WESTERTERP-PLANTENGA M S, SARIS W H, MELANSON K J, GOOSSENS I, GEURTEN P and BROUNS F (2002), 'Associations between spontaneous meal initiations and blood glucose dynamics in overweight men in negative energy balance', *Br J Nutr*, **87** (1), 39–45.

LAVIN J H, WITTERT G, SUN W M, HOROWITZ M, MORLEY J E and READ N W (1996), 'Appetite regulation by carbohydrate: role of blood glucose and gastrointestinal hormones', *Am J Physiol*, **271** (2 Pt 1), E209–E214.

LISSNER L, LEVITSKY D A, STRUPP B J, KALKWARF H J and ROE D A (1987), 'Dietary fat and the regulation of energy intake in human subjects', *Am J Clin Nutr*, **46** (6), 886–892.

LIU Y, GAO J, LIU H and FOX P (2000), 'The temporal response of the brain after eating revealed by functional MRI', *Nature*, **405** (6790), 1058–1062.

MAAS M I, HOPMAN W P, KATAN M B and JANSEN J B (1998), 'Release of peptide YY and inhibition of gastric acid secretion by long-chain and medium-chain triglycerides but not by sucrose polyester in men', *Eur J Clin Invest*, **28** (2), 123–130.

MACINTOSH C G, ANDREWS J M, JONES K L, WISHART J M, MORRIS H A, JANSEN J B, MORLEY J E, HOROWITZ M and CHAPMAN I M (1999), 'Effects of age on concentrations of plasma cholecystokinin, glucagon-like peptide 1, and peptide YY and their relation to appetite and pyloric motility', *Am J Clin Nutr*, **69** (5), 999–1006.

MACINTOSH C G, HOROWITZ M, VERHAGEN M A, SMOUT A J, WISHART J, MORRIS H, GOBLE E, MORLEY J E and CHAPMAN I M (2001), 'Effect of small intestinal nutrient infusion on appetite, gastrointestinal hormone release, and gastric myoelectrical activity in young and older men', *Am J Gastroenterol*, **96** (4), 997–1007.

MARLETT J A, MCBURNEY M I and SLAVIN J L (2002), 'Position of the American Dietetic Association: health implications of dietary fiber', *J Am Diet Assoc*, **102** (7), 993–1000.

MATSUDA M, LIU Y, MAHANKALI S, PU Y, MAHANKALI A, WANG J, DEFRONZO R A, FOX P T and GAO J H (1999), 'Altered hypothalamic function in response to glucose ingestion in obese humans', *Diabetes*, **48** (9), 1801–1806.

MATTES R D (1997), 'Physiologic responses to sensory stimulation by food: nutritional implications', *J Am Diet Assoc*, **97** (4), 406–413.

POPPITT S D and PRENTICE A M (1996), 'Energy density and its role in the control of food intake: evidence from metabolic and community studies', *Appetite*, **26** (2), 153–174.

RABEN A, VASILARAS T H, MOLLER A C and ASTRUP A (2002), 'Sucrose compared with artificial sweeteners: different effects on ad libitum food intake and body weight after 10 wk of supplementation in overweight subjects', *Am J Clin Nutr*, **76** (4), 721–729.

RABEN A, AGERHOLM-LARSEN L, FLINT A, HOLST J J and ASTRUP A (2003), 'Meals with similar energy densities but rich in protein, fat, carbohydrate, or alcohol have different effects on energy expenditure and substrate metabolism but not on appetite and energy intake', *Am J Clin Nutr*, **77** (1), 91–100.

RIZKALLA S W, BELLISLE F and SLAMA G (2002), 'Health benefits of low glycaemic index foods, such as pulses, in diabetic patients and healthy individuals', *Br J Nutr*, **88** (Suppl 3), S255–S262.

ROLLS B, CASTELLANOS V, HALFORD J, KILARA A, PANYAM D, PELKMAN C, SMITH G and THORWART M (1998), 'Volume of food consumed affects satiety in men', *Am J Clin Nutr*, **67** (6), 1170–1177.

ROLLS B J and HAMMER V A (1995), 'Fat, carbohydrate, and the regulation of energy intake', *Am J Clin Nutr*, **62** (5S), 1086–1095.

ROLLS B J, KIM-HARRIS S, FISCHMAN M W, FOLTIN R W, MORAN T H and STONER S A (1994), 'Satiety after preloads with different amounts of fat and carbohydrate: implications for obesity', *Am J Clin Nutr*, **60** (4), 476–487.

ROMON M, LEBEL P, VELLY C, MARECAUX N, FRUCHART J C and DALLONGEVILLE J (1999), 'Leptin response to carbohydrate or fat meal and association with subsequent satiety and energy intake', *Am J Physiol*, **277** (5 Pt 1), E855–E861.

SHIIYA T, NAKAZATO M, MIZUTA M, DATE Y, MONDAL M S, TANAKA M, NOZOE S, HOSODA H, KANGAWA K and MATSUKURA S (2002), 'Plasma ghrelin levels in lean and obese humans and the effect of glucose on ghrelin secretion', *J Clin Endocrinol Metab*, **87** (1), 240–244.

SINHA M, OHANNESIAN J, HEIMAN M, KRIAUCIUNAS A, STEPHENS T, MAGOSIN S, MARCO C and CARO J (1996), 'Nocturnal rise of leptin in lean, obese, and non-insulin-dependent diabetes mellitus subjects', *J Clin Invest*, **97** (5), 1344–1347.

SMEETS P A M, VAN OSCH M J P, DE GRAAF C, STAFLEU A and VAN DER GROND J (2005a), 'Functional MRI of human hypothalamic responses following glucose ingestion', *NeuroImage*, **24** (2), 363–368.

SMEETS P A M, DE GRAAF C, STAFLEU A, VAN OSCH M J P and VAN DER GROND J (2005b), Functional magnetic resonance imaging of human hypothalamic responses to sweet taste and calories', *Am J Clin Nutr*, **82** (5), 1011–1016.

STUBBS J, FERRES S and HORGAN G (2000), 'Energy density of foods: effects on energy intake', *Crit Rev Food Sci Nutr*, **40** (6), 481–515.

TORDOFF M G and ALLEVA A M (1990), 'Effect of drinking soda sweetened with aspartame or high-fructose corn syrup on food intake and body weight', *Am J Clin Nutr*, **51** (6), 963–969.

VAN ERK M J, BLOM W A M, VAN OMMEN B and HENDRIKS H F J (2006), High protein and high carbohydrate breakfasts differentially change the transcriptome of human blood cells', *Am J Clin Nutr*, **84**, 1233–1241.

WERF M J, SCHUREN F H J, BIJLSMA S, TAS A C and OMMEN B V (2001), 'Nutrigenomics: application of genomics technologies in nutritional sciences and food technology', *J Food Sci*, **66** (6), 772–780.

WREN A M, SEAL L J, COHEN M A, BRYNES A E, FROST G S, MURPHY K G, DHILLO W S, GHATEI M A and BLOOM S R (2001), 'Ghrelin enhances appetite and increases food intake in humans', *J Clin Endocrinol Metab*, **86** (12), 5992.

ZEMEL M B (2005), 'The role of dietary calcium in weight management', *J Am Coll Nutr*, **24** (6), 537S–546S.

# 3

# Glycaemic control, insulin resistance and obesity

**I. Aeberli and M. Zimmermann, ETH Zürich, Switzerland**

## 3.1 Introduction

Of all dietary factors, high fat intake in a population has been suggested to be the main contributor to the increasing prevalence of obesity (Astrup & Raben, 1992; Golay & Bobbioni, 1997). However, studies of the US population over the last few decades have reported that, despite the steady increase in the prevalence of overweight and obesity, fat intake has actually fallen from 42 to 34% of total energy, whereas carbohydrate intake has increased (Allred, 1995; Nicklas, 1995). Brand-Miller *et al.* (2002) suggested that current dietary recommendations to increase the percentage of daily energy as carbohydrate may be counterproductive to weight control, as many high-carbohydrate, low-fat diets markedly increase postprandial hyperglycaemia and hyperinsulinaemia. Not only the amount, but also the form of the recommended dietary carbohydrate must be considered, as both the quantity and quality of a carbohydrate can influence postprandial glycaemia (Brand-Miller *et al.*, 2002).

Dietary carbohydrates are digested and absorbed at different rates and to different extents in the gastrointestinal tract, depending on their botanical source and the physical form of the food (Cummings *et al.*, 1997). Diets that contain large amounts of easily digested carbohydrate, which rapidly increase blood glucose and stimulate a large insulin response, may be detrimental to health (Englyst *et al.*, 1999). Several studies have found an association between this type of diet and obesity and type 2 diabetes mellitus (Salmeron *et al.*, 1997a, b; Ludwig *et al.*, 1999). Foods containing easily digested carbohydrates that produce a rapid rise in blood glucose are termed 'high glycaemic index (GI) foods'. The GI will be discussed in detail later in this chapter.

Low-GI foods are generally associated with greater satiety compared with high-GI foods (Haber *et al.*, 1977; Holt *et al.*, 1992; Holt & Miller, 1994; Liljeberg *et al.*, 1999; Ludwig *et al.*, 1999). The characteristic postprandial effects of high-GI foods – including rapid carbohydrate absorption, large fluctuations in blood glucose and insulin levels, together with reduced satiety – may contribute to overweight in the long run (Haber *et al.*, 1977).

## 3.2 The glycaemic index of foods and its effect on insulin response and glycaemia

The glycaemic response to a food, which in turn affects the insulin response, depends on the rate of gastric emptying, as well as on the rate of digestion and absorption of carbohydrates from the small intestine (Jenkins *et al.*, 1987). Traditionally, carbohydrates were classified as 'simple' and 'complex' based on their degree of polymerization. Sugars (which are mono- and disaccharides) were therefore classified as simple, whereas starches (polysaccharides) were classified as complex. However, carbohydrates might be better classified on the basis of their physiological effects, for example their ability to increase blood glucose. The glycaemic response depends both on the type of sugar (e.g. glucose, fructose, galactose) and the physical form of the carbohydrate (e.g. particle size, degree of polymerization) (Augustin *et al.*, 2002).

In 1981, Jenkins *et al.* (1981) proposed the concept of the GI to characterize the rate of carbohydrate absorbed after a meal. The GI was meant to supplement information about chemical composition given in food tables, to help understand and better predict the physiological effects of whole diets. Unexpected differences between the GI values of different foods highlighted the importance of food characteristics not provided in food composition tables. These include food form, particle size, the nature of the starch, food processing and interfering factors, all which may have large effects on the physiological properties of foods.

The GI is defined as the area under the glucose response curve after consumption of 50 g available carbohydrate from a test food divided by the area under the curve after consumption of 50 g available carbohydrate from a control food. The control food can be either white bread or glucose (Wolever *et al.*, 1991). Foods with a high GI produce, per gram of available carbohydrate, a higher peak in postprandial blood glucose and a greater overall blood glucose response during the first 2 h after consumption than the peak for foods with a low GI (Foster-Powell *et al.*, 2002). A higher blood glucose response increases insulin demand and insulin secretion by the pancreas. Repeated episodes of hyperinsulinemia may, over the long term, lead to downregulation of insulin receptors and insulin resistance (Virkamaki *et al.*, 1999). This may in turn increase postprandial blood glucose concentrations and insulin secretion (Fig. 3.1). Insulin resistance is a central characteristic of type 2 diabetes mellitus (Reaven, 1993). Low-GI diets tend to delay glucose absorption and reduce peak insulin concentrations and overall insulin demand. Several studies have found improvements in glycaemic control with low-GI diets in healthy subjects as well as those with coronary heart disease or diabetes (Burke *et al.*, 1982; Jenkins *et al.*, 1987, 1988; Brand *et al.*, 1991; Frost *et al.*, 1996). In addition, low-GI foods are generally associated with greater satiety compared with high-GI foods, delaying hunger and potentially reducing food intake. Examples of the GI values of different foods are given in Table 3.1.

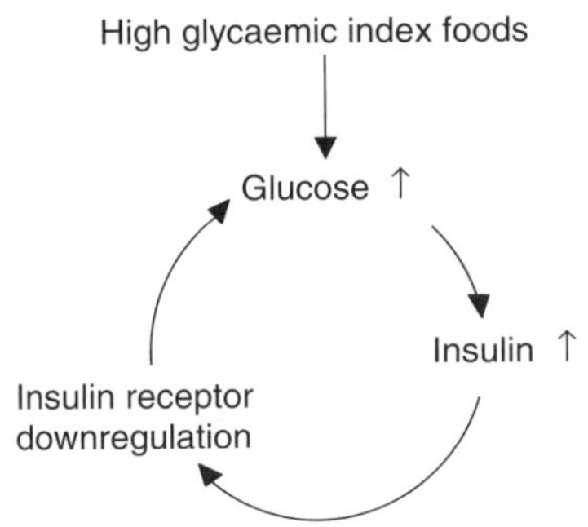


**Fig. 3.1** Potential mechanism for the relationship between high GI foods and insulin resistance [adapted from Jenkins *et al.* (2000)].

**Table 3.1** Examples of the GI and GL[1] of some foods (Foster-Powell *et al.*, 2002)

| Product | GI (glucose = 100) | Carbohydrate (g/100 g) | GL (g/100 g) |
|---|---|---|---|
| Glucose | 100 | 100 | 100 |
| Cornflakes | 81 | 86 | 70 |
| White bread | 70 | 47 | 33 |
| Mars bar | 65 | 66 | 43 |
| Porridge | 58 | 9 | 5 |
| Coca Cola | 58 | 10 | 6 |
| Rice, long grain | 56 | 27 | 15 |
| Mango | 51 | 14 | 7 |
| Whole-grain bread | 51 | 43 | 22 |
| Spaghetti white (cooked) | 44 | 27 | 12 |
| Peach | 42 | 10 | 4 |
| Apple juice | 40 | 10 | 4 |
| Apple | 38 | 13 | 5 |
| Yogurt | 36 | 6 | 2 |

[1]glycaemic load

## 3.3 The effect of food processing on the glycaemic index

Available carbohydrates are those absorbed via the small intestine and used in the metabolism (Livesey, 2005). Indigestible carbohydrates, on the other hand, are considered to be dietary fibre, which include non-starch polysaccharides (mostly of plant and algal origin), resistant starches (RS), oligosaccharides and sugar alcohols (polyols) (Champ *et al.*, 2003). Older methods for measuring dietary fibre did not measure these indigestible carbohydrates completely, leading to an underestimation of the true content of unavailable carbohydrates in foods, and this may have led to inaccuracies in published GI values for foods (Foster-Powell *et al.*, 2002). However, the majority of commercial foods included in the international GI tables contain low levels of these sources of indigestible carbohydrates.

In addition to these problems with analysis, the amount of RS in foods can be influenced by several factors, including processing and preparation methods. Starch can be indigestible due to its botanical structure, or become resistant during processing by retrogradation (the formation of indigestible crystalline structures). The degree of ripening of fruits and vegetables is another variable. For example, a green banana has a very high content of RS, but only negligible amounts remain after ripening (Brouns *et al.*, 2005).

Today, most of the variables that contribute to differences in GI between foods have been identified, and can be used to optimize the GI of commercial food products (see Table 3.2). Some of these factors are related to the choice of raw material and others to the processing conditions. In general, the structure of the food is important. The gross structure can be influenced by grinding or heat treatment; the more homogenized the food, the higher the GI. Cell wall integrity and/or cellular structure changes during the ripening process, and the GI increases with increased ripeness. With respect to starchy foods, a high degree of crystallinity within the starch substrate will favour a lowered rate of amylolysis, and hence a lower GI. A highly ordered starch structure can be obtained by preserving the starch crystallinity present in native granules, i.e. avoiding gelatinization. In most ready-to-eat food items, the starch crystallinity is generally lost as the commonly applied food processing conditions result in more or less complete gelatinization. A tool to increase the crystallinity of processed foods is to promote retrogradation of gelatinized starch. In this respect, the genotype of the raw material can influence the glycaemic response. In starches, the retrogradation of the amylose component but not the amylopectin component can be readily obtained under commonly used conditions of food processing. This makes starches containing high amounts of amylose particularly interesting in this regard.

An enzymatic barrier may be induced by a highly organized food form such as that found in pasta at the molecular level or at the tissue level in leguminous and kernel-based products. The presence of viscous dietary fibre may also reduce the glycaemic response to a carbohydrate meal; the

**Table 3.2** Variables affecting the GI of foods and meals (Arvidsson-Lenner *et al.*, 2004)

| Food variable | Examples of influencing factors | Effect |
|---|---|---|
| **Structure** | | |
| Gross structure | Grinding, heat treatment | Higher GI when homogenized |
| Cellular structure (cell wall integritiy) | Ripeness | Higher GI with increased ripeness |
| **Starch** | | |
| Granular structure (intact or gelatinized) | Heat treatment | Higher GI when gelatinized |
| Amylose (unbranched) | Genotype of raw material | Lower GI compared with amylopectin |
| Amylopectin (branched) | Genotype of raw material | Higher GI compared with amylose |
| **Other factors** | | |
| Gel-forming types of dietary fibre | Genotype of raw material, added fibres | Lowers GI |
| Organic acids | Fermentation, added acids | Lowers GI |
| Amylase inhibitor | Heat treatment | Lowers GI |
| Fructose: glucose ratio | Genotype of raw material, type of added sugar | Lower GI with increased ratio |

mechanism is likely to be due more to reduced gastrointestinal motility than to a reduced rate of starch digestion. Certain organic acids, such as those produced upon sourdough fermentation, may reduce glycaemia either by reducing gastric emptying rate or by reducing the rate of starch digestion. This effect of organic acids has renewed interest in the nutritional benefits of food fermentation. A reduction of the GI for starchy food products appears to be accompanied by a higher content of resistant starch. Food factors that reduce the rate of starch digestion, such as retrogradation of the amylose component or encapsulation within botanical structures, may render a starch fraction resistant to amylase.

For foods high in simple sugars, GI is strongly influenced by the fructose:glucose ratio; the higher the ratio of fructose:glucose, the lower the GI. The GI of sugary foods can therefore be modified by the choice of raw material or through the type of added sugar. The addition of fructose (GI = 19) will lower the GI of a food, whereas addition of glucose (GI = 100) will elevate it (Björck *et al.*, 2000; Arvidsson-Lenner *et al.*, 2004). Fat, by slowing gastric emptying, and protein, by increasing insulin secretion, may both modify the glycaemic response to a carbohydrate food. However, it appears that fat and protein in the amounts found in most foods (with the exception of peanuts and most nuts) do not significantly alter the glycaemic response to the carbohydrate (Wolever *et al.*, 1994).

## 3.4 The glycaemic load

The GI of foods is determined using a food portion containing 50 g available carbohydrate. Although they have the same GI, a portion of two different foods with varying carbohydrate contents per 100 g may have a different impact on glycaemic response (Table 3.1). Therefore the concept of glycaemic load (GL) was introduced to help understand the relationship between the glycaemic response to foods and health outcomes in epidemiological studies (Salmeron *et al.*, 1997a,b). GL is formally the product of the available carbohydrate content and the GI of a food. It is a measure of the quantity and quality of the carbohydrate in the food item and has units of weight (g). Foods with the same GL will theoretically produce the same glycaemic response even if their GI is different (Livesey, 2003).

Which foods should be considered high GI and which should be considered low GI? Professor J. Brand-Miller and her team from the University of Sydney have proposed the following cut-off levels, where the reference food is glucose, with a GI of 100 (www.glycemicindex.com):

- Low GI = 55 or less.
- Medium GI = 56 to 69.
- High GI = 70 or more.

In order to calculate the glycaemic effect of the whole diet, the GL is used. The GL of the diet of one day can be calculated by adding together the individual GLs of all meals consumed over the day. A typical diet of one day will have a GL of about 100. A diet with a daily GL of less than 80 would be considered as low GI and one with a GL of above 120 as high GI.

## 3.5 Association of glycaemic response with satiety and food intake

Satiety signals are physiological responses that follow food consumption and they are believed to terminate eating and/or maintain inhibition of further intake. Many different meal factors – including volume, weight, energy content, macronutrient composition and energy density – may lead to different satiety signals. Cholecystokinin (CCK) is a hormone secreted into the bloodstream by cells in the proximal small intestine after ingestion of food. CCK has been identified as an important satiety signal influenced by the quality of food. It regulates gut motor activity, gallbladder contraction and pancreatic enzyme secretion. It also inhibits gastric emptying thereby enhancing digestion and absorption of nutrients (Bray & James, 1998). Holt *et al.* (1992) studied the effect of meals with different GI but the same macronutrient composition on glycaemic, insulin and CKK response, as well as on satiety. They found that glycaemic and insulin responses to carbohydrate foods are inversely proportional to the CCK response and satiety. High-GI foods, which lead to a high glycaemic and insulin response but a low CCK response, may thereby result in reduced satiety. These data suggest that low-GI foods may enhance satiety in two ways. First, many low-GI foods are rich in dietary fibre and have lower energy density and higher food volume. This may increase satiety and reduce food intake during meals. Second, the low-GI foods increase CCK response, and thereby may increase satiety over a longer period of time.

The rate of hydrolysis of ingested carbohydrate and the rate of gastric emptying are determinants of the rate of glucose absorption, which, in turn, determines the extent and duration of the glucose rise after consumption of a food or meal. Circulating insulin levels are directly determined by β-cell stimulation by absorbed glucose or amino acids. As explained above, the insulin demand is determined not only by the amount of carbohydrate ingested but also by its quality, which will determine the rate of absorption. The GI of foods or meals provides an indication of the rate at which their carbohydrates are digested. Low-GI foods may be considered potential dietary tools to reduce glucose absorption rate and insulin response (Augustin *et al.*, 2002). Slowly digested carbohydrates, which are low GI, may be used to prolong satiety compared with high-GI foods. Studies that have investigated this relationship are summarized in Table 3.3. In one study, the effect of different rice types on satiety and subsequent food intake was measured. Quick-cooking rice and low-amylose rice have a higher GI than ordinary rice and high-amylose rice, respectively. These two low-GI rices induced higher satiety compared with the high-GI ones, and resulted in lower food intake in the 2-hour period after the test meal (Holt & Miller, 1995). Holt and Miller (1994) investigated the blood glucose response and satiety after four test meals of equivalent nutritional composition based on four different grades of wheat. The test meal that caused the highest blood glucose response, fine flour meal, produced the lowest satiety. In contrast, the cracked grain meals caused the lowest blood glucose response and the highest satiety. Warren *et al.* (2003) examined the effect of three different breakfasts on *ad libitum* lunch intake and satiety in children. The different breakfast were low GI, low GI with 10% added sucrose, and high GI. Lunch intake after the high-GI breakfast was significantly higher compared with that after both the low-GI and the low-GI with 10% added sucrose breakfasts. Overall, nearly all of these studies have demonstrated decreased hunger or increased satiety after the ingestion of isoenergetic, low-GI meals compared with high-GI meals (Augustin *et al.*, 2002).

One characteristic response to high-GI foods, termed 'the hypoglycaemic undershot', may induce hunger. High-GI foods trigger high insulin and low blood glucagon concentrations. This postprandial profile normally stimulates glucose uptake and inhibits lipolysis. If this response is exaggerated or prolonged, blood glucose concentration may fall below normal (hypoglycaemic undershot). This may then trigger glucagon release and hunger signals. Low-GI foods on the other hand maintain glucose and insulin at a

**Table 3.3** Studies comparing glycaemic response with changes in hunger, satiety or energy intake [adapted from Ludwig (2000)]

| Reference | Modified dietary factor | Effect of low-GI food |
|---|---|---|
| Haber *et al.* (1977) | Apple, whole or processed | Increased satiety |
| Krotkiewski (1984) | Guar gum | Decreases hunger |
| Spitzer and Rodin (1987) | Fructose or glucose | Lower voluntary energy intake |
| Rodin *et al.* (1988) | Fructose or glucose | Lower voluntary energy intake |
| Leathwood and Pollet (1988) | Bean or potato | Decreased hunger |
| Rodin (1991) | Fructose or glucose | Lower voluntary energy intake |
| Holt *et al.* (1992) | Breakfast cereal | Increased satiety |
| van Amelsvoort and Weststrate (1992) | Amylose or amylopectin | Increased satiety |
| Holt and Miller (1994) | Different grades of wheat | Increased satiety |
| Benini *et al.* (1995) | Fibre added to meal | Decreased hunger |
| Gustafsson *et al.* (1995a) | Vegetable type | Increased satiety |
| Gustafsson *et al.* (1995b) | Raw or cooked carrots | Increased satiety |
| Holt and Miller (1995) | Rice type | Lower voluntary energy intake |
| Lavin and Read (1995) | Guar gum | Decreased hunger |
| Holt *et al.* (1996) | 38 individual foods | No change in satiety |
| Rigaud *et al.* (1998) | Psyllium fibre | Lower voluntary energy intake |
| Ludwig *et al.* (1999) | Oatmeal type | Lower voluntary energy intake |
| Ball *et al.* (2003) | Breakfast meal replacement | Prolonged satiety |
| Warren *et al.* (2003) | Breakfast type | Lower voluntary energy intake |

moderate level and therefore are less likely to produce reactive hypoglycaemia (Augustin *et al.*, 2002).

## 3.6 Carbohydrate type, glycaemic response and weight control

It has been debated whether excess dietary carbohydrate can increase adipose stores. Although test animals are able to convert significant amounts of ingested carbohydrate into body fat, in humans, *de novo* lipogenesis from carbohydrate appears to be limited (Strawford *et al.*, 2004). Despite this, excess dietary carbohydrate may indirectly increase body fat stores. Dietary carbohydrate, in the form of starch or sucrose, increases blood insulin levels, which in turn increase activity of the enzyme lipoprotein lipase. Lipoprotein lipase mediates storage of dietary fat in adipose cells. At the same time, insulin decreases the activity of hormone-sensitive triglyceride lipase, an enzyme that regulates the release of fatty acids from stored fat. Thus, excess dietary carbohydrate increases the amount of dietary fat that is stored, and decrease fat turnover (Allred, 1995).

Short- and long-term studies in humans and animals indicate that high-GI diets affect appetite and nutrient partitioning to promote fat storage. However, human studies showing reduced bodyweight after consumption of low-GI diets need to be interpreted with caution. The outcome can rarely be attributed solely to the GI, because interventions designed to modify the GI of a diet usually also modify other variables that influence bodyweight (e.g. fibre content, palatability, energy density). Pawlak *et al.* (2004) assigned rats and mice either to a low- or a high-GI diet. The carbohydrate portion of the low-GI diet consisted of 60% amylose:40% amylopectin starch, whereas the carbohydrate in the high-GI diet was 100% amylopectin starch. Other than this, the two diets were similar in nutrient and energy content. In both mice and rats, animals consuming the high-GI diet had more body fat and less lean body mass than those on the low-GI diet. The rats on the high-GI diet required less food to gain the same amount of weight than the low-GI group. The high-GI group also showed a greater increase over time in the area-under-the-curve of blood glucose and insulin after an oral glucose load. The authors suggested hyperinsulinaemia resulting from the high-GI diet altered nutrient partitioning in favour of fat deposition, shifting metabolic fuels from oxidation in muscle to storage in fat. Overall, the findings indicate the consumption of a high-GI diet *per se* adversely affects body composition in rodents (Pawlak *et al.*, 2004).

Ludwig *et al.* (1999) examined the effect of isoenergetic low-, medium- and high-GI breakfast and lunch meals on *ad libitum* food intake during the 5 hours after lunch. Compared with the low- and medium-GI groups, ratings of hunger were higher in the high-GI group during the postprandial period. In addition, voluntary energy intake after the high-GI lunch was 53% and 81% higher than after the medium-GI and the low-GI lunches, respectively. In addition, compared with the other two meals, the high-GI meal induced hormonal changes, including higher serum insulin and lower plasma glucagon levels. The combination of hyperinsulinaemia and hypoglucagonaemia tends to promote glucose uptake in muscle and liver, restrain hepatic glucose production and suppress lipolysis (Ludwig *et al.*, 1999).

In order to analyze the effect of low-GI or low-GL diets on weight loss, two different kinds of studies need to be distinguished: studies of isoenergetic low- versus high-GI diets, and *ad libitum* low- versus high-GI diets. Livesey (2005) reviewed 14 isoenergetic diets and 7 *ad libitum* studies and found that only in *ad libitum* studies could an effect of GI or GL on bodyweight be determined. A 12-week pilot study in children, which reduced the

GI of the diet by giving brief instructions and a handout about dietary changes to the parents, resulted in a reduction of body mass index (BMI) Z-scores of the children (Young *et al.*, 2004). A 5-week study in healthy men allocated to a high- or a low-GI diet reported both groups experienced an increase in lean body mass but no changes in BMI after the low-GI period (Bouche *et al.*, 2002). A more marked effect was reported in a study of men with abdominal obesity given an *ad libitum* low glycaemic load or low-fat diet for 6 days; there was a reduction in energy intake, bodyweight, and waist and hip circumference with the low glycemic load diet, but not with the low-fat diet (Dumesnil *et al.*, 2001). Although these findings suggest a potential advantage of low-GI or low-GL diets, the definitive long-term study, where *ad libitum* intake is permitted but diets are similar in all aspects except the GI, has not yet been done.

## 3.7 Future trends

More research is needed on the potential benefits of a low-GI diet for weight control. The ideal design would be a long-term study where *ad libitum* food intake and fluctuations in bodyweight are permitted, and where the diets are similar in all aspects except GI.

Although it appears there may a beneficial effect of low-GI diets for weight control (Ludwig, 2000; Brouns *et al.*, 2005), for consumers it is difficult to make the right choices. Information is often hidden in international tables containing only a limited number of products. Moreover, as explained earlier in this chapter, it is not always easy to measure the GI of a product accurately. To facilitate consumer choice, the food industry could provide information on the GI of their products, preferably directly on the package. An example of this approach is the GI Symbol Program in Australia (www.gisymbol.com). In this food labelling programme, producers can obtain certificates stating the GI for their products, provided the food has been properly tested for GI with a standard method. All products that contain a minimum amount of 10 g carbohydrates per serving and meet a set of nutritional criteria – including, for example, sodium, fat and fibre content – can be certified. So far this programme is only operating in Australia, but other countries may follow.

Many processed foods on the market have a high GI. For cereal products, in particular, the food industry has several different choices for processing, and thus may be able to produce lower-GI options. As mentioned in Section 3.3, the starch structure is important for the GI, and the less the structure of the grain is changed, the lower the GI. Therefore, 'whole-grain' products should be preferred to 'wholemeal' products (where the whole grain is included, but usually finely milled). Another important decision for the food industry is the choice of raw material. If cereals containing a higher amount of gel-forming dietary fibre, or a higher fructose: glucose ratio were used more frequently, the choice of low-GI foods for the consumer could be expanded.

Overall, the food industry could put greater effort into producing truly low-GI foods rather than foods that only appear to be low GI. Some examples of foods that might appear to be low GI but are not are several types of wholemeal, bran-flake breakfast cereals (GI = 74) and certain cereal bars (GI = 78). A labelling system such as the one in Australia would give additional impetus to producers, as they would be able to market their products as low GI with the support of a recognizable and trustworthy label.

Compared with glucose (GI = 100) or sucrose (GI = 68), the GI of fructose is very low (GI = 19). Therefore, it might be expected that to exchange fructose for glucose or sucrose, and thereby reduce the GI of a food product, might be beneficial in relation to weight control. However, this may not be true. Ingested disaccharides such as sucrose, maltose or lactose, are cleaved by disaccharidases as soon as they enter the small intestine. Released glucose then leads to an insulin response and enters the cells via an insulin-dependent mechanism (Glut-4). Once inside the cells, glucose is phosphorylated to glucose-6-phosphate, from which the intracellular metabolism of glucose begins. In contrast, fructose increases blood insulin levels only slightly and enters the cells via the Glut-5 transporter, which is not insulin dependent. This transporter, however, is absent from the brain, and therefore fructose may not send satiety signals to the brain as glucose does. Furthermore, the secretion of leptin, which is important in inhibiting food intake, is mediated by insulin. As fructose only increases insulin levels slightly, leptin levels may not rise much after fructose consumption. This could lead to decreased satiety and increased food intake (Mayes, 1993).

Another issue that argues against the use of large quantities of fructose in an effort to lower GI, is its effect on *de novo* lipogenesis. While only a small percentage (1–3%) of glucose carbon enters *de novo* lipogenesis and is incorporated into triglycerides in normal individuals, a proportionally much greater amount of carbon from fructose is metabolized to triglyceride. Thus, the positive effect of a lower GI with fructose-containing foods might be unfavourably balanced by the negative effects of lower satiety and a potential increase in *de novo* lipogenesis (Bray *et al.*, 2004; Havel, 2005).

## 3.8 Sources of further information and advice

The group of Professor J. Brand-Miller at the University of Sydney has done extensive research in the area of GI and GL and has tested a wide variety of foods. They have assembled a comprehensive list of tested foods, first published in 1995 as the 'International tables of glycemic index' (Foster-Powell & Miller, 1995). In 2002 a revised table was published, including all the data published between 1981 and 2001, as well as unpublished data from their laboratory and from others where the quality of the data could be verified on the basis of the method used. In its 2002 edition, the table contained nearly 1300 entries, representing over 750 different types of foods (Foster-Powell *et al.*, 2002). This database is continuously updated and is available online on the following site: http://www.glycemicindex.com. On this site, products can be located with the aid of a specific search engine. Furthermore, additional information on GI and GL can be found in several books written by Professor J. Brand-Miller on this subject.

Additional information about glycaemic carbohydrates and their effect on bodyweight regulation are provided in a recent review by Saris (2003). The different effects of fat and carbohydrates on the thermogenic response and fat deposition are also discussed in this review.

Several reviews on the association between GI and chronic disease have been published by Jenkins and colleagues (e.g. Jenkins *et al.*, 2002). They conclude that, despite inconsistencies in the data, overall findings suggest that dietary GI is of potential importance in the treatment and prevention of chronic diseases. On the other hand, a recent comprehensive review by Raben (2002) examined 31 short-term and 20 longer-term published human intervention studies comparing the effects of high- and low-GI diets on appetite, food intake, energy expenditure and bodyweight. The author suggested that the data were not conclusive that low-GI foods are superior to high-GI foods in regard to long-term control of bodyweight.

## 3.9 References

ALLRED J B (1995), 'Too much of a good thing? An overemphasis on eating low-fat foods may be contributing to the alarming increase in overweight among US adults', *J Am Diet Assoc*, **95** (4), 417–418.

ARVIDSSON-LENNER R A, ASP N-G, AXELSEN M, BRYNGELSSON S, HAAPA E, JÄRVI A, KERLSTRÖM B, RABEN A, SOHLSTRÖM A, THORSDOTTIR I and VESSBY B (2004), 'Glycaemic index', *Scand J Nutr*, **48** (2), 84–94.

ASTRUP A and RABEN A (1992), 'Obesity: an inherited metabolic deficiency in the control of macronutrient balance?' *Eur J Clin Nutr*, **46** (9), 611–620.

AUGUSTIN L S, FRANCESCHI S, JENKINS D J, KENDALL C W and LA VECCHIA C (2002), 'Glycemic index in chronic disease: a review', *Eur J Clin Nutr*, **56** (11), 1049–1071.

BALL S D, KELLER K R, MOYER-MILEUR L J, DING Y W, DONALDSON D and JACKSON W D (2003), 'Prolongation of satiety after low versus moderately high glycemic index meals in obese adolescents', *Pediatrics*, **111** (3), 488–494.

BENINI L, CASTELLANI G, BRIGHENTI F, HEATON K W, BRENTEGANI M T, CASIRAGHI M C, SEMBENINI C, PELLEGRINI N, FIORETTA A, MINNITI G, *et al.* (1995), 'Gastric emptying of a solid meal is accelerated by the removal of dietary fibre naturally present in food', *Gut*, **36** (6), 825–830.

BJÖRCK I L, LILJEBERG H and ÖSTMAN E (2000), 'Low glycaemic-index foods', *Br J Nutr*, **83** (Suppl. 1), S149–S155.

BOUCHE C, RIZKALLA S W, LUO J, VIDAL H, VERONESE A, PACHER N, FOUQUET C, LANG V and SLAMA G (2002), 'Five-week, low-glycemic index diet decreases total fat mass and improves plasma lipid profile in moderately overweight nondiabetic men', *Diabetes Care*, **25** (5), 822–828.

BRAND J C, COLAGIURI S, CROSSMAN S, ALLEN A, ROBERTS D C and TRUSWELL A S (1991), 'Low-glycemic index foods improve long-term glycemic control in NIDDM', *Diabetes Care*, **14** (2), 95–101.

BRAND-MILLER J C, HOLT S H, PAWLAK D B and MCMILLAN J (2002), 'Glycemic index and obesity', *Am J Clin Nutr*, **76** (1), 281S–285S.

BRAY G A, NIELSEN S J and POPKIN B M (2004), 'Consumption of high-fructose corn syrup in beverages may play a role in the epidemic of obesity', *Am J Clin Nutr*, **79** (4), 537–543.

BRAY G A, BOUCHARD C and JAMES W P T (Eds) (1998), *Handbook of Obesity*. New York: Marcel Dekker Inc.

BROUNS F, BJORCK I, FRAYN K, GIBBS A, LANG V, SLAMA G and WOLEVER T (2005), 'Glycaemic index methodology', *Nutr Res Rev*, **18** (1), 145–171.

BURKE B J, HARTOG M, HEATON K W and HOOPER S (1982), 'Assessment of the metabolic effects of dietary carbohydrate and fibre by measuring urinary excretion of C-peptide', *Hum Nutr Clin Nutr*, **36** (5), 373–380.

CHAMP M, LANGKILDE A, BROUNS F, KETTLITZ B and COLLET Y (2003), 'Advances in dietary fibre characterisation. 1. Definition of dietary fibre, physiological relevance, health benefits and analytical aspects', *Nutr Res Rev*, **16** (1), 71–82.

CUMMINGS J H, ROBERFROID M B, ANDERSSON H, BARTH C, FERRO LUZZI A, GHOOS Y, GIBNEY M, HERMONSEN K, JAMES W P, KORVER O, LAIRON D, PASCAL G and VORAGEN A G (1997), 'A new look at dietary carbohydrate: chemistry, physiology and health. Paris Carbohydrate Group', *Eur J Clin Nutr*, **51** (7), 417–423.

DUMESNIL J G, TURGEON J, TREMBLAY A, POIRIER P, GILBERT M, GAGNON L, ST-PIERRE S, GARNEAU C, LEMIEUX I, PASCOT A, BERGERON J and DESPRES J P (2001), 'Effect of a low-glycaemic index–low-fat–high protein diet on the atherogenic metabolic risk profile of abdominally obese men', *Br J Nutr*, **86** (5), 557–568.

ENGLYST K N, ENGLYST H N, HUDSON G J, COLE T J and CUMMINGS J H (1999), 'Rapidly available glucose in foods: an in vitro measurement that reflects the glycemic response', *Am J Clin Nutr*, **69** (3), 448–454.

FOSTER-POWELL K, HOLT S H and BRAND-MILLER J C (2002), 'International table of glycemic index and glycemic load values: 2002', *Am J Clin Nutr*, **76** (1), 5–56.

FOSTER-POWELL K and MILLER J B (1995), 'International tables of glycemic index', *Am J Clin Nutr*, **62** (4), 871S–890S.

FROST G, KEOGH B, SMITH D, AKINSANYA K and LEEDS A (1996), 'The effect of low-glycemic carbohydrate on insulin and glucose response in vivo and in vitro in patients with coronary heart disease', *Metabolism*, **45** (6), 669–672.

GOLAY A and BOBBIONI E (1997), 'The role of dietary fat in obesity', *Int J Obes Relat Metab Disord*, **21** (Suppl 3), S2–11.

GUSTAFSSON K, ASP N G, HAGANDER B and NYMAN M (1995a), 'Satiety effects of spinach in mixed meals: comparison with other vegetables', *Int J Food Sci Nutr*, **46** (4), 327–334.

GUSTAFSSON K, ASP N G, HAGANDER B, NYMAN M and SCHWEIZER T (1995b), 'Influence of processing and cooking of carrots in mixed meals on satiety, glucose and hormonal response', *Int J Food Sci Nutr*, **46** (1), 3–12.

HABER G B, HEATON K W, MURPHY D and BURROUGHS L F (1977), 'Depletion and disruption of dietary fibre. Effects on satiety, plasma-glucose, and serum-insulin', *Lancet*, **2** (8040), 679–682.

HAVEL P J (2005), 'Dietary fructose: implications for dysregulation of energy homeostasis and lipid/carbohydrate metabolism', *Nutr Rev*, **63** (5), 133–157.

HOLT S, BRAND J, SOVENY C and HANSKY J (1992), 'Relationship of satiety to postprandial glycaemic, insulin and cholecystokinin responses', *Appetite*, **18** (2), 129–141.

HOLT S H and MILLER J B (1994), 'Particle size, satiety and the glycaemic response', *Eur J Clin Nutr*, **48** (7), 496–502.

HOLT S H and MILLER J B (1995), 'Increased insulin responses to ingested foods are associated with lessened satiety', *Appetite*, **24** (1), 43–54.

HOLT S H, BRAND MILLER J C and PETOCZ P (1996), 'Interrelationships among postprandial satiety, glucose and insulin responses and changes in subsequent food intake', *Eur J Clin Nutr*, **50** (12), 788–797.

JENKINS D J, AXELSEN M, KENDALL C W, AUGUSTIN L S, VUKSAN V and SMITH U (2000), 'Dietary fibre, lente carbohydrates and the insulin-resistant diseases', *Br J Nutr*, **83** (Suppl 1), S157–163.

JENKINS D J, KENDALL C W, AUGUSTIN L S, FRANCESCHI S, HAMIDI M, MARCHIE A, JENKINS A L and AXELSEN M (2002), 'Glycemic index: overview of implications in health and disease', *Am J Clin Nutr*, **76** (1), 266S–273S.

JENKINS D J, WOLEVER T M, BUCKLEY G, LAM K Y, GIUDICI S, KALMUSKY J, JENKINS A L, PATTEN R L, BIRD J, WONG G S and JOSSE R G (1988), 'Low-glycemic-index starchy foods in the diabetic diet', *Am J Clin Nutr*, **48** (2), 248–254.

JENKINS D J, WOLEVER T M, COLLIER G R, OCANA A, RAO A V, BUCKLEY G, LAM Y, MAYER A and THOMPSON L U (1987), 'Metabolic effects of a low-glycemic-index diet', *Am J Clin Nutr*, **46** (6), 968–975.

JENKINS D J, WOLEVER T M, TAYLOR R H, BARKER H, FIELDEN H, BALDWIN J M, BOWLING A C, NEWMAN H C, JENKINS A L and GOFF D V (1981), 'Glycemic index of foods: a physiological basis for carbohydrate exchange', *Am J Clin Nutr*, **34** (3), 362–366.

KROTKIEWSKI M (1984), 'Effect of guar gum on body-weight, hunger ratings and metabolism in obese subjects', *Br J Nutr*, **52** (1), 97–105.

LAVIN J H and READ N W (1995), 'The effect on hunger and satiety of slowing the absorption of glucose: relationship with gastric emptying and postprandial blood glucose and insulin responses', *Appetite*, **25** (1), 89–96.

LEATHWOOD P and POLLET P (1988), 'Effects of slow release carbohydrates in the form of bean flakes on the evolution of hunger and satiety in man', *Appetite*, **10** (1), 1–11.

LILJEBERG H G, AKERBERG A K and BJORCK I M (1999), 'Effect of the glycemic index and content of indigestible carbohydrates of cereal-based breakfast meals on glucose tolerance at lunch in healthy subjects', *Am J Clin Nutr*, **69** (4), 647–655.

LIVESEY G (2003), 'Health potential of polyols as sugar replacers, with emphasis on low glycaemic properties', *Nutr Res Rev*, **16** (2), 163–191.

LIVESEY G (2005), 'Low-glycaemic diets and health: implications for obesity', *Proc Nutr Soc*, **64** (1), 105–113.

LUDWIG D S (2000), 'Dietary glycemic index and obesity', *J Nutr*, **130** (2S Suppl), 280S–283S.

LUDWIG D S, MAJZOUB J A, AL-ZAHRANI A, DALLAL G E, BLANCO I and ROBERTS S B (1999), 'High glycemic index foods, overeating, and obesity', *Pediatrics*, **103** (3), E26.

MAYES P A (1993), 'Intermediary metabolism of fructose', *Am J Clin Nutr*, **58** (5 Suppl), 754S–765S.

NICKLAS T A (1995), 'Dietary studies of children: the Bogalusa Heart Study experience', *J Am Diet Assoc*, **95** (10), 1127–1133.

PAWLAK D B, KUSHNER J A and LUDWIG D S (2004), 'Effects of dietary glycaemic index on adiposity, glucose homoeostasis, and plasma lipids in animals', *Lancet*, **364** (9436), 778–785.

RABEN A (2002), 'Should obese patients be counselled to follow a low-glycaemic index diet? No', *Obes Rev*, **3** (4), 245–256.

REAVEN G M (1993), 'Role of insulin resistance in human disease (syndrome X): an expanded definition', *Annu Rev Med*, **44**, 121–131.

RIGAUD D, PAYCHA F, MEULEMANS A, MERROUCHE M and MIGNON M (1998), 'Effect of psyllium on gastric emptying, hunger feeling and food intake in normal volunteers: a double blind study', *Eur J Clin Nutr*, **52** (4), 239–245.

RODIN J (1991), 'Effects of pure sugar vs. mixed starch fructose loads on food intake', *Appetite*, **17** (3), 213–219.

RODIN J, REED D and JAMNER L (1988), 'Metabolic effects of fructose and glucose: implications for food intake', *Am J Clin Nutr*, **47** (4), 683–689.

SALMERON J, ASCHERIO A, RIMM E B, COLDITZ G A, SPIEGELMAN D, JENKINS D J, STAMPFER M J, WING A L and WILLETT W C (1997a), 'Dietary fiber, glycemic load, and risk of NIDDM in men', *Diabetes Care*, **20** (4), 545–550.

SALMERON J, MANSON J E, STAMPFER M J, COLDITZ G A, WING A L and WILLETT W C (1997b), 'Dietary fiber, glycemic load, and risk of non-insulin-dependent diabetes mellitus in women', *JAMA*, **277** (6), 472–477.

SARIS W H (2003), 'Glycemic carbohydrate and body weight regulation', *Nutr Rev*, **61** (5 Pt 2), S10–16.

SPITZER L and RODIN J (1987), 'Effects of fructose and glucose preloads on subsequent food intake', *Appetite*, **8** (2), 135–145.

STRAWFORD A, ANTELO F, CHRISTIANSEN M and HELLERSTEIN M K (2004), 'Adipose tissue triglyceride turnover, de novo lipogenesis, and cell proliferation in humans measured with $^2H_2O$', *Am J Physiol Endocrinol Metab*, **286** (4), E577–588.

VAN AMELSVOORT J and WESTSTRATE J (1992), 'Amylose-amylopectin ratio in a meal affects postprandial variables in male volunteers', *Am J Clin Nutr*, **55**, 712–718.

VIRKAMAKI A, UEKI K and KAHN C R (1999), 'Protein–protein interaction in insulin signaling and the molecular mechanisms of insulin resistance', *J Clin Invest*, **103** (7), 931–943.

WARREN J M, HENRY C J and SIMONITE V (2003), 'Low glycemic index breakfasts and reduced food intake in preadolescent children', *Pediatrics*, **112** (5), e414.

WOLEVER T, KATZMANRELLE L, JENKINS A, VUKSAN V, JOSSE R and JENKINS D (1994), 'Glycemic index of 102 complex carbohydrate foods in patients with diabetes', *Nutr Res*, **14** (5), 651–669.

WOLEVER T M, JENKINS D J, JENKINS A L and JOSSE R G (1991), 'The glycemic index: methodology and clinical implications', *Am J Clin Nutr*, **54** (5), 846–854.

YOUNG P C, WEST S A, ORTIZ K and CARLSON J (2004), 'A pilot study to determine the feasibility of the low glycemic index diet as a treatment for overweight children in primary care practice', *Ambul Pediatr*, **4** (1), 28–33.

# 4

# Controlling lipogenesis and thermogenesis and the use of ergogenic aids for weight control

**A. Palou and M. L. Bonet, University of the Balearic Islands, Spain**

## 4.1 Introduction

Body weight management implies tuning of energy intake to energy requirement, while avoiding accumulating energy storage as fat. Key targets for body weight management strategies are hunger and satiety, intestinal nutrient absorption, thermogenesis, fat oxidation, lipogenesis and body composition.[1,2] These targets represent highly controlled and interconnected biochemical processes that are influenced by the interplay between genetic makeup and environmental factors, including the amount and composition of the diet and physical activity.

Achieving a negative energy balance is the essential component and a *sine qua non* of weight loss, but conventional strategies simply based on caloric restriction and increased physical activity are difficult to follow and have been ineffective in preventing the obesity epidemic. At the same time, it is becoming increasingly clear that specific nutrients and other food components influence one or more of the above-mentioned targets in such a way that they may facilitate negative energy balance or a preferential partitioning of energy towards lean body mass. This knowledge constitutes the basis for the development of nutritional strategies for weight management based on the selection of traditional foods (e.g. intake of specific foods or of specific macronutrient balances), novel foods (i.e. designed foods that incorporate one or more functional ingredients) or nutraceuticals (purified functional food components or food extracts presented in capsular or non-food format). In this chapter, we will focus on fat oxidation/thermogenesis, lipogenesis and body composition as potential targets of nutritional aids for weight management. Some of these aids are also marketed as ergogenic aids, purported to enhance exercise performance.

## 4.2 Overview of nutrition and thermogenesis

Total body energy expenditure represents the conversion of oxygen and food (or stored forms of energy) to carbon dioxide, water, biological work and heat, the production of which is inherent to net biochemical reactions in energy metabolism. Energy expenditure at rest can be measured directly as heat produced, hence the term thermogenesis, or indirectly as the amount of oxygen consumed.

Total energy expenditure can be broken down into three components: (a) obligatory energy expenditure required for normal functioning of cells and organs (represented by the basal metabolic rate, which is defined as the amount of energy expended when an adult organism is awake but resting, not actively digesting food and at thermoneutrality); (b) physical activity; (c) adaptive thermogenesis, which is physiologically regulated and is usually defined operationally as heat production in response to environmental factors including temperature and diet. Adaptive thermogenesis has received a lot of attention in the context of weight-control management strategies because it comprises a set of unconscious mechanisms that lead to the regulated dissipation of part of the energy of foods as heat, thus reducing energy efficiency and opposing weight gain.

### 4.2.1 Sites and mechanisms of adaptive thermogenesis

In rodents, a major site of adaptive thermogenesis is brown adipose tissue (BAT). The main mechanism behind BAT thermogenesis relies on the activity of uncoupling protein 1 (UCP1), a mitochondrial inner membrane protein that is uniquely and abundantly expressed in brown adipocytes, which are mitochondria-rich cells (reviewed in references 3–5). When active, UCP1 leaks protons across the mitochondrial inner membrane, allowing dissipation of the proton electrochemical gradient generated by the respiratory chain during fuel oxidation. In this way, the energy that had been stored in the proton gradient is released as heat instead of protons being channeled through the ATP synthase and the energy used in ATP synthesis (Fig. 4.1). Together with the expression of UCP1, a low expression of ATP synthase and a high expression of fatty acid oxidation enzymes and respiratory chain components make brown adipocytes well equipped for inefficient substrate (mainly fat) oxidation. Even in BAT, however, UCP1-independent thermogenic mechanisms are likely to exist, because whereas transgenic mice with toxigene-mediated reduction of BAT are cold sensitive and obese,[6] UCP1-deficient (knockout) mice are sensitive to cold exposure but are not obese or especially prone to diet-induced obesity.[7]

In humans, as in rodents, energy expenditure increases in response to cold exposure and after feeding. The latter phenomenon, which accounts for approximately 10% of total daily energy expenditure, is referred to as the thermic effect of food and comprises two conceptually different

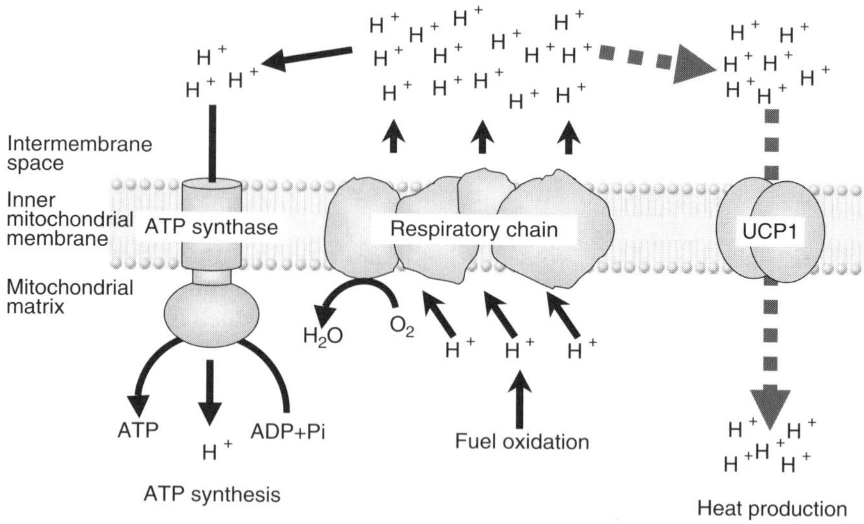


**Fig. 4.1** Functioning of the UCP1 in BAT mitochondria. UCP1 dissipates the proton gradient generated by the respiratory chain during nutrient oxidation, leading to the release of energy as heat; Pi, inorganic phosphate (Modified from reference 3).

components: the obligatory cost of nutrient utilization (digestion, absorption, processing and storage) and an adaptive component linked to oropharyngeal stimulation that typically constitutes 30–40% of the thermic effect of food and is under the control of the sympathetic nervous system (SNS) (see reference 8). The sites and mechanisms of adaptive thermogenesis in humans are unclear. Unlike rodents, adult humans do not have large, well-defined BAT depots, but both rodents and humans have varying numbers of brown adipocytes dispersed within white adipose tissue (WAT) depots, which can be recruited under appropriate stimulation (see reference 9). Skeletal muscle, which represents up to 40% of total body weight and is endowed with significant mitochondrial capacity, may be an important contributor to adaptive thermogenesis; in fact, it has been shown that a significant portion of the variation in metabolic rate between humans can be accounted for by differences in skeletal muscle energy expenditure at rest.[10] Other tissues, such as liver and WAT, may also contribute to adaptive thermogenesis.

Apart from UCP1 activity, other mechanisms of adaptive thermogenesis are poorly understood. One possibility is the activity of mitochondrial uncoupling proteins other than UCP1. In fact, UCP1 homologues with a wider tissue distribution, such as UCP2 and UCP3, have been identified both in rodents and humans (reviewed in references 11–13). UCP2 is expressed in most tissues at varying levels and UCP3 is expressed predominantly in skeletal muscle and BAT. Several studies have shown that these UCP1 homologues have proton transport activity, and a strong linkage between markers in the vicinity of human UCP2 and UCP3 genes (which are adjacent genes in both the human and rat genome) and resting metabolic rate was reported. However, the expression of UCP2 and UCP3 increases with starvation,[11,13,14] a state associated with decreased energy expenditure, and neither UCP2-[15] nor UCP3-[16,17] deficient (knockout) mice are obese or especially sensitive to developing diet-induced obesity. Thus, a primary function of the UCP homologues in regulating whole-body energy expenditure seems unlikely.

Adaptive thermogenesis in mammalian tissues may also depend on mechanisms connected to increased utilization of ATP, rather than to uncoupling. Enhanced operation of the so-called 'futile cycles', which imply ATP consumption not linked to the performance of net biological work, may be one of such mechanisms. Examples of potentially important futile cycles include the synthesis and degradation of proteins, the pumping and leakage of ions across membranes, and the esterification and lipolysis of fatty acid/triacylgycerol.[18] Increased non-exercise activity thermogenesis (associated with fidgeting, maintenance of posture and other physical activities of daily life) may be another mechanism of adaptive thermogenesis, also based on increased ATP utilization. There are physiological studies in humans suggesting that non-exercise activity thermogenesis is modulated with changes in energy balance, so that it increases with overfeeding and decreases with underfeeding, although the mechanisms behind this regulation are unknown.[19]

Thermogenesis and substrate oxidation are tightly linked processes. Substrate oxidation drives thermogenesis and thermogenesis favors further substrate oxidation to meet cellular ATP demands. Remarkably in this context, there is increasing evidence that the uncoupling activity of the UCPs may serve primarily to assist oxidative metabolism, and particularly fat oxidation, by facilitating fatty acid handling by mitochondria[20–23] and reducing reactive oxygen species (ROS) production in mitochondria.[15,16] Facilitation of oxidative metabolism at the expense of a small loss of energy could have been the main ancestral role of the UCPs. The molecular basis for a role of the UCPs in mitochondrial fatty acid handling is the capacity of UCPs to uncouple respiration acting as fatty acid cyclers, rather than as proton transporters;[24] their role in reducing ROS is related to the fact that the higher the coupling of respiration, the higher the ROS production in the mitochondria.[25] The connection of the UCPs with both thermogenesis and oxidative metabolism makes these proteins an interesting target for up-regulation in the context of weight-management strategies.

### 4.2.2 The contribution of reduced thermogenesis and fat oxidation to obesity and its metabolic complications

In rodents, there is compelling evidence that obesity may develop as a result of a deficit in energy expenditure and more specifically in adaptive thermogenesis. A feature of most animal models of obesity, whether genetic- or lesion-induced, is a decreased energy expenditure and an abnormally low BAT thermogenic response to cold or feeding;[26] in these models, even when food intake is restricted to that of wild-type or control animals (a maneuver termed pair feeding) marked obesity still develops.

The contribution of reduced energy expenditure to human obesity is less clear. The concept was supported by early epidemiological studies showing that obese subjects maintained their obese state with self-reported energy intakes that were on average less than those of lean subjects, but has been challenged by more recent studies – using the doubly labeled water method, which allows capturing of total energy expenditure for long periods of time with the individual under free-living conditions – indicating that obese subjects have a greater average energy expenditure than do lean and normal-weight subjects (reviewed in reference 27). The increase of total energy expenditure with increasing weight or body mass index is dramatic, and is probably a consequence of a parallel increase of fat-free mass, which is the single best determinant of resting energy expenditure.[28]

Nevertheless, there is evidence that a reduced rate of energy expenditure is a risk factor for both body weight gain and resistance to weight loss in humans. In a now classic study conducted in Pima Indians, it was found that low 24h energy expenditure, normalized for lean body mass, predicted future weight gain during follow-up.[29] In another study, activation of non-exercise activity thermogenesis proved to be the principal mediator of resistance to fat gain during overfeeding, so that individuals that failed to activate this component of energy expenditure were those that gained more weight.[30] There are also studies suggesting that specifically a deficit in the thermic response to food, as a consequence of a reduced sympathetic response to feeding, may contribute to human obesity, although this is a highly controversial issue (reviewed in references 31 and 32).

A low capacity to oxidize fat may also contribute to obesity, particularly when dietary fat is in large supply. In fact, human epidemiological studies point to a reduced rate of fat oxidation as a risk marker for body weight gain, independent of low energy expenditure.[33,34] Moreover, formerly obese individuals of normal weight have been shown to have a lower rate of fat oxidation compared with control, never-obese subjects.[35,36]

Besides and beyond contributing to increased fat mass (obesity), decreased fat oxidation and thermogenesis may result in an excess of available fatty acids to muscle, liver, pancreatic β cells and other non-adipose cells. Lipid accumulation can lead to functional impairments in these cells (lipotoxicity), and has been related to the development of insulin resistance, type 2 diabetes and other pathologies linked to obesity and the metabolic syndrome (reviewed in references 37 and 38). Because the activity of the UCPs may facilitate fat oxidation in the organism (see Section 4.2.1), it may help avoiding lipid accumulation in non-adipose cells and derived lipotoxicity. For instance, intramyocellular fat accumulation is highly correlated with insulin resistance and may be prevented through the activity of muscle UCP3, which is normally up-regulated under conditions of high fatty acid supply to muscles.[39] Also in this context, it has been suggested that brown fat function may be important for the modulation of systemic insulin sensitivity, because a reduced expression of genes involved in brown adipogenesis was found in subcutaneous WAT of non-obese, insulin-resistant human subjects compared with non-obese, insulin-sensitive subjects.[40,41]

### 4.2.3 Central and nutritional control of adaptive thermogenesis

Adaptive thermogenesis is under central control. Exposure to cold and diet is detected by the brain, resulting in the activation of efferent pathways controlling energy dissipation. The SNS, which heavily innervates thermogenic targets such as BAT and skeletal muscle, appears to be the main effector of this response (reviewed in references 4 and 42). The sympathoadrenergic control of BAT thermogenesis is well understood (Fig. 4.2). In BAT, the noradrenaline released by the activated SNS endings interacts with β-adrenoceptors on the brown adipocyte cell membrane promoting lipolysis of the stored triacylglycerols and mitochondrial oxidation of the released fatty acids to fuel thermogenesis, UCP1 synthesis and activity, and tissue recruitment (reviewed in references 5 and 43).

The brain also affects energy expenditure by means of the hypothalamic–pituitary–thyroid axis. The mechanism by which thyroid hormone stimulates thermogenesis is not established, but it seems to be due to multiple effects on various aspects of energy metabolism such as substrate cycling, ion cycling and mitochondrial proton leaks.[44] Thyroid hormone levels seem not to be modulated during cold exposure or consumption of high-calorie diets, but they do drop during starvation, and this may contribute to starvation-induced decreases in thermogenesis (see reference 4).

Signals involved in the long-term regulation of energy balance that convey information to the brain about the size of body fat stores (the so-called 'adiposity signals'), besides affecting food intake, modulate energy expenditure through effects on the activity of the SNS and the pituitary–thyroid axis, and also through direct effects on the oxidative and thermogenic capacity/activity of peripheral tissues. This is the case for leptin, the paradigm of the adiposity signal, which suppresses appetite, and enhances energy expenditure and fat oxidation in peripheral tissues (reviewed in reference 45). In human obesity, leptin deficiency is rare, but leptin resistance is common.

Although feeding in general stimulates thermogenesis, not all macronutrients are equally effective in triggering this response. The thermic effect of protein is 20–35% of energy consumed, and this number falls to 5–15% for carbohydrates; the thermic effect associated with fat is generally even lower than that associated with carbohydrate (see reference 46). The differences are attributed mainly to the fixed component of the thermic effect

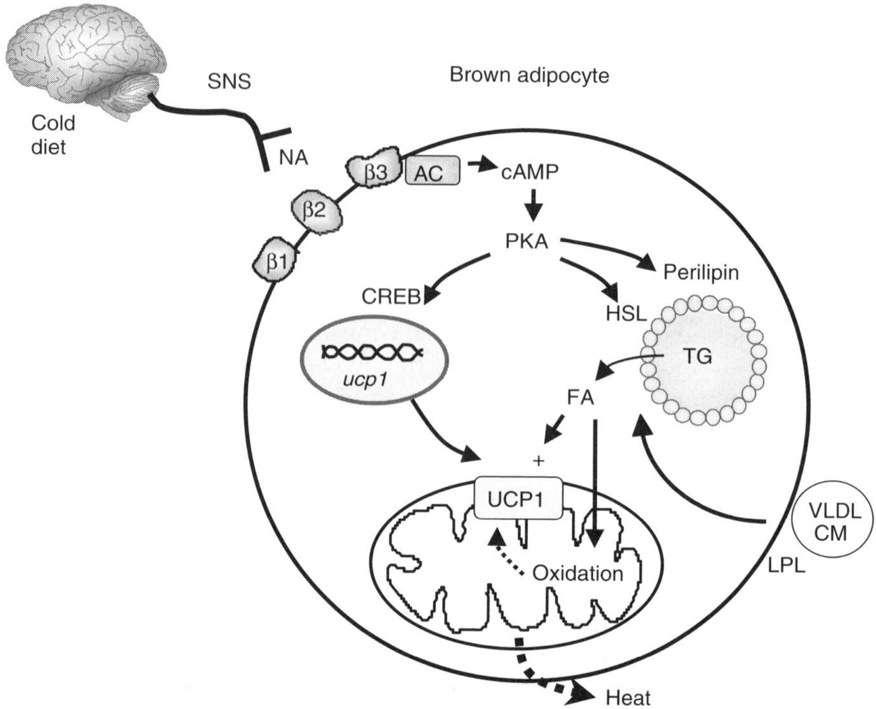


**Fig. 4.2** Adrenergic control of BAT thermogenesis. Noradrenaline (NA) released by the activated SNS acts on β-adrenoceptors, primarily the β3, which are coupled to adenylyl cyclase (AC) through stimulatory G proteins, and thus stimulates the generation of cAMP, which in turn activates protein kinase A (PKA). PKA catalyzes the phosphorylation of cAMP regulatory element binding protein (CREB), which leads to increased ucp1 gene expression. PKA also catalyzes the phosphorylation of hormone sensitive lipase (HSL) and perilipin (the protein that covers the intracellular lipid droplets) triggering activation of the former and dissociation of the latter from the lipid droplets, thus activating lipolysis of triacylglycerol (TG) stores. Released fatty acids (FA) are channeled to the mitochondria where they enter the β-oxidation pathway and then the citric acid cycle, leading to the formation of reduced electron carriers ($FADH_2$ and NADH) which are then oxidized by the respiratory chain. UCP1 dissipates the proton gradient generated by the respiratory chain, leading to a release of energy as heat (thermogenesis). CM, chylomicrons; VLDL, very low density lipoproteins; LPL, lipoprotein lipase.

of food, that representing the obligatory cost of nutrient utilization (digestion, absorption, processing and storage): because the body has no storage capacity for protein, protein needs to be metabolically processed immediately, with a high ATP cost associated with protein synthesis and peptide bond formation, urea production and gluconeogenesis from amino acids.

In addition, evidence is accumulating as to the effects of particular food components on the thermogenic system, thus supporting our hypothesis for developing thermogenic foods (i.e. foods enriched in thermogenic active ingredients) to combat obesity (see references 47 and 48). On the one hand, there are a number of food components (e.g. caffeine, catechin polyphenols, ephedrine) known to stimulate the activity of the sympathoadrenergic system or the release of noradrenaline from the adrenals (e.g. capsaicin). On the other hand, certain nutrients/foods – such as vitamin A, carotenoids, olive oil, medium-chain triacylglycerols, polyunsaturated fatty acids (PUFAs) and dietary protein – have been shown to have the potential to stimulate the expression of the UCPs in tissues. For instance, rats adapted to medium and high protein exposure have increased expression levels of UCP2 in liver and UCP1 in BAT, this correlating with a higher energy expenditure and oxygen consumption in the dark period and a lower feed energy efficiency.[49] Replacement of habitual foods with others that may enhance energy expenditure may be a practical way to maintain a stable body weight or to help achieve weight loss. The effects of specific foods and food components on the thermogenic system are discussed in more detail in Section 4.5.

## 4.3 Overview of nutrition and lipogenesis

Lipogenesis encompasses the processes of fatty acid synthesis and subsequent triacylglycerol synthesis, mainly from excess carbohydrate in the diet. The main sites of lipogenesis are liver and adipose tissue. A detailed overview of lipogenesis and other processes of lipid metabolism is presented in Chapter 1 and here only some specific aspects will be addressed.

In humans, the main site of *de novo* synthesis of fatty acids is the liver. Fatty acid synthesis requires NADPH, acetyl coenzyme A (CoA) and ATP, all of which are obtained by the liver in the postprandial state (i.e. after meals), mainly from glucose metabolism (through the pentose phosphate pathway, glycolysis plus the pyruvate dehydrogenase reaction, and complete oxidation, respectively) (Fig. 4.3). Newly synthesized fatty acids (as acyl-CoA) are esterified to glycerol-3-phosphate, forming triacylglycerols that, to a large extent, abandon the liver as part of liver-born lipoproteins (mainly very low density lipoproteins, VLDL). These fatty acids eventually would reach adipocytes for storage. Therefore, enhanced lipogenesis over fatty acid oxidation in the liver may favor WAT enlargement.

In human WAT, *de novo* synthesis of fatty acids is quantitatively less important than in the liver. Rather, in the postprandial state, adipocytes synthesize triacylglycerol from fatty acids – derived from the action of lipoprotein lipase (LPL) on the lipoprotein (chylomicron, VLDL)-containing triacylglycerols – and glucose, which enters the adipocyte through insulin-regulated glucose transporter GLUT4 and whose intracellular metabolism produces the glycerol-3-phosphate needed for triacylglycerol synthesis (Fig. 4.3). Triacylglycerols are stored in the adipocytes,

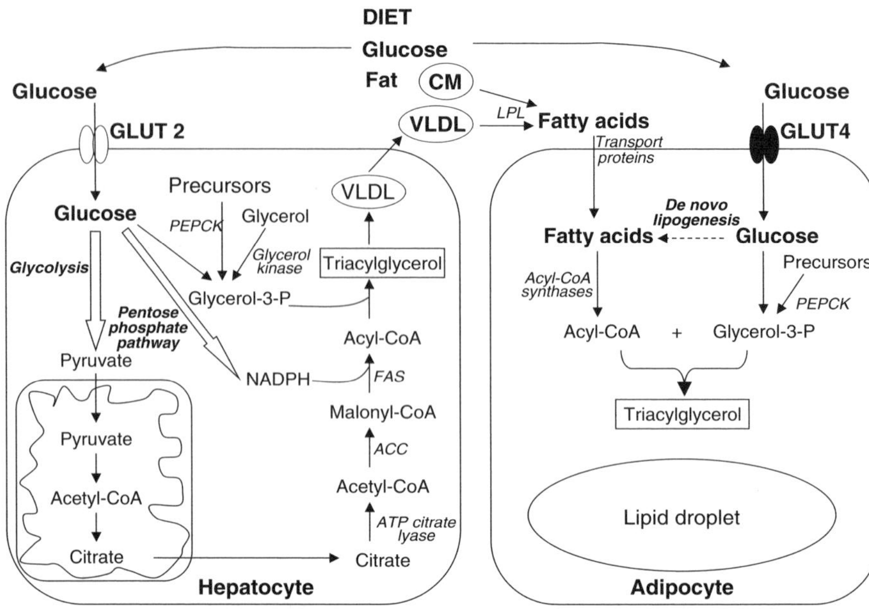


**Fig. 4.3** Overview of lipogenesis in hepatocytes and adipocytes. See Section 4.3 for details. PEPCK, phosphoenolpyruvate carboxykinase; ACC, acetyl-CoA carboxylase; FAS, fatty acid synthase; GLUT4, glucose-transporter 4.

contributing to adipocyte hypertrophy, and are mobilized in situations of energy deficit, such as fasting.

The traditional view is that low activity of the enzyme glycerol kinase in adipocytes ensures that triacylglycerol formation in these cells is dependent on an optimal supply of glucose, avoiding re-esterification under conditions in which fatty acids are to be exported, such as fasting. However, cycles of triacylglycerol hydrolysis and re-esterification do occur within the adipocytes, even during fasting, because glycerol-3-phosphate can be produced from precursors (other than glucose or glycerol) through glyceroneogenesis, which is an abbreviated version of gluconeogenesis that occurs both in liver and adipose tissue.[50,51] Disregulation of glyceroneogenesis in WAT can contribute to obesity (reviewed in reference 52). Overactivity, due to WAT-specific overexpression of the rate-limiting enzyme of the pathway (phosphoenolpyruvate carboxykinase, PEPCK), results in obesity without insulin resistance in transgenic mice.[52,53]

### 4.3.1 Hormonal and nutritional control of lipogenesis

Carbohydrate-rich diets stimulate lipogenesis in the liver by providing the energy and carbons required for it, because insulin secreted after carbohydrate-rich meals triggers the activation of key enzymes in the glycolytic and lipogenic pathways, and because both glucose (independent of insulin) and insulin favor an increment in the concentration of glycolytic and lipogenic enzymes, and hence of liver lipogenic capacity, through the up-regulation of the expression levels and activity of key transcription factors controlling the transcription of the genes encoding these enzymes. Transcription factors are proteins that, in their active form, modulate the transcription of target genes by binding to specific nucleotide sequences contained in the corresponding gene promoter; from there, they facilitate or impair the consti-tution of the RNA pol II transcriptional initiation complex and hence transcription. Two key transcription factors promoting the expression of glycolytic and lipogenic genes in the liver are sterol regulatory element binding protein 1 (SREBP-1) and carbohydrate response element binding protein (ChREBP) (reviewed in references 54 and 55) (Fig. 4.4). ChREBP is activated as a transcription factor by dephosphorylation of specific serine residues when glucose is abundant in the hepatocyte (a secondary metabolite of glucose, xylulose-5-phosphate, is believed to alosterically activate the protein phosphatase catalyzing ChREBP dephosphorylation). SREBP-1 is both induced at the transcriptional level and activated (through controlled proteolysis of an inactive precursor) in response to insulin.

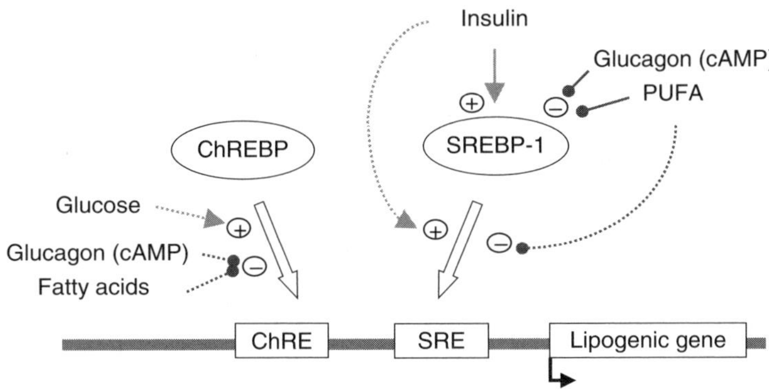


**Fig. 4.4** Transcriptional control of lipogenic genes in hepatocytes. Most lipogenic enzyme genes contain in their gene promoter response elements (ChRE, SRE) for the binding of ChREBP and SREBP-1. These two factors work synergistically to induce transcription of the lipogenic enzyme genes in the presence of glucose and insulin. Insulin induces the expression of SREBP-1 and favors its activation as a transcription factor for lipogenic genes; glucose favors ChREBP activation. Glucagon, through its intracellular mediator cAMP, inhibits ChREBP activity and suppresses SREBP-1 expression. Excess free fatty acids inhibit ChREBP activity, and PUFAs specifically repress the expression and activity of SREBP-1. In this manner, the output of lipogenic enzyme production is integrated to multiple hormonal and nutritional signals. Solid lines indicate effects on transcription of the gene encoding the transcription factor; dotted lines indicate effects on transcription factor activity (adapted from reference 56).

Glucose and insulin also favor lipogenesis in WAT. Glucose serves as precursor for glycerol-3-phosphate in adipocytes and it may have an insulin-independent effect stimulating LPL activity in WAT.[57] Insulin enhances LPL activity in WAT, promotes GLUT4 translocation to the adipocyte cell membrane and induces the expression of two key lipogenic transcription factors in adipocytes, the above-mentioned SREBP-1 and peroxisome proliferator-activated receptor gamma (PPARγ) (reviewed in refernce 58). PPARγ is an important stimulator of lipogenesis in differentiated WAT and also plays a pivotal role in adipocyte differentiation.[59]

On the other hand, dietary fats, and particularly PUFAs, decrease lipogenesis and lipogenic capacity in the liver (Fig. 4.4) and probably also in WAT. This is discussed in more detail in Section 4.5.

## 4.4 Nutrition and development of lean body mass and body fat mass

Because lean body mass is the main single determinant of resting energy expenditure, methods to possibly increase lean body mass at the expense of fat body mass are of great relevance in the context of weight-management strategies. Preservation of lean body mass during weight loss helps further weight loss, and a preferential regain of lean body mass over fat mass helps body weight maintenance after weight loss. Body composition is very much dependent on the balance between lipogenesis and fat oxidation/thermogenesis (see Sections 4.2 and 4.3). Other important determinants are nutrient partitioning between fat and muscle, adipocyte hyperplasia and the balance between protein synthesis and breakdown in muscle. These processes, like lipogenesis and thermogenesis, are influenced by the nutritional status and the composition of the diet.

### 4.4.1 Nutrient partitioning between fat and muscle

Adipose tissue hypertrophy is enhanced when fatty acids and glucose are preferentially channeled to adipose tissue rather than to other tissues, and particularly to muscle, where their main metabolic fate is oxidation. Two important players in nutrient partitioning between fat and muscle are LPL and GLUT4, both of which are highly expressed in the two tissues. Disregulation or imbalances of these two activities in muscle and adipose tissue may contribute to obesity, or may even cause it. Muscle LPL activity is inversely correlated with percentage body fat and body mass index in humans,[60,61] and moderate overexpression of LPL selectively in skeletal muscle prevents the development of diet-induced obesity in transgenic mice.[62] In mice, transgenic overexpression of GLUT4 in adipose tissue results in an obese phenotype,[63,64] whereas lack of GLUT4 in adipose tissue (through tissue-specific knockout) results in reduced adiposity.[65]

LPL activity in adipose tissue changes during the day according to the nutritional state: it decreases during short-term fasting, by means of a post-translational mechanism,[66] and recovers upon refeeding. Failure to decrease adipose tissue LPL activity in the post-absorptive state may contribute to increased fat deposition in obesity,[66] as suggested by the finding of a higher LPL activity in adipose tissue during fasting in obese subjects compared with lean controls.[67] LPL activity in adipose tissue is affected not only by the nutritional state, but also by specific nutrients: it is stimulated by glucose, by post-transcriptional mechanisms,[57] and inhibited by fatty acids and high-fat diets, which however induce the transcription of the LPL gene in adipocytes.[68,69] GLUT4 expression is also subject to dietary modulation: it increases with high-fat diets more in adipose tissue than in muscle, whereas in the unfed state it is markedly down-regulated in adipose tissue and up-regulated in muscle (reviewed in reference 70).

### 4.4.2 Adipocyte hyperplasia

Besides adipocyte hypertrophy, another process that favors WAT enlargement is adipocyte hyperplasia, i.e. the increment of adipocyte number. Adipocytes are formed through proliferation of committed precursor cells (pre-adipocytes) residing in fat depots and subsequent differentiation of the progeny into cells capable of regulating fat accumulation and release. This differentiation process, called adipogenesis, implies the concerted induction and activation of a series of adipogenic transcription factors, among which PPARγ plays a key role in terminal differentiation.[59] In mice, the knockout of cyclin-dependent kinase inhibitors (p21 and p27), normally required for pre-adipocyte exit from the cell cycle, results in marked adipocyte hyperplasia and massive spontaneous obesity.[71]

Both in humans and rodents, adipose tissue retains the capacity to generate new adipocytes at all ages, but basic adipocyte number is established by adolescence. Adipocyte hyperplasia is characteristic of some forms of extreme adult human obesity and is particularly relevant in childhood obesity, which typically involves both hyperplasia and hypertrophy of adipocytes. The frequent persistence of childhood obesity into adulthood suggests that the increased adipocyte number in these individuals may predispose them to lasting obesity or even be causative for obesity.

Proliferation of pre-adipocytes and adipogenesis are influenced by nutrients. Long-chain fatty acids, both saturated and unsaturated, promote adipogenesis (probably through activation of PPARs, which are lipid-activated transcription factors), providing a molecular link between excess lipid intake, enhanced flux of fatty acids entering adipose tissue and increased fat mass.[72] Linoleic acid and arachidonic acid (both n-6 PUFAs) appear to have additional pro-adipogenic effects (see Section 4.5.1). Another nutrient known to affect the differentiation of pre-adipose cells in culture is vitamin A; retinoic acid, its acidic form, promotes adipogenesis at low doses, but dramatically inhibits adipogenesis at relatively high doses, mainly through blockage of the transcriptional activity of an early adipogenic transcription factor, CCAAT/enhancer binding protein (C/EBP)β, mediated by retinoic acid-activated retinoid receptors (reviewed in reference 73). Local glucose levels may also be of importance: it has been suggested that excess glucose in adipocytes may favor adipocyte hyperplasia through a glucose metabolite-induced down-regulation of a late adipogenic transcription factor, C/EBPα, that is critical for the loss of the proliferative capacity during terminal differentiation;[74] consistent with this idea, hyperplasic obesity was reported in transgenic mice overexpressing GLUT4 in adipose tissue.[63]

### 4.4.3 Muscle protein synthesis and breakdown

The balance between protein synthesis and breakdown in muscle is influenced by energy balance and exercise. A negative energy balance favors the loss of both fat body mass and lean body mass. Resistance training favors a net increase of lean body mass provided that the individual is at energy balance, so that diet is supporting the exercise she/he is performing. In fact, it has been pointed out that nutritional interventions in athletes may have their biggest impact on performance by supporting consistent intensive training and thus promoting the physiological and biochemical adaptations that will, in turn, lead to muscle hypertrophy and improved performance.[75]

There is some evidence that a high protein intake may favor a preferential loss of fat *versus* lean body mass during weight loss, by favoring muscle protein deposition, among other mechanisms (see Section 4.5.2). Likewise, there is some evidence that protein intake shortly after resistance training may facilitate exercise-induced muscle hypertrophy,[76] although, overall, there is little evidence to support the premise that extra protein intake is essential for maximal performance in the athletes.[77]

The amino acid leucine has specifically been implicated in the promotion of net muscle protein anabolism, through effects on protein synthesis and/or protein breakdown (see references 78 and 79). In rats, it is well established that leucine promotes protein synthesis in muscle, mainly via activation of mTOR (mammalian target of rapamycin) kinases, which leads to the activation and increased expression of key translational factors and other proteins involved in protein synthesis (reviewed in reference 80). In humans, it appears that the main effect of leucine is on muscle protein breakdown, reducing breakdown without increasing muscle protein synthesis (reviewed in reference 79). The mechanism behind leucine-induced reduction of protein breakdown is not known, but it is noteworthy that synthetic leucine aldehyde peptides – such as *N*-acetyl-leucyl-leucyl-norleucinal (LLN) and CBZ-leucyl-leucyl-leucinal (MG132) – are commonly used inhibitors of an important component of the cell machinery for protein breakdown, the proteosome.

## 4.5 Using food and food components to control lipogenesis and thermogenesis

In this section, foods and food components that have the potential to assist weight loss/maintenance due to effects on lipogenesis, thermogenesis and/or body composition are presented.

### 4.5.1 Dietary fats

Dietary fat is related to the etiology of obesity because of its high energy density, high hedonic value, delayed satiating capacity thus promoting passive overconsumption, low associated thermic effect and efficient storage capacity. This has fueled the market for low-fat and fat-free foods for weight management. However, there is evidence that not all fats are equally *bad*.[81] Some specific fats and fat types, when consumed in replacement of other, less convenient, fats, may help prevent body weight gain, or may even enhance body weight loss in the context of more rigorous weight-loss plans. These fats are presented below.

*Polyunsaturated fatty acids*

For many years it has been known that PUFAs have a certain capacity of lowering adiposity and plasma triacylglycerol levels, mainly due to their effects of inhibiting lipogenic capacity and activating fatty acid catabolism in the liver (reviewed in references 82–84; see also Chapter 13).

In the liver, PUFAs repress the expression of the key lipogenic transcription factor SREBP-1 (by binding to and blocking the activity of a transcription factor, liver X receptor, needed for efficient SREBP-1 gene transcription) and inhibit the proteolytic process leading to SREBP-1 activation (reviewed in references 82–84) (Fig. 4.4). PUFAs also inhibit, by a post-transcriptional mechanism, the hepatic expression of glucose-6-phosphate-dehydrogenase, a key enzyme in the pentose phosphate pathway,[85] thus compromising NADPH availability for *de novo* fatty acid synthesis. On the other hand, PUFAs and PUFA-derivatives enhance fatty acid oxidation and fatty acid oxidation capacity in the liver. This enhancement is achieved through: (1) suppression of the expression of the lipogenic enzyme acetyl-CoA carboxylase (ACC) and subsequent reduction of the hepatic levels of its product, malonyl-CoA (which is both a substrate in fatty acid syntheis and a powerful inhibitor of fatty acyl-CoA uptake by mitochondria, the rate-limiting step in mitochondrial fatty acid oxidation); and (2) through activation of PPARα, a lipid-activated transcription factor abundantly expressed in hepatocytes that up-regulates the expression of a collection of genes for proteins involved in mitochondrial, peroxisomal and microsomal fatty acid catabolism (reviewed in reference 83).

PUFAs also have potential anti-adiposity effects targeting tissues other than the liver, such as WAT and muscle. Dietary n-3 PUFAs were shown to depress lipogenesis and down-regulate the expression levels of a collection of lipogenic genes, to up-regulate mitochondrial biogenesis and to induce beta-oxidation of fatty acids in visceral WAT depots of rodents.[86,87] PUFA may also enhance fatty acid oxidation in muscle,[88] although the effect appears to be less marked than in the liver (reviewed in reference 83). PUFA-induced increases in fatty acid oxidation may be linked to increased thermogenesis, since PUFAs were shown to up-regulate the expression of uncoupling proteins, including UCP1 in BAT,[89] UCP3 in skeletal muscle[88] and UCP2 in liver and WAT.[90,91] Both the UCP1 gene and the UCP3 gene contain a PPAR response element in their promoter, which may explain their sensitivity to PUFAs (PPARs are activated as transcription factors after binding certain fatty acids or fatty acid derivatives) (see reference 73).

### Biological activities of n-3 and n-6 PUFAs

PUFAs active in the regulation of gene expression and lipid metabolism are highly unsaturated fatty acids of 20 and 22 carbons of both the n-3 and the n-6 series, such as arachidonic acid (20:4, n-6), docosahexaenoic acid (DHA, 22:6, n-3) and eicosapentaenoic acid (EPA, 20:5, n-3). These fatty acids can be produced endogenously from linoleic acid (18:2, n-6), which is the precursor of arachidonic acid, and linolenic acid (18:3, n-3), which is the precursor of EPA and DHA, through the action of delta-5 and delta-6 desaturases. Linolenic acid is present predominantly in flaxseed, soybean and canola oils, and in English walnuts. Linoleic acid is found in most vegetable oils (such as corn oil and sunflower oil) and most nuts. However, only small amounts of linoleic and linolenic acids undergo delta-desaturation in the body. Therefore, foods rich in fatty acids that are the *products* of delta-desaturases, that bypass the regulated and required steps of further desaturation and elongation, are much more effective suppressors of hepatic lipogenesis and inducers of fatty acid oxidation than are foods rich in linoleic acid or linolenic acid, the *substrates* of delta-desaturases.[3] This is the case of fish oils, which are rich in long-chain highly polyunsaturated fatty acids of the n-3 series (DHA and EPA).

In other aspects, PUFAs of the n-3 and the n-6 series appear to have different biological activities. For instance, n-6 PUFAs have a greater hypocholesterolemic effect than n-3 PUFAs,[92] while n-3 PUFAs, due to the particular eicosanoids to which they give rise, appear to have beneficial effects on vascular endothelial function that are not displayed by the n-6 PUFAs, from which a different set of eicosanoids is produced (reviewed in reference 93). Together with their marked hypotriglycerydemic effect, this may explain the reduced risk of cardiovascular disease associated with fish and fish oil consumption that has been repeatedly observed in human epidemiologic studies and clinical intervention trials (reviewed in references 92 and 94).

PUFAs of the n-6 and n-3 series also differ in their effects on adipogenesis. Linoleic acid and arachidonic acid (both n-6 PUFAs) may be particularly pro-adipogenic, because they serve as precursors in pre-adipocytes of prostacyclins which, in a paracrine/autocrine fashion, through activation of a specific cell surface receptor, trigger early adipogenic events in these cells (reviewed in reference 95). Interestingly, n-3 PUFAs inhibit the above process, and in this sense can be considered as anti-adipogenic.[95] It has been suggested that a high dietary n-6 PUFA/n-3 PUFA ratio during early life and infancy may favor increased adipocyte numbers and future obesity, and it is remarkable that this ratio has continuously and markedly increased in human breast milk over recent decades.[95]

Studies in rodents have consistently reported that intake of n-3 PUFAs reduces adipose mass, preferentially visceral fat, in general without affecting body weight (see references in reference 87). Some studies in humans also reported an effect of dietary fish oil consumption increasing whole-body lipid oxidation and decreasing total body fat content,[96] and specifically abdominal fat content.[97] Most human studies, however, have so far examined the effect of PUFA intake on end-points related to cardiovascular health and insulin sensitivity, rather than to body weight and body fat control. There is a paucity of human studies specifically designed to ascertain whether the intake of PUFAs (or PUFA-rich foods such as fish oils and nuts) can assist in weight loss and/or in weight maintenance after weight loss in the long-term.

*Monounsaturated fatty acids*

Monounsaturated fatty acids (MUFAs), and particularly oleic acid, appear to have beneficial effects regarding cardiovascular health and insulin sensitivity (reviewed in references 98 and 99). MUFAs may also be beneficial in the context of weight-management strategies. For instance, MUFAs induce a lower increase of postprandial triglyceridemia than saturated fats[100] and may favor energy expenditure and thermogenic function. In a rodent study in which the influence of four dietary lipid sources (olive oil, sunflower oil, palm oil and beef tallow) were compared, it was found that total-body oxygen consumption was higher in rats fed olive oil than in those fed the other three diets, and that olive oil feeding induced the highest uncoupling protein expression in BAT and skeletal muscle.[101]

These and other results have prompted considerable interest in the use of *modified fat* diets rich in MUFAs for weight management. To date, however, there is no evidence from *ad libitum* dietary intervention studies that a normal-fat, high-MUFA diet is similar to a low-fat diet in preventing weight gain.[102] Likewise, there is no evidence that energy-restricted, moderate-fat diets rich in MUFAs are better than isoenergetic diets with mixed dietary fats[103] or a low fat content[104,105] for weight loss, although in some studies the MUFA-rich diets did improve the cardiovascular disease risk profile relative to the low-fat diets.[105,106]

*Medium-chain triacylglycerols*

Medium-chain triacylglycerols (MCTs) are triacylglycerols composed of fatty acids that contain 6–12 carbon atoms (see also Chapter 14). Medium-chain fatty acids (MCFAs) formed upon digestion of MCTs behave in a metabolically different way to long-chain fatty acids (LCFAs, of more than 12 carbon atoms) derived from long-chain tricylglycerols (LCTs). LCFAs require chylomicron formation for their absorption and transport. MCFAs, in contrast, are transported in the portal blood directly to the liver, thus bypassing peripheral tissues such as adipose tissue, making them less susceptible to the action of LPL and to deposition into adipose tissue stores. The structure-based differences continue through the processes of fat utilization: thus, unlike LCFAs, MCFAs enter the mitochondria independently of the carnitine transport system, so that they may be more easily oxidized.[107]

Studies in animals and humans have shown that MCTs have a greater thermogenic effect than LCTs in the short term, probably due to their rapid oxidation (reviewed in reference 108). Longer studies in animals and humans have shown that consumption of MCTs instead of LCTs can result in less body weight gain and decreased size of fat depots.[108–110] Coconut oil is particularly rich in MCTs, and we found in rats that a coconut-oil enriched diet was particularly effective in stimulating BAT UCP1 expression during *ad libitum* feeding and in preventing UCP1 down-regulation during food restriction, and that these effects went hand in hand with a decrease in the mass of white fat stores.[111] Furthermore, data suggest that MCT consumption increases satiety more than LCT consumption.[108,109]

The above results indicate the potential for MCTs to act as dietary adjuncts for improved body weight maintenance or even possibly weight loss. However, evidence for the latter role is not compelling from the human studies conducted so far. In one study, hypocaloric feeding in obese women with a diet containing 24% of calories as MCTs did not result in increased rate or amount of weight loss (compared with LCTs) after 12 weeks.[112] In another study, MCTs as part of a very low calorie diet supported higher weight and fat loss than LCTs during the first two weeks, accompanied by less intense hunger feelings and increased satiety, but the effects gradually declined during the third and fourth weeks of treatment, indicating subsequent metabolic adaptation.[113] In addition, there are some concerns regarding the cardiovascular effects of MCTs, because MCT consumption was found to result in increased total cholesterol, LDL-cholesterol, triacylglycerol and glucose concentrations in plasma.[114] MCTs appear to increase hepatic *de novo* lipogenesis and to enhance insulin sensitivity.[112,115] Thus, findings in support of a potential slimming effect of MCTs (lower energy density, control of satiety, rapid intrahepatic delivery and oxidation rates, poor adipose tissue incorporation) may be invalidated by counteracting effects (stimulation of insulin secretion and of anabolic-related processes, increased *de novo* fatty acid synthesis and induced hypertriglyceridemia).[116]

*Diacylglycerols*
Substitution of triacylglycerols in the diet by diacylglycerols has also been proposed to be of potential value in the prevention and management of obesity, probably because of effects of diacylglycerols that are similar to those of MCTs. Whereas triacylglycerols are catabolized to two fatty acid molecules and a 2-monoacylglycerol molecule that in the enterocyte acts as a backbone for the reformation of triacylglycerol molecules for packaging into chylomicrons, diacylglycerols of the 1,3 conformation are catabolized to two fatty acids and a glycerol moiety, which may be diverted through the portal circulation directly to the liver. Thus, fatty acids derived from diacylglycerol may be less available to adipose tissue and more easily oxidized in the liver.

Reported effects of the intake of diacylglycerol compared with triacylglycerol of a similar fatty acid composition include, in animals, lowering of plasma triacylglycerol levels and decreasing postprandial hyperlipidemia, increasing energy expenditure, increasing lipid oxidation capacity in liver and intestinal cells, and reducing diet-induced obesity[117,118] (reviewed in reference 119). The serum triglyceride-lowering effect of diacylglycerol compared with triacylglycerol intake can be related to an impairment of chylomicron assembly and subsequent release into the blood through the lymph, because reacylation to triacylglycerol in small intestinal cells was found to be slower with diacylglycerol feeding than triacylglycerol feeding.[119] Stimulation of enzyme activities responsible for beta-oxidation in the small intestine and liver may also contribute to reduced postprandial hyperlipidemia as well as to increased energy expenditure, which result in suppression of diet-induced obesity.[119] A decrease in triacylglycerol content in the chylomicron lipoprotein fraction following acute diacylglycerol-oil *versus* triacylglycerol-oil intake was also shown in humans;[120] other reported acute effects of diacylglycerol consumption in humans include lowering parameters of appetite and increasing fat oxidation and ketone body formation.[121]

Studies in humans support the potential value of diacylglycerol for the management of excess body weight and related disorders. In one study, carried out in 38 healthy non-obese and slightly overweight men, supplementation for 16 weeks with dietary diacylglycerol (provided at breakfast in the form of bread, mayonnaise and shortbread as part of an otherwise self-selected diet) resulted in decreases of body mass index, waist circumference, and visceral and subcutaneous adipose tissue greater than with triacylglycerol supplementation.[122] In a weight-loss study carried out in 131 obese men and women, it was found that consumption of diacylglycerol oil as part of a reduced-energy diet enhanced loss of body weight and fat in comparison with consumption of a triacylglycerol control oil.[123] Moreover, dietary diacylglycerol has been shown to suppress postprandial increases in serum lipid levels and to produce a higher postprandial energy expenditure and lipid oxidation compared with dietary triacylglycerol in humans,[124,125] and evidence has been obtained that diacylglycerol may be useful in the management of obesity and lipid abnormalities in both type 2 diabetic subjects and non-diabetic subjects with insulin resistance.[126,127]

Diacylglycerol has been approved by the Japanese Government as a food for specific health use to control postmeal blood lipids and body fat[128] and has recently been introduced in the EU as a novel food. Diacylglycerols occur naturally in small concentrations in several edible oils, cottonseed being among the richest. A diacylglycerol-rich cooking oil has been produced that contains about 80% diacylglycerols,[128] the oil can be incorporated into foods or consumed as a salad dressing.

### 4.5.2 Dietary protein and amino acids

High-protein diets for weight management have being revisited in recent years (reviewed in references 46 and 129). Proteins are more thermogenic (see Section 4.2.3) and satiating (see Chapter 2) than fats and carbohydrates. There is convincing evidence from human intervention studies that a higher protein intake (25% or more of the total energy as protein) increases thermogenesis and satiety, and reduces subsequent energy intake in the short-term compared with diets having the usually recommended protein content (15% or less of total energy as protein).[46,129] There is also evidence that higher-protein diets can result in an increased weight loss and fat loss as compared with diets lower in protein, probably due to reduced perceived hunger and energy intake.[46,129,130] Higher fat loss with high-protein diets is evident, however, even under isocaloric conditions, where total weight loss is not affected, pointing to a metabolic effect of protein favoring energy repartitioning towards lean body mass. Increasing the protein intake (from 15 to 18% total energy) has also been shown to limit weight regain and favor the regaining of fat-free mass at the cost of fat mass during weight maintenance after weight loss, under *ad libitum* energy intake conditions.[131]

How can a higher protein intake affect body composition? Layman *et al.*[132] reported that substituting dietary protein for carbohydrate in energy-restricted diets brought about endocrine changes (maintenance of thyroid hormones T3 and T4 and reduced insulin response to a test meal) consistent with higher rates of lipolysis. In addition, an increased amount of dietary protein has been shown to reduce nitrogen losses associated with very low energy diets and to sustain muscle protein anabolism during catabolic conditions (reviewed in reference 78). Hence, the changes in body composition associated with the higher protein diets may be associated with either targeting of body fat or sparing of muscle protein or both.[132]

A high intake of branched-chain amino acids (BCAAs: leucine, valine and isoleucine), and specifically of leucine, may be of special interest in the context of body weight-loss strategies, because of the effects of BCAAs on glycemic control and the specific effects of leucine in promoting muscle protein synthesis and/or inhibiting muscle protein breakdown (see Section 4.4.3) (reviewed in references 78 and 133). These metabolic roles for BCAAs can only be sustained by diets that provide them at levels exceeding the requirements for BCAAs as substrates for protein synthesis, which is their primordial metabolic destiny.[78] Of note, the BCAAs are the only amino acids not degraded in the liver, so that dietary intake directly impacts plasma levels and concentrations in peripheral tissues. BCAAs account for 15–25% of the total protein intake, with whey protein and dairy products being particularly rich sources.

Major concerns about using higher-protein diets, particularly those rich in animal products, are an increased risk of renal failure and the association of cholesterol and, especially, saturated fatty acids with cardiovascular disease. There is little evidence for adverse effects of high-protein diets on renal function in individuals without established renal disease,[134] although it is obvious that caution should be exerted in the case of susceptible groups. Likewise, it appears that moderately high protein diets are not harmful to cardiovascular health and may indeed be beneficial.[135–137] In any case, although recent evidence supports potential benefits, rigorous longer-term studies are needed to investigate the safety and effects of high-protein diets on weight loss and weight maintenance.

It is important to emphasize that a high-protein diet does not necessarily mean a very low carbohydrate, high-fat Atkins diet (the latter diets having ~10% of the energy as carbohydrate and ~60% as fat). Various studies have found greater fat losses with diets consisting, for instance, of 25–30% protein, 40–45% carbohydrate, 30% fat compared with diets close to the usually recommended 15% protein, 60% carbohydrate, 25% fat macronutrient balance (see reference 46).

### 4.5.3 Micronutrients

*Calcium*

Anti-obesity effects of dietary calcium have been demonstrated in rodents, in which calcium supplementation attenuates the development of high-fat diet-induced obesity, accelerates weight and fat loss under energy restriction conditions, and limits weight and fat gain during refeeding after weight loss (reviewed in reference 138). Dairy products were found to be more potent than supplemental calcium in these animal studies.

In humans, observational studies have noted an inverse relationship between dietary calcium intake, and specifically of dairy products intake, and body mass index or body fat,[138] but these effects could be due to other characteristics of high-calcium/dairy consumers. A systematic review of randomized trials of calcium/dairy supplementation (which were designed to analyze end-points related to bone health, but included information on changes in body weight/composition) concluded that the data available provide little support for an effect of calcium in reducing body weight or fat mass,[139] but other reviews (not systematic) have reached the opposite conclusion.[140] Some studies found that a high calcium (and especially a high dairy) intake increased weight and fat loss in response to caloric restriction in obese people,[141–143] but others failed to detect any effect of high calcium/dairy intake beyond that seen with energy restriction alone.[144–146] Thus, there is evidence that calcium intake may help to reduce body weight or adiposity, but the evidence is not conclusive and further weight-loss and weight-maintenance studies assessing long-term effects of calcium and dairy supplementation are needed.[147]

A mechanism by which dietary calcium intake might affect body weight/adiposity is by reducing dietary fat absorption (see reference 147). In addition, a metabolic mechanism for the effect of dietary calcium on adiposity has been proposed, based on studies in cultured human adipocytes and animal studies (reviewed in references 138 and 147). This mechanism involves effects of dietary calcium intake on the levels of calcitrophic hormones, and the subsequent effect of these hormones on calcium uptake by adipocytes and pancreatic beta cells, which leads to changes in intracellular calcium concentration that impact on adipocyte metabolism and insulin secretion. Low-calcium diets favor high circulating levels of 1,25-dihydroxyvitamin D (active vitamin D), which was demonstrated to stimulate calcium entry into adipocytes (through activation of a membrane receptor different from the nuclear vitamin D receptor) and is assumed to stimulate calcium entry into pancreatic beta cells. Within the adipocytes, increased intracellular calcium concentration was shown to enhance lipogenesis and inhibit lipolysis, by inducing fatty acid synthase transcription and stimulating cAMP phosphodiesterase activity, respectively. Within the pancreas, intracellular calcium is known to stimulate insulin release, which will further act to stimulate lipogenesis and inhibit lipolysis. Thus, suppression of 1,25-dihydroxyvitamin D, as occurs during high-calcium diets, would result in reduced lipogenesis and increased lipo-lysis – and possibly increased fat oxidation and thermogenesis – in adipocytes.

The augmented anti-obesity effect of dairy products relative to supplemental calcium found in many animal and human studies may be due to differences in the bioavailability of calcium, or to the presence of additional bioactive compounds in whey or whole milk, such as BCAAs or conjugated linoleic acid (see Section 4.6), which may act synergistically with calcium to attenuate adiposity (see reference 138).

### *Vitamin A*

A possible involvement of vitamin A in the modulation of body adiposity is suggested by cell and animal studies (reviewed in reference 73). In rodents, acute treatment with pharmacological doses of retinoic acid (RA), the carboxylic form of vitamin A, causes a reduction of body weight and adiposity that is not dependent on reduced energy intake and correlates with an increased thermogenic potential in BAT (with increased expression of UCP1 and UCP2) and muscle (with increased expression of UCP3) and a depressed adipogenic/lipogenic potential and the acquisition of BAT features in white fat depots.[148–151] Reduction of adiposity after *in vivo* RA treatment supports effects of RA in inhibiting adipogenesis, promoting apoptosis of fat cells and triggering transcriptional activation of the genes encoding uncoupling proteins, all of which have been demonstrated in cell culture systems (reviewed in reference 73). Both the UCP1 and the UCP3 gene contain an RA response element in their promoter for the binding of specific transcription factors (the retinoid receptors) capable of enhancing transcription after their interaction with an RA molecule (see reference 73). Dietary pro-vitamin A carotenoids also induce UCP1 expression in cultured brown adipocytes, an effect that could be due, at least in part, to local conversion into RA.[152]

As with acute RA treatment, dietary vitamin A supplementation (with retinyl palmitate, at 40- to 50-fold the usual dose, over 8–18 weeks) also increases thermogenic potential in BAT and muscle of rodents, and appears to confer some resistance to the development of high-fat diet-induced obesity in mice[153] and to modestly but significantly reduce adiposity in rats fed normal chow.[154] A poor vitamin A status, on the other hand, favors in mice an increment of adiposity, independent of changes of energy intake, that correlates with an increased adipogenic/lipogenic potential in WAT depots and a depressed thermogenic potential in BAT.[149,150] The latter result agrees with the observation that diets poor in vitamin A favor adipose tissue formation in sirloin (the so-called 'bovine marbling').[155]

RA treatment and dietary vitamin A supplementation also affect the secretory function of adipose tissues in rodents, triggering a marked down-regulation of the expression and circulating levels of two adipocyte-secreted proteins, the excess of which has been related to insulin resistance – namely resistin[156] and leptin.[154,157,158]

Together, the results of these animal studies point to a relationship between vitamin A status and body adiposity and systemic insulin sensitivity that deserves further investigation in humans. Of note, there are studies linking a low dietary intake of vitamin A with high incidence of obesity in certain human populations.[159,160] Subclinical deficiency in vitamin A is common in industrialized countries[161] and, on the top of energy-dense diets, may be a factor contributing to the obesity epidemics.

### 4.5.4 Plant ingredients interfering with the sympathoadrenal system

Because thermogenesis and fat oxidation are to a large extent under the control of the SNS, approaches that mimic or interfere with the SNS and its neurotransmitter noradrenaline offer a rational approach for obesity management. Current interest in the nutritional/nutraceutical arenas has focused on plant ingredients capable of enhancing the release of noradrenaline from presynaptic neurons (ephedrine), prolonging the half-life of noradrenaline in the synaptic cleft (catechin polyphenols), potentiating the actions of noradrenaline in postsynaptic cells (caffeine and other methylxanthines), or having adrenergic agonist activity (ephedrine, synephrine).

*Combinations of caffeine and ephedrine*
Caffeine (and other methylxanthines, abundant in coffee and teas) inhibits cAMP phosphodiesterases, thus prolonging the half-life of cAMP, which is a critical intracellular mediator for the lipolytic and thermogenic effects of catecholamines. Ephedrine, the principle alkaloid found in shrubs of plants of the genus *Ephedra*, and other *Ephedra* alkaloids, promote the release of noradrenaline from SNS terminals and possess adrenoceptor agonist activity, thus favoring thermogenesis, vasoconstriction and increased blood pressure; in addition, *Ephedra* alkaloids have amphetamine-like effects in the central nervous system, promoting appetite suppression, mood elevation and resistance to fatigue (reviewed in reference 162). Combinations of ephedrine and caffeine are marketed both as pure compounds in capsular form and as herbal preparations sold under the category of dietary supplements.

Ephedrine and *Ephedra* alkaloids, alone and especially when combined with caffeine or caffeine-containing herbs, have been repeatedly demonstrated to promote a modest but significant short-term weight loss (approximately 0.9 kg/month more than placebo, without caloric restriction) in human trials, as concluded in a recent meta-analysis.[163] This meta-analysis also concluded, however, that the intake is associated with a 2.2- to 3.6-fold increase in the likelihood of psychiatric, autonomic or gastrointestinal symptoms, and heart palpitations.[163] Some authors consider that the benefits of mixtures of ephedrine and caffeine in treating obesity may outweigh the associated risks, because side effects, when the products are used under controlled conditions, are usually mild and transient.[164,165] However, individual susceptibility to adverse effects associated with the consumption of combinations of ephedrine and caffeine cannot be ignored; similarly, it is essential not to ignore the fact that the side effects may be particularly inappropriate for obese individuals, who often already have hypertension and other cardiovascular risk factors. Moreover, there have been case reports of serious adverse effects (such as death, myocardial infarction, hypertension and stroke) attributed to the consumption of ephedrine and *Ephedra*.[162,166] Because of safety concerns, the US Food and Drug Administration (FDA) banned *Ephedra* and ephedrine-containing drugs and dietary supplements in April 2004.

*Bitter orange (Citrus aurantium)*
Following the withdrawal of ephedrine from the dietary supplement marketplace, sales of products containing *Citrus aurantium* (bitter orange or Seville orange) for weight loss are believed to have increased dramatically. *Citrus aurantium* contains a number of constituents speculated to lead to

weight loss, of which the most frequently cited constituents are synephrine and octopamine, which are structural analogs of adrenaline and noradrenaline, respectively, that can act as adrenoceptor agonists.

An increase in the thermic effect of food in women by adrenergic amines extracted from *Citrus aurantium* has been described, but this acute response may not translate into a chronic effect or a clinically significant weight loss over time.[167] Synephrine has lipolytic effects in human fat cells only at high doses, and octopamine does not have lipolytic effects in human adipocytes.[168] The only randomized placebo-controlled clinical trial of *Citrus aurantium* for weight loss conducted so far tested a combination product with high levels of caffeine (in addition to energy restriction and physical exercise over 6 weeks) and did not find an effect superior to placebo on body weight loss; reduction of body fat mass was higher in the treated group, but this effect cannot be attributed to *Citrus aurantium* alone (see references 169 and 170). In addition, concerns have been raised about the safety of products containing synephrine, since this compound increases blood pressure in humans and other species, and has the potential to increase the incidence of adverse cardiovascular events (see references 169 and 170).

*Catechin polyphenols and teas containing them*

Catechin polyphenols inhibit the enzyme catechol-*O*-methyl-transferase, which normally degrades noradrenaline at the synaptic junctions. Catechin polyphenols are found in large quantities in non-fermented teas, which also contain caffeine, and considerable interest has focused on the potential use of these teas, green tea and oolong tea (or extracts of them), in assisting in weight management. Acutely, oral administration of green tea extract was shown to increase 24h energy expenditure and fat oxidation in humans,[171] and administration of green tea extract over 12 weeks, as part of a regular self-selected diet, was claimed to result in a 4.6% reduction of body weight and a 4.5% reduction of body circumference.[172] The few studies examining the effects of oolong and green tea as a beverage did find modest effects on energy expenditure and fat oxidation, but were studies of very short duration.[173,174] Therefore, whether these slight increases in energy expenditure and fat oxidation persist over a long period, or are subject to dietary compensation to offset the slight energy imbalance, remains to be established. In addition, the quantity of tea (as a beverage) that must be consumed to obtain an effect has not been established, and may be disproportionately high.[108] Thus, the potential of green tea and oolong tea as functional foods for weight management remains to be established.

### 4.5.5 Other food and food components of interest

*Capsaicin and capsaicin-rich foods*

Capsaicin is the major pungent component in fruits of *Capsium*. In experimental animals it was reported to enhance adrenal catecholamine secretion, activate BAT function, enhance energy expenditure and suppress body fat accumulation upon long-term treatment (see references 175 and 176). Capsaicin-rich foods (e.g. chilli peppers and red peppers) have been shown to stimulate fat oxidation and thermogenesis in humans,[177,178] although the effects appear to be weaker in obese subjects.[179] Non-pungent capsaicin analogs found in some pepper varieties, which may be more suitable than capsaicin for functional food and nutraceutical developments, also increase thermogenesis and energy consumption in humans and mice.[175,176]

*Anthocyanins*

Anthocyanins are phenolic phytochemicals used for the coloring of foods and widely distributed in human diets through crops, beans, fruits, vegetables and red wine. In one study,[180] it was found that dietary supplementation with anthocyanins (cyanidin 3-*O*-β-D-glucoside-rich purple corn color) suppressed the development of high-fat-diet-induced obesity and insulin resistance in mice; the effect was not due to reduced energy intake or fat absorption, and was accompanied by reduced expression of key enzymes and transcription factors for fatty acid and triacylglycerol synthesis in both liver and WAT. These results suggest that anthocyanins may constitute functional food factors of benefit in the prevention of obesity and diabetes, probably by targeting lipogenesis (effects on energy expenditure/thermogenesis were not addressed in the above study, and remain to be investigated).

*Hydroxycitric acid (HCA)* (*Garcinia cambogia*)

HCA is the active ingredient of fruit rinds of *Garcinia cambogia*, a plant native to India. HCA is a potent inhibitor of ATP citrate lyase, which catalyzes the extramitochondrial cleavage of citrate to oxaloacetate and acetyl-CoA (see Fig. 4.3). The inhibition of this reaction limits the availability of acetyl-CoA units required for fatty acid synthesis and lipogenesis during a lipogenic diet (reviewed in reference 181). Animal studies have shown that dietary HCA can suppress *de novo* fatty acid synthesis and food intake, and decrease body weight gain. Clinical studies in humans conducted so far have shown controversial findings, and evidence of a weight-loss effect of *Garcinia cambogia* or HCA in humans is not compelling (reviewed in references 182 and 183). A recent randomized, double-blind placebo-controlled study concluded, however, that a novel calcium/potassium salt of HCA, in addition to a moderate caloric restriction and exercise program, is a highly effective adjunct to weight control.[184]

*Oleoyl-estrone*

Oleoyl-estrone is a natural hormone derivative found in plasma and tissues, and also in milk and dairy products.[185] Oleoyl-estrone administration (as a drug) was shown to induce a dose-dependent loss of body fat in a variety of rodent models.[186–188] This slimming effect is due to both a decrease in food intake and the maintenance of energy expenditure, creating an energy gap that is filled with internal fat stores while preserving body protein.[189] Recently, weight loss in a patient with morbid obesity under treatment with oleoyl-estrone was reported.[190] Human phase I clinical studies of oleoyl-estrone administration as an anti-obesity therapy are currently underway in the United States.[191]

*Tungstate*

Tungstate, first studied as a potential antidiabetic agent, was recently shown to have an anti-obesity effect in a rodent model of diet-induced obesity.[192] In this study, in obese rats, oral administration of tungstate significantly decreased body weight gain and adiposity without modifying caloric intake, intestinal fat absorption or growth rate. These effects were mediated by an increase in whole-body energy dissipation and by changes in the expression of genes involved in the oxidation of fatty acids and mitochondrial uncoupling in adipose tissue. Furthermore, treatment increased the number of small adipocytes with a concomitant induction of apoptosis. These results indicate a potential value of tungstate in obesity treatment. Further clinical studies are needed to test the efficacy and safety of tungstate for weight loss.

*Yerba mate*

Yerba mate (*Ilex paraguariensis*) is an evergreen tree that is native to South America, and contains relatively large amounts of caffeine. In a combination preparation with guarana (*Paullinia cupana*, also rich in caffeine) and damiana (*Turnera diffusa*) it was tested in a double-blind, placebo-controlled trial in obese patients, who were instructed not to change their eating habits during the treatment; the combination was found to delay gastric emptying, reducing the time to perceived gastric fullness and to produce substantial weight loss.[193] Further clinical studies are needed to test the efficacy and safety of yerba mate for weight loss.

*Yohimbe*

Yohimbe (*Pausinystalia yohimbe*) is an evergreen tree that is native to Central Africa. The rationale for its use in weight-management strategies relies on the fact that yohimbine, the main active constituent of the ground bark of yohimbe, is an antagonist of alpha-2 adrenoceptors and there is evidence that antagonism of these receptors may lead to increased lipolysis. However, the results of three double-blind, randomized clinical trials using yohimbine to achieve weight loss have been conflicting, and at present it is unclear whether yohimbine is effective in reducing body weight (reviewed in reference 182).

*Licorice*

Licorice, the root of the *Glycyrrhiza* species, is one of the most frequently employed botanicals in traditional medicines. Some animal studies reported suppression of abdominal fat accumulation after dietary supplementation with licorice[194] and, in a human trial, licorice administration was found to reduce body fat mass, without changing body mass index, in 15 normal-weight subjects under free-living conditions (no caloric restriction).[195] The mechanism of action, safety and efficacy of licorice for weight loss is unknown.

## 4.6 Using ergogenic aids for weight control

A comprehensive definition of the use of nutritional ergogenic aids is 'dietary manipulation to improve physical and sports performance'. Nutritional ergogenic aids are a growing market and are increasing in popularity and variety. There are a large number of products marketed as nutritional ergogenic aids that also claim to assist in weight management, by virtue of a purported capability to affect some aspects of energy metabolism or, more often, body composition, increasing lean body (muscle) mass and/or reducing fat mass. These include protein and amino acid supplements, and combinations of ephedrine and caffeine, already presented in the preceding section. Caffeine has been proven to have ergogenic effects in a number of human studies, although the mechanism(s) behind these effects are largely unknown: the popular view is that caffeine, by virtue of its capability to inhibit cAMP phosphodiesterases, increases fat supply to the muscle, which in turn can increase fat oxidation, spare glycogen and thus extend exercise time, but there are other ways in which caffeine may impact positively on exercise performance, including effects on Na/K ATPase and intracellular calcium distribution in muscle cells (reviewed in references 75, 196 and 197). Evidence for ergogenic effects of *Ephedra* alkaloids – or of their combination with caffeine, beyond the effect brought about by the latter – is weak and insufficient,[163,197,198] as is the evidence for ergogenic effects of protein and amino acid supplements.[77,199]

Other supplements marketed both as ergogenic aids and weight-loss aids, by virtue of purported effects on body composition, are presented below.

### 4.6.1 Conjugated linoleic acid (CLA)

CLA is the acronym that describes a group of octadecadienoic acids (18:2) that are isomers of the essential fatty acid linoleic (C18:2, n-6) but whose double bonds are not separated by a methylene group but are conjugated. CLA is naturally present in certain foods, such as the meat of ruminants (e.g. beef, lamb) and dairy products (e.g. milk, cheese) where they can represent 0.5–2% of the fatty acids. In these products the predominant isomer (about 75–90%) is *cis*-9,*trans*-11 CLA. Three other isomers (trans-7,*cis*-9

CLA, *trans*-9,*cis*-11 CLA and *trans*-11,*cis*-13 CLA) are usually present in intermediate concentrations, whereas there are approximately 20 other isomers that can be present in smaller quantities. The CLA chemically produced for commercialization and used in dietetic complements or foods is usually a relatively rich CLA mixture containing about equal proportions of two isomers, *trans*-10,*cis*-12 CLA and *cis*-9,*trans*-11 CLA, with a minor presence of other isomers.

Interest in CLA arose, initially, in its anticarcinogenic action. However, CLA may have several other health benefits, including the reduction of body fat and an improvement of blood lipid profile in relation to the risk of cardiovascular diseases and diabetes (see reference 200). However, conflicting results on the effects of CLA have been reported depending on days of treatment, dose, animal species used and proportion of each isomer (reviewed in reference 201). Most of the experiments have used a mixture of different isomers, while it is increasingly evident that different CLA isomers have different or even opposite biological effects (e.g. see references 200 and 202). There is substantial evidence that the *trans*-10,*cis*-12 CLA isomer is responsible for the effects on body composition and lipid metabolism, whereas anticarcinogenic properties are mostly associated with the *cis*-9,*trans*-11 CLA isomer.[203]

In different animal models, CLA has been shown to reduce substantially the amount of body fat and to increase relatively the proportion of lean body mass, without substantially reducing body weight (reviewed in references 204–206). Reduction of fat accretion is mainly explained by the effects of *trans*-10,*cis*-12 CLA inhibiting lipoprotein lipase activity in adipose tissue *in vivo*, thereby reducing lipid uptake into adipocytes and inhibiting adipogenesis (reviewed in reference 200). In humans, the available information indicates that CLA can produce, among other effects, a moderate reduction in body fat content and a relative, very modest, increase in lean body mass (reviewed in references 201 and 207). The conclusion of the longest double-blind, placebo-controlled study conducted to date has been that daily supplementation with a 1:1 mixture of the CLA isomers *trans*-10,*cis*-12 and *cis*-9,*trans*-11, administered in either the triacylglycerol or free fatty acid form for 12 months reduced body fat mass by approximately 8% without affecting lean mass in overweight subjects consuming an *ad libitum* diet.[208] In an extension of the latter study, it was found that the reduction of body fat mass persisted after one more year of daily CLA supplementation,[209] suggesting that CLA helps prevent regain of body fat. In fact, in a human study designed to analyze the effect of CLA on body weight gain after weight loss, CLA supplementation for 13 weeks did not affect the percentage of body weight regain, but favored the regain of lean body mass instead of fat mass.[210]

In most human studies no safety problems have been described with the currently used daily doses of CLA (1.5–7 g/day). However, different reports by the Riserus and Vessby group have described significant increases in lipid peroxidation parameters and insulin resistance, as well as in blood glucose and serum lipid concentrations, in obese patients treated with CLA (see reference 211). The longest human studies on CLA supplementation performed to date concluded that CLA is well tolerated and safe for use in overweight humans for 1–2 years.[208,209,212] In one of these studies, the groups treated with CLA had higher values of lipoprotein(a), trombocytes and leucocytes, suggesting that CLA may increase cardiovascular disease risk and may promote an inflammatory response, even though the observed changes were within the normal range and were not considered clinically relevant.[208]

In summary, CLA (i.e. some combinations of isomers) appears to be a potentially interesting ingredient of functional foods to combat obesity or, to be more precise, to prevent excess fat gain. However, additional studies are needed in both animal models (to select appropriate combinations, looking at mechanistic aspects) and in humans (to address and qualify risk/benefits) regarding potential effects on inflammation and the insulin system.

### 4.6.2 Chromium and chromium picolinate

Chromium is an essential trace mineral and cofactor to insulin. Chromium picolinate is an organic compound of trivalent chromium and picolinic acid (a naturally occurring derivative of tryptophan), which is better absorbed than dietary chromium. Reported effects of chromium in connection with body weight management found in some clinical trials include an increase in lean body mass, a decrease in percentage body fat and an increase in basal metabolic rate (reviewed in reference 182). However, there is no conclusive evidence of positive effects of chromium supplementation on body composition of healthy humans, even when taken in combination with an exercise training program.[213] A 2003 meta-analysis of ten randomized, double-blind, placebo-controlled studies assessing chromium picolinate supplementation without energy restriction for a period of 6–14 weeks in obese subjects found a small but significant effect of the supplement in reducing body weight; however, this effect was largely dependent on the results of a single trial and was much lower than the effect brought about by moderate energy restriction.[214] Very recently, a randomized, double-blind, placebo-controlled trial lasting 6 months similarly concluded that there is no evidence that high-dose chromium picolinate treatment is effective in reducing body mass index or improving metabolic parameters in obese patients with type 2 diabetes.[215] Additionally, some trials reported adverse effects, and cell and animal studies have indicated that chromium picolinate is mutagenic and may generate oxidative damage to DNA and lipids (see reference 213). Thus, the efficacy and long-term safety of chromium and chromium picolinate for weight loss and as an ergogenic aid are uncertain.

### 4.6.3 Hydroxymethylbutyrate

Beta-hydroxy-beta-methylbutyrate (HMB) is a leucine metabolite that has shown anticatabolic actions through inhibiting ubiquitin-proteosome-mediated protein breakdown[216] and that may prevent exercise-induced muscle damage.[217] It is primarily used by bodybuilders as a supportive measure to induce changes in body composition, and could be a potential dietary supplement for body weight reduction.[182] Randomized clinical trials conducted to assess the potential for HMB as an ergogenic aid reported modest effects in reducing fat mass and increasing lean body mass, and no apparent adverse effects (reviewed in references 199 and 218).

### 4.6.4 Carnitine

Carnitine is a trimethylamine molecule that plays an important role in the transport of long-chain fatty acids into mitochondria for oxidation. There is some evidence for a beneficial effect of carnitine supplementation in training, competition and recovery from strenuous exercise and in regenerative athletics (reviewed in reference 219). The rationale for carnitine supplementation as a weight-loss agent is based on the assumption that regular oral ingestion of the substance increases its intracellular concentration, thus favoring fat oxidation. However, studies have shown that oral carnitine ingestion does not change muscle carnitine concentration in healthy non-obese humans, and that carnitine supplementation does not promote weight loss in moderately overweight humans.[220,221]

## 4.7 Future trends

Obesity – with its associated co-morbidities such as the metabolic syndrome and also its health costs – is one of the major biomedical problems of recent decades, and effective and satisfying preventive strategies and treatments are necessary. Compliance with conventional weight-management programs is notoriously poor, and there is room for innovation.

A plethora of over-the-counter dietary supplements to treat obesity are currently marketed worldwide. Many of them have not been tested in randomized controlled trials in humans.[183] For those that have been tested in this way, evidence for effectiveness and safety is not compelling (reviewed in references 182 and 183). Products for which there actually is a scientific rationale have in general only minor weight-reducing effects, so that they must be considered to have at most an adjuvant role within the framework of more strict weight-loss regimens.[222] Moreover, the risk/benefit balance is unfavorable for some supplements of proven effectiveness, because of adverse effects associated with their consumption, as is the case with supplements containing *Ephedra* or ephedrine.

Functional foods that affect energy metabolism and fat partitioning may also serve as adjuncts to a dietary approach to body weight control, when incorporated in a healthy and balanced diet. Some traditional foods – such as tea, milk and nuts – might be of value in this sense, as might be designed foods with saturated fat replaced by n-3 PUFA or CLA, with long-chain triacylglycerols replaced by medium-chain triacylglycerols or diacylglycerols, or enriched in thermogenic ingredients or certain amino acids, among other emerging possibilities.

Another important aspect to be considered is the macronutrient balance of the diet. Negative energy balance produces weight loss independently of the macronutrient composition of the diet (see references 99 and 223), but there is increasing evidence that the latter can affect weight loss/maintenance, by virtue of distinct effects of proteins, fats and carbohydrates on processes involved in body weight and body fat control. Elevated protein intake, for instance, might assist body weight management through increased satiety and reduced subsequent energy intake, increased diet-induced thermogenesis, its contribution to storage of fat-free mass and its low energy efficiency during overfeeding (due to the increased diet-induced thermogenesis and to the composition of the body mass gained, with more fat-free mass) (see reference 129). The results of human studies using high-protein diets that have been conducted so far – together with the evidence pointing to undesirable effects associated with high levels of consumption of refined carbohydrates, such as decreased satiety and increased carbohydrate-induced hypertriglyceridemia – suggest that, in dietary practice, it may be beneficial to partially replace refined carbohydrate with protein sources that are low in saturated fat for weight-management purposes.[46] However, longer-term studies are needed to establish the safety and efficacy of high-protein diets in the long-term.

The system of body weight control is highly complex and redundant, and very often intended changes in one pathway are compensated for by non-intended changes in another one. Because of this, strategies/developments that affect different targets are of special interest. The combination of different bioactive ingredients in a unique dietary supplement or nutraceutical is already a common practice, and, likewise, multi-factorial functional foods for weight management may become commonplace in the near future. For instance, a functional food product containing low-glycemic index carbohydrates, 5-hydroxytryptophan, green tea extract and chromium has already been developed and is undergoing clinical testing;[224] the first two nutrients are purported to decrease appetite, while green tea is purported to increase energy expenditure and chromium to promote the composition of the weight loss to be fat rather than lean tissue.

With the advancing sciences of nutrition and nutrigenomics (which studies nutrient–gene interactions globally using post-genomic approaches) new developments in the functional foods and nutraceutical arenas are envisaged for obesity control based on an increasing knowledge of how specific nutrients and other food components affect hunger and satiety, thermogenesis, fat oxidation, lipogenesis or body composition. Hand in hand with this, increasing knowledge of how the individual's genetic background influences his/her response to nutrients/diets and drugs will lead to more individualized approaches for weight management.

Nutritional strategies and dietary patterns for obesity management become increasingly important as we recognize from previous experience the value of promoting positive behaviors rather than using a prohibitive approach to accomplish a given health outcome. Most probably, however, these measures will still have to be combined with energy restriction and increased physical activity to achieve significant weight loss. In any case, knowledge of the molecular mechanisms and mechanistic aspects explaining the biological activity/effects, assessment of long-term efficacy and safety in well-designed human trials, proper risk/benefit evaluation and, where appropriate, product quality (e.g. absence of contamination, accuracy of labeling), are aspects that will become progressively more important if weight-loss claims are to be made for a given food/product, or if dietary patterns are to be recommended for weight-management purposes.

## 4.8 Sources of further information and advice

The reader is referred to other chapters in this book for more detailed information on:

- lipogenesis and other processes of lipid metabolism (Chapter 1);
- satiety and its modulation by specific nutrients (Chapter 2);
- dietary calcium and body weight control (Chapter 11);
- conjugated linoleic acid (Chapter 12);
- polyunsaturated fatty acids (Chapter 13);
- medium-chain triacylglycerols (Chapter 14).

Websites of interest:

- http://www.efsa.eu.int/, home page of the European Food Safety Authority (EFSA);
- http://www.cfsan.fda.gov/~dms/ds-info.html, US Food and Drug Administration (FDA), pages on dietary supplements;

- http://www.nceff.com.au/regulatory/reg-japan.htm, FOSHU system;
- http://www.wisc.edu/fri/clarefs.htm, for current citations of the published scientific literature on CLA.

## 4.9 References


1 PALOU A, SERRA F, BONET M L and PICO C (2000), Obesity: molecular bases of a multifactorial problem, *Eur J Nutr* **39**, 127–144.

2 PALOU A, BONET M L and PICÓ C, The integrated system of body weight control, in *Study on Obesity and Functional Foods in Europe* (PALOU A., BONET M., and SERRA F., *EDS*), pp. 40–54, European commission, Directorate General for Research, Luxembourg, 2002.

3 PALOU A, PICO C, BONET M L and OLIVER P (1998), The uncoupling protein, thermogenin, *Int J Biochem Cell Biol* **30**, 7–11.

4 LOWELL B B and SPIEGELMAN B M (2000), Towards a molecular understanding of adaptive thermogenesis, *Nature* **404**, 652–660.

5 CANNON B and NEDERGAARD J (2004), Brown adipose tissue: function and physiological significance, *Physiol Rev* **84**, 277–359.

6 LOWELL B B, SUSULIC V S V, HAMANN A, LAWITTS J A, HIMMS-HAGEN J, BOYER B B, KOZAK L P and FLIER J S (1993), Development of obesity in transgenic mice after genetic ablation of brown adipose tissue, Nature **366**, 740–742.

7 ENERBACK S, JACOBSSON A, SIMPSON E M, GUERRA C, YAMASHITA H, HARPER M E and KOZAK L P (1997), Mice lacking mitochondrial uncoupling protein are cold-sensitive but not obese, *Nature* **387**, 90–94.

8 PERSEGHIN G (2001), Pathogenesis of obesity and diabetes mellitus: insights provided by indirect calorimetry in humans, *Acta Diabetol* **38**, 7–21.

9 CINTI S (2002), Adipocyte differentiation and transdifferentiation: plasticity of the adipose organ, *J Endocrinol Invest* **25**, 823–835.

10 ZURLO F, LARSON K, BOGARDUS C and RAVUSSIN E (1990), Skeletal muscle metabolism is a major determinant of resting energy expenditure, *J Clin Invest* **86**, 1423–1427.

11 RICQUIER D and BOUILLAUD F (2000), The uncoupling protein homologues: UCP1, UCP2, UCP3, StUCP and AtUCP, *Biochem J* **345**, Pt 2 161–179.

12 RICQUIER D and BOUILLAUD F (2000), Mitochondrial uncoupling proteins: from mitochondria to the regulation of energy balance, *J Physiol* **529**, Pt 1 3–10.

13 ERLANSON-ALBERTSSON C (2003), The role of uncoupling proteins in the regulation of metabolism, *Acta Physiol Scand* **178**, 405–412.

14 WEIGLE D S, SELFRIDGE L E, SCHWARTZ M W, SEELEY R J, CUMMINGS D E, HAVEL P J, KUIJPER J L and BELTRANDELRIO H (1998), Elevated free fatty acids induce uncoupling protein 3 expression in muscle: a potential explanation for the effect of fasting, *Diabetes* **47**, 298–302.

15 ARSENIJEVIC D, ONUMA H, PECQUEUR C, RAIMBAULT S, MANNING B S, MIROUX B, COUPLAN E, ALVES-GUERRA M C, GOUBERN M, SURWIT R, BOUILLAUD F, RICHARD D, COLLINS S and RICQUIER D (2000), Disruption of the uncoupling protein-2 gene in mice reveals a role in immunity and reactive oxygen species production, *Nat Genet* **26**, 435–439.

16 VIDAL-PUIG A J, GRUJIC D, ZHANG C Y, HAGEN T, BOSS O, IDO Y, SZCZEPANIK A, WADE J, MOOTHA V, CORTRIGHT R, MUOIO D M and LOWELL B B (2000), Energy

metabolism in uncoupling protein 3 gene knockout mice, *J Biol Chem* **275**, 16258–16266.

17 GONG D W, MONEMDJOU S, GAVRILOVA O, LEON L R, MARCUSSAMUELS B, CHOU C J, EVERETT C, KOZAK L P, LI C, DENG C, HARPER M E and REITMAN M L (2000), Lack of obesity and normal response to fasting and thyroid hormone in mice lacking uncoupling protein-3, *J Biol Chem* **275**, 16251–16257.

18 ROLFE D F and BROWN G C (1997), Cellular energy utilization and molecular origin of standard metabolic rate in mammals, *Physiol Rev* **77**, 731–758.

19 LEVINE J A (2002), Non-exercise activity thermogenesis (NEAT), *Best Pract Res Clin Endocrinol Metab* **16**, 679–702.

20 SCHRAUWEN P, HOEKS J, SCHAART G, KORNIPS E, BINAS B, VAN DE VUSSE G J, VAN BILSEN M, LUIKEN J J, COORT S L, GLATZ J F, SARIS W H and HESSELINK M K (2003), Uncoupling protein 3 as a mitochondrial fatty acid anion exporter, *FASEB J* **17**, 2272–2274.

21 SCHRAUWEN P, SARIS W H and HESSELINK M K (2001), An alternative function for human uncoupling protein 3: protection of mitochondria against accumulation of nonesterified fatty acids inside the mitochondrial matrix, *FASEB J* **15**, 2497–2502.

22 HIMMS-HAGEN J and HARPER M E (2001), Physiological role of UCP3 may be export of fatty acids from mitochondria when fatty acid oxidation predominates: an hypothesis, *Exp Biol Med (Maywood)* **226**, 78–84.

23 GOGLIA F and SKULACHEV V P (2003), A function for novel uncoupling proteins: antioxidant defense of mitochondrial matrix by translocating fatty acid peroxides from the inner to the outer membrane leaflet, *FASEB J* **17**, 1585–1591.

24 JEZEK P, ENGSTOVA H, ZACKOVA M, VERCESI A E, COSTA A D, ARRUDA P and GARLID K D (1998), Fatty acid cycling mechanism and mitochondrial uncoupling proteins, *Biochim Biophys Acta* **1365**, 319–327.

25 SKULACHEV V P (1998), Uncoupling: new approaches to an old problem of bioenergetics, *Biochim Biophys Acta* **1363**, 100–124.

26 HIMMS-HAGEN J (1989), Brown adipose tissue thermogenesis and obesity, *Prog Lipid Res* **28**, 67–115.

27 SCHOELLER D A (2001), The importance of clinical research: the role of thermogenesis in human obesity, *Am J Clin Nutr* **73**, 511–516.

28 RAVUSSIN E, LILLIOJA S, ANDERSON T E, CHRISTIN L and BOGARDUS C (1986), Determinants of 24-hour energy expenditure in man. Methods and results using a respiratory chamber, *J Clin Invest* **78**, 1568–1578.

29 RAVUSSIN E, LILLIOJA S, KNOWLER W C, CHRISTIN L, FREYMOND D, ABBOTT W G, BOYCE V, HOWARD B V and BOGARDUS C (1988), Reduced rate of energy expenditure as a risk factor for body-weight gain, *N Engl J Med* **318**, 467–472.

30 LEVINE J A, EBERHARDT N L and JENSEN M D (1999), Role of nonexercise activity thermogenesis in resistance to fat gain in humans, *Science* **283**, 212–214.

31 GRANATA G P and BRANDON L J (2002), The thermic effect of food and obesity: discrepant results and methodological variations, *Nutr Rev* **60**, 223–233.

32 DE JONGEL and BRAY G A (1997), The thermic effect of food and obesity: a critical review, *Obes Res* **5**, 622–631.

33 ZURLO F, LILLIOJA S, ESPOSITO-DEL PUENTE A, NYOMBA B L, RAZ I, SAAD M F, SWINBURN B A, KNOWLER W C, BOGARDUS C and RAVUSSIN E (1990), Low ratio of fat to carbohydrate oxidation as predictor of weight gain: study of 24-h RQ, *Am J Physiol* **259**, E650–657.

34 TREUTH M S, BUTTE N F and SORKIN J D (2003), Predictors of body fat gain in nonobese girls with a familial predisposition to obesity, *Am J Clin Nutr* **78**, 1212–1218.

35 ASTRUP A, BUEMANN B, CHRISTENSEN N J and TOUBRO S (1994), Failure to increase lipid oxidation in response to increasing dietary fat content in formerly obese women, *Am J Physiol* **266**, E592–599.

36 FILOZOF C M, MURUA C, SANCHEZ M P, BRAILOVSKY C, PERMAN M, GONZALEZ C D and RAVUSSIN E (2000), Low plasma leptin concentration and low rates of fat oxidation in weight-stable post-obese subjects, *Obes Res* **8**, 205–210.

37 UNGER R H (2002), Lipotoxic diseases, *Annu Rev Med* **53**, 319–336.

38 UNGER R H and ORCI L (2002), Lipoapoptosis: its mechanism and its diseases, *Biochim Biophys Acta* **1585**, 202–212.

39 SCHRAUWEN P and HESSELINK M K (2004), Oxidative capacity, lipotoxicity, and mitochondrial damage in type 2 diabetes, *Diabetes* **53**, 1412–1417.

40 YANG X, ENERBACK S and SMITH U (2003), Reduced expression of FOXC2 and brown adipogenic genes in human subjects with insulin resistance, *Obes Res* **11**, 1182–1191.

41 HAMMARSTEDT A, JANSSON P A, WESSLAU C, YANG X and SMITH U (2003), Reduced expression of PGC-1 and insulin-signaling molecules in adipose tissue is associated with insulin resistance, *Biochem Biophys Res Commun* **301**, 578–582.

42 LOWELL B B and BACHMAN E S (2003), Beta-adrenergic receptors, diet-induced thermogenesis, and obesity, *J Biol Chem* **278**, 29385–29388.

43 CANNON B, JACOBSSON A, REHNMARK S and NEDERGAARD J (1996), Signal transduction in brown adipose tissue recruitment: noradrenaline and beyond, *Int J Obes Relat Metab Disord* **20**, Suppl 3 S36–42.

44 SILVA J E (1995), Thyroid hormone control of thermogenesis and energy balance, *Thyroid* **5**, 481–492.

45 AHIMA R S and FLIER J S (2000), Leptin, *Annu Rev Physiol* **62**, 413–437.

46 HALTON T L and HU F B (2004), The effects of high protein diets on thermogenesis, satiety and weight loss: a critical review, *J Am Coll Nutr* **23**, 373–385.

47 PALOU A, BONET M L and SERRA F (Eds), *Study on Obesity and Functional Foods in Europe*, European comission, Directorate General for Research, Luxembourg, 2002.

48 PALOU A, PICO C and BONET M L (2004), Food safety and functional foods in the European Union: obesity as a paradigmatic example for novel food development, *Nutr Rev* **62**, S169–181.

49 PETZKE K J, FRIEDRICH M, METGES C C and KLAUS S (2005), Long-term dietary high protein intake up-regulates tissue specific gene expression of uncoupling proteins 1 and 2 in rats, *Eur J Nutr* **44**, 414–421.

50 RESHEF L, OLSWANG Y, CASSUTO H, BLUM B, CRONIGER C M, KALHAN S C, TILGHMAN S M and HANSON R W (2003), Glyceroneogenesis and the triglyceride/fatty acid cycle, *J Biol Chem* **278**, 30413–30416.

51 BEALE E G, ANTOINE B and FOREST C (2003), Glyceroneogenesis in adipocytes: another textbook case, *Trends Biochem Sci* **28**, 402–403.

52 BEALE E G, HAMMER R E, ANTOINE B and FOREST C (2004), Disregulated glyceroneogenesis: PCK1 as a candidate diabetes and obesity gene, *Trends Endocrinol Metab* **15**, 129–135.

53 FRANCKHAUSER S, MUNOZ S, PUJOL A, CASELLAS A, RIU E, OTAEGUI P, SU B and BOSCH F (2002), Increased fatty acid re-esterification by PEPCK overexpression in adipose tissue leads to obesity without insulin resistance, *Diabetes* **51**, 624–630.

54 FOUFELLE F and FERRE P (2002), New perspectives in the regulation of hepatic glycolytic and lipogenic genes by insulin and glucose: a role for the transcription factor sterol regulatory element binding protein-1c, *Biochem J* **366**, 377–391.
55 UYEDA K, YAMASHITA H and KAWAGUCHI T (2002), Carbohydrate responsive element-binding protein (ChREBP): a key regulator of glucose metabolism and fat storage, *Biochem Pharmacol* **63**, 2075–2080.
56 TOWLE H C (2001), Glucose and cAMP: adversaries in the regulation of hepatic gene expression, *Proc Natl Acad Sci U S A* **98**, 13476–13478.
57 ONG J M and KERN P A (1989), The role of glucose and glycosylation in the regulation of lipoprotein lipase synthesis and secretion in rat adipocytes, *J Biol Chem* **264**, 3177–3182.
58 KERSTEN S (2002), Peroxisome proliferator activated receptors and obesity, *Eur J Pharmacol* **440**, 223–234.
59 ROSEN E D, WALKEY C J, PUIGSERVER P and SPIEGELMAN B M (2000), Transcriptional regulation of adipogenesis, *Genes Dev* **14**, 1293–1307.
60 YOST Y, JENSEN D R and ECKEL R H (1993), Tissue-specific lipoprotein lipase: relationships to body composition and body fat distribution in normal weight humans, *Obes Res* **1**, 1–4.
61 RICHELSEN B, PEDERSEN S B, MOLLER-PEDERSEN T, SCHMITZ O, MOLLER N and BORGLUM J D (1993), Lipoprotein lipase activity in muscle tissue influenced by fatness, fat distribution and insulin in obese females, *Eur J Clin Invest* **23**, 226–233.
62 JENSEN D R, SCHLAEPFER I R, MORIN C L, PENNINGTON D S, MARCELL T, AMMON S M, GUTIERREZ-HARTMANN A and ECKEL R H (1997), Prevention of diet-induced obesity in transgenic mice overexpressing skeletal muscle lipoprotein lipase, *Am J Physiol* **273**, R683–689.
63 SHEPHERD P R, GNUDI L, TOZZO E, YANG H, LEACH F and KAHN B B (1993), Adipose cell hyperplasia and enhanced glucose disposal in transgenic mice overexpressing GLUT4 selectively in adipose tissue, *J Biol Chem* **268**, 22243–22246.
64 GNUDI L, SHEPHERD P R and KAHN B B (1996), Over-expression of GLUT4 selectively in adipose tissue in transgenic mice: implications for nutrient partitioning, *Proc Nutr Soc* **55**, 191–199.
65 TSAO T S, STENBIT A E, LI J, HOUSEKNECHT K L, ZIERATH J R, KATZ E B and CHARRON M J (1997), Muscle-specific transgenic complementation of GLUT4-deficient mice. Effects on glucose but not lipid metabolism, *J Clin Invest* **100**, 671–677.
66 BERGO M, WU G, RUGE T and OLIVECRONA T (2002), Down-regulation of adipose tissue lipoprotein lipase during fasting requires that a gene, separate from the lipase gene, is switched on, *J Biol Chem* **277**, 11927–11932.
67 ONG J M and KERN P A (1989), Effect of feeding and obesity on lipoprotein lipase activity, immunoreactive protein, and messenger RNA levels in human adipose tissue, *J Clin Invest* **84**, 305–311.
68 AMRI E Z, TEBOUL L, VANNIER C, GRIMALDI P A and AILHAUD G (1996), Fatty acids regulate the expression of lipoprotein lipase gene and activity in preadipose and adipose cells, *Biochem J* **314**, Pt 2 541–546.
69 SADUR C N, YOST T J and ECKEL R H (1984), Fat feeding decreases insulin responsiveness of adipose tissue lipoprotein lipase, *Metabolism* **33**, 1043–1047.
70 KAHN B B (1994), Dietary regulation of glucose transporter gene expression: tissue specific effects in adipose cells and muscle, *J Nutr* **124**, 1289S-1295S.

71 NAAZ A, HOLSBERGER D R, IWAMOTO G A, NELSON A, KIYOKAWA H and COOKE P S (2004), Loss of cyclin-dependent kinase inhibitors produces adipocyte hyperplasia and obesity, *FASEB J* **18**, 1925–1927.

72 AMRI E Z, AILHAUD G and GRIMALDI P A (1994), Fatty acids as signal transducing molecules: involvement in the differentiation of preadipose to adipose cells, *J Lipid Res* **35**, 930–937.

73 BONET M L, RIBOT J, FELIPE E and PALOU A (2003), Vitamin A and the regulation of fat reserves, *Cell Mol Life Sci* **60**, 1311–1321.

74 WANG Y, LEE-KWON W, MARTINDALE J L, ADAMS L, HELLER P, EGAN J M and BERNIER M (1999), Modulation of CCAAT/enhancer-binding protein-alpha gene expression by metabolic signals in rodent adipocytes, *Endocrinology* **140**, 2938–2947.

75 MAUGHAN R (2002), The athlete's diet: nutritional goals and dietary strategies, *Proc Nutr Soc* **61**, 87–96.

76 ESMARCK B, ANDERSEN J L, OLSEN S, RICHTER E A, MIZUNO M and KJAER M (2001), Timing of postexercise protein intake is important for muscle hypertrophy with resistance training in elderly humans, *J Physiol* **535**, 301–311.

77 SCIENTIFIC COMMITTEE on FOOD (SCF), Report of the SCF on composition and specification of food intended to meet the expenditure of intense muscular effort, especially for sportsmen. SCF/CS/NUT/SPORT/5 Final. 28 February 2001, http://europa.eu.int/comm/food/fs/sc/scf/out64_en.pdf.

78 LAYMAN D K (2003), The role of leucine in weight loss diets and glucose homeostasis, *J Nutr* **133**, 261S–267S.

79 MATTHEWS D E (2005), Observations of branched-chain amino acid administration in humans, *J Nutr* **135**, 1580S–1584S.

80 ANTHONY J C, ANTHONY T G, KIMBALL S R and JEFFERSON L S (2001), Signaling pathways involved in translational control of protein synthesis in skeletal muscle by leucine, *J Nutr* **131**, 856S–860S.

81 WESTERTERP-PLANTENGA M S (2004), Fat intake and energy-balance effects, *Physiol Behav* **83**, 579–585.

82 DUPLUS E, GLORIAN M and FOREST C (2000), Fatty acid regulation of gene transcription, *J Biol Chem* **275**, 30749–30752.

83 CLARKE S D, GASPERIKOVA D, NELSON C, LAPILLONNE A and HEIRD W C (2002), Fatty acid regulation of gene expression: a genomic explanation for the benefits of the mediterranean diet, *Ann N Y Acad Sci* **967**, 283–298.

84 JUMP D B (2002), Dietary polyunsaturated fatty acids and regulation of gene transcription, *Curr Opin Lipidol* **13**, 155–164.

85 TAO H, SZESZEL-FEDOROWICZ W, AMIR-AHMADY B, GIBSON M A, STABILE L P and SALATI L M (2002), Inhibition of the splicing of glucose-6-phosphate dehydrogenase precursor mRNA by polyunsaturated fatty acids, *J Biol Chem* **277**, 31270–31278.

86 RACLOT T, GROSCOLAS R, LANGIN D and FERRE P (1997), Site-specific regulation of gene expression by n-3 polyunsaturated fatty acids in rat white adipose tissues, *J Lipid Res* **38**, 1963–1972.

87 FLACHS P, HORAKOVA O, BRAUNER P, ROSSMEISL M, PECINA P, FRANSSEN-VAN HAL N, RUZICKOVA J, SPONAROVA J, DRAHOTA Z, VLCEK C, KEIJER J, HOUSTEK J and KOPECKY J (2005), Polyunsaturated fatty acids of marine origin upregulate mitochondrial biogenesis and induce beta-oxidation in white fat, *Diabetologia* **48**, 2365–2375.

88 BAILLIE R A, TAKADA R, NAKAMURA M and CLARKE S D (1999), Coordinate induction of peroxisomal acyl-CoA oxidase and UCP-3 by dietary fish oil: a mechanism for decreased body fat deposition, *Prostaglandins Leukot Essent Fatty Acids* **60**, 351–356.

89 SADURSKIS A, DICKER A, CANNON B and NEDERGAARD J (1995), Polyunsaturated fatty acids recruit brown adipose tissue: increased UCP content and NST capacity, *Am J Physiol* **269**, E351–360.
90 TSUBOYAMA-KASAOKA N, TAKAHASHI M, KIM H and EZAKI O (1999), Up-regulation of liver uncoupling protein-2 mRNA by either fish oil feeding or fibrate administration in mice, *Biochem Biophys Res Commun* **257**, 879–885.
91 HUN C S, HASEGAWA K, KAWABATA T, KATO M, SHIMOKAWA T and KAGAWA Y (1999), Increased uncoupling protein2 mRNA in white adipose tissue, and decrease in leptin, visceral fat, blood glucose, and cholesterol in KK-Ay mice fed with eicosapentaenoic and docosahexaenoic acids in addition to linolenic acid, *Biochem Biophys Res Commun* **259**, 85–90.
92 HU F B, MANSON J E and WILLETT W C (2001), Types of dietary fat and risk of coronary heart disease: a critical review, *J Am Coll Nutr* **20**, 5–19.
93 BROWN A A and HU F B (2001), Dietary modulation of endothelial function: implications for cardiovascular disease, *Am J Clin Nutr* **73**, 673–686.
94 BUCHER H C, HENGSTLER P, SCHINDLER C and MEIER G (2002), N-3 polyunsaturated fatty acids in coronary heart disease: a meta-analysis of randomized controlled trials, *Am J Med* **112**, 298–304.
95 AILHAUD G and GUESNET P (2004), Fatty acid composition of fats is an early determinant of childhood obesity: a short review and an opinion, *Obes Rev* **5**, 21–26.
96 COUET C, DELARUE J, RITZ P, ANTOINE J M and LAMISSE F (1997), Effect of dietary fish oil on body fat mass and basal fat oxidation in healthy adults, *Int J Obes Relat Metab Disord* **21**, 637–643.
97 SUMMERS L K, FIELDING B A, BRADSHAW H A, ILIC V, BEYSEN C, CLARK M L, MOORE N R and FRAYN K N (2002), Substituting dietary saturated fat with polyunsaturated fat changes abdominal fat distribution and improves insulin sensitivity, *Diabetologia* **45**, 369–377.
98 MASSARO M and DE CATERINA R (2002), Vasculoprotective effects of oleic acid: epidemiological background and direct vascular antiatherogenic properties, *Nutr Metab Cardiovasc Dis* **12**, 42–51.
99 LARA-CASTRO C and GARVEY W T (2004), Diet, insulin resistance, and obesity: zoning in on data for Atkins dieters living in South Beach, *J Clin Endocrinol Metab* **89**, 4197–4205.
100 WILLIAMS C M (2001), Beneficial nutritional properties of olive oil: implications for postprandial lipoproteins and factor VII, *Nutr Metab Cardiovasc Dis* **11**, 51–56.
101 RODRIGUEZ V M, PORTILLO M P, PICO C, MACARULLA M T and PALOU A (2002), Olive oil feeding up-regulates uncoupling protein genes in rat brown adipose tissue and skeletal muscle, *Am J Clin Nutr* **75**, 213–220.
102 ASTRUP A (2005), The role of dietary fat in obesity, *Semin Vasc Med* **5**, 40–47.
103 PIETERSE Z, JERLING J C, OOSTHUIZEN W, KRUGER H S, HANEKOM S M, SMUTS C M and SCHUTTE A E (2005), Substitution of high monounsaturated fatty acid avocado for mixed dietary fats during an energy-restricted diet: effects on weight loss, serum lipids, fibrinogen, and vascular function, *Nutrition* **21**, 67–75.
104 CLIFTON P M, NOAKES M and KEOGH J B (2004), Very low-fat (12%) and high monounsaturated fat (35%) diets do not differentially affect abdominal fat loss in overweight, nondiabetic women, *J Nutr* **134**, 1741–1745.

105 PELKMAN C L, FISHELL V K, MADDOX D H, PEARSON T A, MAUGER D T and KRIS-ETHERTON P M (2004), Effects of moderate-fat (from monounsaturated fat) and low-fat weight-loss diets on the serum lipid profile in overweight and obese men and women, *Am J Clin Nutr* **79**, 204–212.
106 GUMBINER B, LOW C C and REAVEN P D (1998), Effects of a monounsaturated fatty acid-enriched hypocaloric diet on cardiovascular risk factors in obese patients with type 2 diabetes, *Diabetes Care* **21**, 9–15.
107 PAPAMANDJARIS A A, MACDOUGALL D E and JONES P J (1998), Medium chain fatty acid metabolism and energy expenditure: obesity treatment implications, *Life Sci* **62**, 1203–1215.
108 ST-ONGE M P (2005), Dietary fats, teas, dairy, and nuts: potential functional foods for weight control? *Am J Clin Nutr* **81**, 7–15.
109 ST-ONGE M P and JONES P J (2002), Physiological effects of medium-chain triglycerides: potential agents in the prevention of obesity, *J Nutr* **132**, 329–332.
110 ST-ONGE M P, ROSS R, PARSONS W D and JONES P J (2003), Medium-chain triglycerides increase energy expenditure and decrease adiposity in overweight men, *Obes Res* **11**, 395–402.
111 PORTILLO M P, SERRA F, SIMON E, DEL BARRIO A S and PALOU A (1998), Energy restriction with high-fat diet enriched with coconut oil gives higher UCP1 and lower white fat in rats, *Int J Obes Relat Metab Disord* **22**, 974–979.
112 YOST T J and ECKEL R H (1989), Hypocaloric feeding in obese women: metabolic effects of medium-chain triglyceride substitution, *Am J Clin Nutr* **49**, 326–330.
113 KROTKIEWSKI M (2001), Value of VLCD supplementation with medium chain triglycerides, *Int J Obes Relat Metab Disord* **25**, 1393–1400.
114 THOLSTRUP T, EHNHOLM C, JAUHIAINEN M, PETERSEN M, HOY C E, LUND P and SANDSTROM B (2004), Effects of medium-chain fatty acids and oleic acid on blood lipids, lipoproteins, glucose, insulin, and lipid transfer protein activities, *Am J Clin Nutr* **79**, 564–569.
115 GEELEN M J (1994), Medium-chain fatty acids as short-term regulators of hepatic lipogenesis, *Biochem J* **302**, Pt 1 141–146.
116 BACH A C, INGENBLEEK Y and FREY A (1996), The usefulness of dietary medium-chain triglycerides in body weight control: fact or fancy? *J Lipid Res* **37**, 708–726.
117 MURATA M, IDE T and HARA K (1997), Reciprocal responses to dietary diacylglycerol of hepatic enzymes of fatty acid synthesis and oxidation in the rat, *Br J Nutr* **77**, 107–121.
118 MURASE T, MIZUNO T, OMACHI T, ONIZAWA K, KOMINE Y, KONDO H, HASE T and TOKIMITSU I (2001), Dietary diacylglycerol suppresses high fat and high sucrose diet-induced body fat accumulation in C57BL/6J mice, *J Lipid Res* **42**, 372–378.
119 TADA N (2004), Physiological actions of diacylglycerol outcome, *Curr Opin Clin Nutr Metab Care* **7**, 145–149.
120 TAGUCHI H, WATANABE H, ONIZAWA K, NAGAO T, GOTOH N, YASUKAWA T, TSUSHIMA R, SHIMASAKI H and ITAKURA H (2000), Double-blind controlled study on the effects of dietary diacylglycerol on postprandial serum and chylomicron triacylglycerol responses in healthy humans, *J Am Coll Nutr* **19**, 789–796.
121 KAMPHUIS M M, MELA D J and WESTERTERP-PLANTENGA M S (2003), Diacylglycerols affect substrate oxidation and appetite in humans, *Am J Clin Nutr* **77**, 1133–1139.

122 NAGAO T, WATANABE H, GOTO N, ONIZAWA K, TAGUCHI H, MATSUO N, YASUKAWA T, TSUSHIMA R, SHIMASAKI H and ITAKURA H (2000), Dietary diacylglycerol suppresses accumulation of body fat compared to triacylglycerol in men in a double-blind controlled trial, *J Nutr* **130**, 792–797.

123 MAKI K C, DAVIDSON M H, TSUSHIMA R, MATSUO N, TOKIMITSU I, D UMPOROWICZ M, DICKLIN M R, FOSTER G S, INGRAM K A, ANDERSON B D, FROST S D and BELL M (2002), Consumption of diacylglycerol oil as part of a reduced-energy diet enhances loss of body weight and fat in comparison with consumption of a triacylglycerol control oil, *Am J Clin Nutr* **76**, 1230–1236.

124 TOMONOBU K, HASE T and TOKIMITSU I (2006), Dietary diacylglycerol in a typical meal suppresses postprandial increases in serum lipid levels compared with dietary triacylglycerol, *Nutrition* **22**, 128–135.

125 SAITO S, TOMONOBU K, HASE T and TOKIMITSU I (2006), Effects of diacylglycerol on postprandial energy expenditure and respiratory quotient in healthy subjects, *Nutrition* **22**, 30–35.

126 YAMAMOTO K, TAKESHITA M, TOKIMITSU I, WATANABE H, MIZUNO T, ASAKAWA H, TOKUNAGA K, TATSUMI T, OKAZAKI M and YAGI N (2006), Diacylglycerol oil ingestion in type 2 diabetic patients with hypertriglyceridemia, *Nutrition* **22**, 23–29.

127 TAKASE H, SHOJI K, HASE T and TOKIMITSU I (2005), Effect of diacylglycerol on postprandial lipid metabolism in non-diabetic subjects with and without insulin resistance, *Atherosclerosis* **180**, 197–204.

128 FLICKINGER B D and MATSUO N (2003), Nutritional characteristics of DAG oil, *Lipids* **38**, 129–132.

129 WESTERTERP-PLANTENGA M S and LEJEUNE M P (2005), Protein intake and body-weight regulation, *Appetite* **45**, 187–190.

130 NICKOLS-RICHARDSON S M, COLEMAN M D, VOLPE J J and HOSIG K W (2005), Perceived hunger is lower and weight loss is greater in overweight premenopausal women consuming a low-carbohydrate/high-protein vs high-carbohydrate/low-fat diet, *J Am Diet Assoc* **105**, 1433–1437.

131 WESTERTERP-PLANTENGA M S, LEJEUNE M P, NIJS I, VAN OOIJEN M and KOVACS E M (2004), High protein intake sustains weight maintenance after body weight loss in humans, *Int J Obes Relat Metab Disord* **28**, 57–64.

132 LAYMAN D K, BOILEAU R A, ERICKSON D J, PAINTER J E, SHIUE H, SATHER C and CHRISTOU D D (2003), A reduced ratio of dietary carbohydrate to protein improves body composition and blood lipid profiles during weight loss in adult women, *J Nutr* **133**, 411–417.

133 LAYMAN D K and BAUM J I (2004), Dietary protein impact on glycemic control during weight loss, *J Nutr* **134**, 968S–973S.

134 EISENSTEIN J, ROBERTS S B, DALLAL G and SALTZMAN E (2002), High-protein weight-loss diets: are they safe and do they work? A review of the experimental and epidemiologic data, *Nutr Rev* **60**, 189–200.

135 HU F B, STAMPFER M J, MANSON J E, RIMM E, COLDITZ G A, SPEIZER F E, HENNEKENS C H and WILLETT W C (1999), Dietary protein and risk of ischemic heart disease in women, *Am J Clin Nutr* **70**, 221–227.

136 ISO H, STAMPFER M J, MANSON J E, REXRODE K, HU F, HENNEKENS C H, COLDITZ G A, SPEIZER F E and WILLETT W C, Prospective study of fat and protein intake and risk of intraparenchymal hemorrhage in women, *Circulation* **103**, 856–863.

137 NOAKES M, KEOGH J B, FOSTER P R and CLIFTON P M (2005), Effect of an energy-restricted, high-protein, low-fat diet relative to a conventional high-carbohydrate, low-fat diet on weight loss, body composition, nutritional status, and

markers of cardiovascular health in obese women, *Am J Clin Nutr* **81**, 1298–1306.
138 ZEMEL M B (2004), Role of calcium and dairy products in energy partitioning and weight management, *Am J Clin Nutr* **79**, 907S–912S.
139 BARR S I (2003), Increased dairy product or calcium intake: is body weight or composition affected in humans? *J Nutr* **133**, 245S–248S.
140 HEANEY R P, DAVIES K M and BARGER-LUX M J (2002), Calcium and weight: clinical studies, *J Am Coll Nutr* **21**, 152S–155S.
141 ZEMEL M B, THOMPSON W, MILSTEAD A, MORRIS K and CAMPBELL P (2004), Calcium and dairy acceleration of weight and fat loss during energy restriction in obese adults, *Obes Res* **12**, 582–590.
142 ZEMEL M B, RICHARDS J, MILSTEAD A and CAMPBELL P (2005), Effects of calcium and dairy on body composition and weight loss in African-American adults, *Obes Res* **13**, 1218–1225.
143 ZEMEL M B, RICHARDS J, MATHIS S, MILSTEAD A, GEBHARDT L and SILVA E (2005), Dairy augmentation of total and central fat loss in obese subjects, *Int J Obes (Lond)* **29**, 391–397.
144 BOWEN J, NOAKES M and CLIFTON P M (2004), A high dairy protein, high-calcium diet minimizes bone turnover in overweight adults during weight loss, *J Nutr* **134**, 568–573.
145 SHAPSES S A, HESHKA S and HEYMSFIELD S B (2004), Effect of calcium supplementation on weight and fat loss in women, *J Clin Endocrinol Metab* **89**, 632–637.
146 THOMPSON W G, ROSTAD HOLDMAN N, JANZOW D J, SLEZAK J M, MORRIS K L and ZEMEL M B (2005), Effect of energy-reduced diets high in dairy products and fiber on weight loss in obese adults, *Obes Res* **13**, 1344–1353.
147 PARIKH S J and YANOVSKI J A (2003), Calcium intake and adiposity, *Am J Clin Nutr* **77**, 281–287.
148 PUIGSERVER P, VÁZQUEZ F, BONET M L, PICÓ C and PALOU A (1996), In vitro and in vivo induction of brown adipocyte uncoupling protein (thermogenin) by retinoic acid, *Biochem J* **317**, 827–833.
149 BONET M L, OLIVER J, PICÓ C, FELIPE F, RIBOT J, CINTI S and PALOU A (2000), Opposite effects of vitamin A deficient diet-feeding and retinoic acid treatment on brown adipose tissue UCP1, UCP2 and leptin expression, *J. Endocrinol* **166**, 511–517.
150 RIBOT J, FELIPE F, BONET M L and PALOU A (2001), Changes of adiposity in response to vitamin A status correlate with changes of PPAR gamma 2 expression, *Obes Res* **9**, 500–509.
151 MERCADER J, RIBOT J, MURANO I, FELIPE F, CINTI S, BONET M L and PALOU A (2006), Remodeling of white adipose tissue after retinoic acid administration in mice, *Endocrinology* **147**, 5325–5332.
152 SERRA F, BONET M L, PUIGSERVER P, OLIVER J and PALOU A (1999), Stimulation of uncoupling protein 1 expression in brown adipocytes by naturally occurring carotenoids, *Int J Obes Relat Metab Disord* **23**, 650–655.
153 FELIPE F, BONET M L, RIBOT J and PALOU A (2003), Up-regulation of muscle uncoupling protein 3 gene expression in mice following high fat diet, dietary vitamin A supplementation and acute retinoic acid-treatment, *Int J Obes Relat Metab Disord* **27**, 60–69.
154 KUMAR M V, SUNVOLD G D and SCARPACE P J (1999), Dietary vitamin A supplementation in rats: suppression of leptin and induction of UCP1 mRNA, *J Lipid Res* **40**, 824–829.
155 KAWADA T, KAMEI Y and SUGIMOTO E (1996), The possibility of active form of vitamin A and D as supressors on adipocyte development via ligand-

dependent transcriptional regulators, *Int J Obes Relat Metab Disord* **20**, S52–S57.
156 FELIPE F, BONET M L, RIBOT J and PALOU A (2004), Modulation of resistin expression by retinoic acid and vitamin A status, *Diabetes* **53**, 882–889.
157 KUMAR M V and SCARPACE P J (1998), Differential effects of retinoic acid on uncoupling protein-1 and leptin gene expression, *J Endocrinol* **157**, 237–243.
158 FELIPE F, MERCADER J, RIBOT J, PALOU A and BONET M L (2005), Effects of retinoic acid administration and dietary vitamin A supplementation on leptin expression in mice: lack of correlation with changes of adipose tissue mass and food intake, *Biochim Biophys Acta* **1740**, 258–265.
159 WOLFE W S and SANJUR D (1988), Contemporary diet and body weight of Navajo women receiving food assistance: an ethnographic and nutritional investigation, *J Am Diet Assoc* **88**, 822–827.
160 VAUGHAN L A, BENYSHEK D C and MARTIN J F (1997), Food acquisition habits, nutrient intakes, and anthropometric data of Havasupai adults, *J Am Diet Assoc* **97**, 1275–1282.
161 STEPHENS D, JACKSON P L and GUTIERREZ Y (1996), Subclinical vitamin A deficiency: a potentially unrecognized problem in the United States, *Pediatr Nurs* **22**, 377–389, 456.
162 ANDRAWS R, CHAWLA P and BROWN D L (2005), Cardiovascular effects of ephedra alkaloids: a comprehensive review, *Prog Cardiovasc Dis* **47**, 217–225.
163 SHEKELLE P G, HARDY M L, MORTON S C, MAGLIONE M, MOJICA W A, SUTTORP M J, RHODES S L, JUNGVIG L and GAGNE J (2003), Efficacy and safety of ephedra and ephedrine for weight loss and athletic performance: a meta-analysis, *JAMA* **289**, 1537–1545.
164 DULLOO A G (2002), Herbal simulation of ephedrine and caffeine in treatment of obesity, *Int J Obes Relat Metab Disord* **26**, 590–592.
165 GREENWAY F L (2001), The safety and efficacy of pharmaceutical and herbal caffeine and ephedrine use as a weight loss agent, *Obes Rev* **2**, 199–211.
166 HALLER C A and BENOWITZ N L (2000), Adverse cardiovascular and central nervous system events associated with dietary supplements containing ephedra alkaloids, *N Engl J Med* **343**, 1833–1838.
167 GOUGEON R, HARRIGAN K, TREMBLAY J F, HEDREI P, LAMARCHE M and MORAIS J A (2005), Increase in the thermic effect of food in women by adrenergic amines extracted from citrus aurantium, *Obes Res* **13**, 1187–1194.
168 CARPENE C, GALITZKY J, FONTANA E, ATGIE C, LAFONTAN M and BERLAN M (1999), Selective activation of beta3-adrenoceptors by octopamine: comparative studies in mammalian fat cells, *Naunyn Schmiedebergs Arch Pharmacol* **359**, 310–321.
169 FUGH-BERMAN A and MYERS A (2004), Citrus aurantium, an ingredient of dietary supplements marketed for weight loss: current status of clinical and basic research, *Exp Biol Med (Maywood)* **229**, 698–704.
170 BENT S, PADULA A and NEUHAUS J (2004), Safety and efficacy of citrus aurantium for weight loss, *Am J Cardiol* **94**, 1359–1361.
171 DULLOO A G, DURET C, ROHRER D, GIRARDIER L, MENSI N, FATHI M, CHANTRE P and VANDERMANDER J (1999), Efficacy of a green tea extract rich in catechin polyphenols and caffeine in increasing 24-h energy expenditure and fat oxidation in humans, *Am J Clin Nutr* **70**, 1040–1045.
172 CHANTRE P and LAIRON D (2002), Recent findings of green tea extract AR25 (Exolise) and its activity for the treatment of obesity, *Phytomedicine* **9**, 3–8.

173 RUMPLER W, SEALE J, CLEVIDENCE B, JUDD J, WILEY E, YAMAMOTO S, KOMATSU T, SAWAKI T, ISHIKURA Y and HOSODA K (2001), Oolong tea increases metabolic rate and fat oxidation in men, *J Nutr* **131**, 2848–2852.
174 KOMATSU T, NAKAMORI M, KOMATSU K, HOSODA K, OKAMURA M, TOYAMA K, ISHIKURA Y, SAKAI T, KUNII D and YAMAMOTO S (2003), Oolong tea increases energy metabolism in Japanese females, *J Med Invest* **50**, 170–175.
175 OHNUKI K, NIWA S, MAEDA S, INOUE N, YAZAWA S and FUSHIKI T (2001), CH-19 sweet, a non-pungent cultivar of red pepper, increased body temperature and oxygen consumption in humans, *Biosci Biotechnol Biochem* **65**, 2033–2036.
176 OHNUKI K, HARAMIZU S, OKI K, WATANABE T, YAZAWA S and FUSHIKI T (2001), Administration of capsiate, a non-pungent capsaicin analog, promotes energy metabolism and suppresses body fat accumulation in mice, *Biosci Biotechnol Biochem* **65**, 2735–2740.
177 HENRY C J and EMERY B (1986), Effect of spiced food on metabolic rate, *Hum Nutr Clin Nutr* **40**, 165–168.
178 YOSHIOKA M, ST-PIERRE S, SUZUKI M and TREMBLAY A (1998), Effects of red pepper added to high-fat and high-carbohydrate meals on energy metabolism and substrate utilization in Japanese women, *Br J Nutr* **80**, 503–510.
179 MATSUMOTO T, MIYAWAKI C, UE H, YUASA T, MIYATSUJI A and MORITANI T (2000), Effects of capsaicin-containing yellow curry sauce on sympathetic nervous system activity and diet-induced thermogenesis in lean and obese young women, *J Nutr Sci Vitaminol (Tokyo)* **46**, 309–315.
180 TSUDA T, HORIO F, UCHIDA K, AOKI H and OSAWA T (2003), Dietary cyanidin 3-O-beta-D-glucoside-rich purple corn color prevents obesity and ameliorates hyperglycemia in mice, *J Nutr* **133**, 2125–2130.
181 JENA B S, JAYAPRAKASHA G K, SINGH R P and SAKARIAH K K (2002), Chemistry and biochemistry of (–)-hydroxycitric acid from *Garcinia*, *J Agric Food Chem* **50**, 10–22.
182 PITTLER M H and ERNST E (2004), Dietary supplements for body-weight reduction: a systematic review, *Am J Clin Nutr* **79**, 529–536.
183 SAPER R B, EISENBERG D M and PHILLIPS R S (2004), Common dietary supplements for weight loss, *Am Fam Physician* **70**, 1731–1738.
184 PREUSS H G, GARIS R I, BRAMBLE J D, BAGCHI D, BAGCHI M, RAO C V and SATYANARAYANA S (2005), Efficacy of a novel calcium/potassium salt of (–)-hydroxycitric acid in weight control, *Int J Clin Pharmacol Res* **25**, 133–144.
185 GARCIA-PELAEZ B, FERRER-LORENTE R, GOMEZ-OLLES S, FERNANDEZ-LOPEZ J A, REMESAR X and ALEMANY M (2004), Technical note: Measurement of total estrone content in foods. Application to dairy products, *J Dairy Sci* **87**, 2331–2336.
186 SANCHIS D, BALADA F, DEL MAR GRASA M, VIRGILI J, PEINADO J, MONSERRAT C, FERNANDEZ-LOPEZ J A, REMESAR X and ALEMANY M (1996), Oleoyl-estrone induces the loss of body fat in rats, *Int J Obes Relat Metab Disord* **20**, 588–594.
187 GRASA M M, VILA R, ESTEVE M, CABOT C, FERNANDEZ-LOPEZ J A, REMESAR X and ALEMANY M (2000), Oleoyl-estrone lowers the body weight of both ob/ob and db/db mice, *Horm Metab Res* **32**, 246–250.
188 REMESAR X, GUIJARRO P, TORREGROSA C, GRASA M M, LOPEZ J, FERNANDEZ-LOPEZ J A and ALEMANY M (2000), Oral oleoyl-estrone induces the rapid loss of body fat in Zucker lean rats fed a hyperlipidic diet, *Int J Obes Relat Metab Disord* **24**, 1405–1412.

189 SANCHIS D, BALADA F, PICO C, GRASA M M, VIRGILI J, FARRERONS C, PALOU A, FERNANDEZ-LOPEZ J A, REMESAR X and ALEMANY M (1997), Rats receiving the slimming agent oleoyl-estrone in liposomes (Merlin-2) decrease food intake but maintain thermogenesis, *Arch Physiol Biochem* **105**, 663–672.

190 ALEMANY M, FERNANDEZ-LOPEZ J A, PETROBELLI A, GRANADA M, FOZ M and REMESAR X (2003), [Weight loss in a patient with morbid obesity under treatment with oleoyl-estrone], *Med Clin (Barc)* **121**, 496–499.

191 MCCARTHY A A (2004), When enough is too much: new strategies to treat obesity, *Chem Biol* **11**, 1025–1026.

192 CLARET M, COROMINOLA H, CANALS I, SAURA J, BARCELO-BATLLORI S, GUINOVART J J and GOMIS R (2005), Tungstate decreases weight gain and adiposity in obese rats through increased thermogenesis and lipid oxidation, *Endocrinology* **146**, 4362–4369.

193 ANDERSEN T and FOGH J (2001), Weight loss and delayed gastric emptying following a South American herbal preparation in overweight patients, *J Hum Nutr Diet* **14**, 243–250.

194 NAKAGAWA K, KISHIDA H, ARAI N, NISHIYAMA T and MAE T (2004), Licorice flavonoids suppress abdominal fat accumulation and increase in blood glucose level in obese diabetic KK-A(y) mice, *Biol Pharm Bull* **27**, 1775–1778.

195 ARMANINI D, DE PALO C B, MATTARELLO M J, SPINELLA P, ZACCARIA M, ERMOLAO A, PALERMO M, FIORE C, SARTORATO P, FRANCINI-PESENTI F and KARBOWIAK I (2003), Effect of licorice on the reduction of body fat mass in healthy subjects, *J Endocrinol Invest* **26**, 646–650.

196 GRAHAM T E (2001), Caffeine and exercise: metabolism, endurance and performance, *Sports Med* **31**, 785–807.

197 MAGKOS F and KAVOURAS S A (2004), Caffeine and ephedrine: physiological, metabolic and performance-enhancing effects, *Sports Med* **34**, 871–889.

198 KEISLER B D and HOSEY R G (2005), Ergogenic aids: an update on ephedra, *Curr Sports Med Rep* **4**, 231–235.

199 NISSEN S L and SHARP R L (2003), Effect of dietary supplements on lean mass and strength gains with resistance exercise: a meta-analysis, *J Appl Physiol* **94**, 651–659.

200 PARIZA M W (2004), Perspective on the safety and effectiveness of conjugated linoleic acid, *Am J Clin Nutr* **79**, 1132S–1136S.

201 LARSEN T M, TOUBRO S and ASTRUP A (2003), Efficacy and safety of dietary supplements containing CLA for the treatment of obesity: evidence from animal and human studies, *J Lipid Res* **44**, 2234–2241.

202 RODRIGUEZ E, RIBOT J and PALOU A (2002), Trans-10, cis-12, but not cis-9, trans-11 CLA isomer, inhibits brown adipocyte thermogenic capacity, *Am J Physiol Regul Integr Comp Physiol* **282**, R1789–1797.

203 PARIZA M W, PARK Y and COOK M E (2001), The biologically active isomers of conjugated linoleic acid, *Prog Lipid Res* **40**, 283–298.

204 RAINER L and HEISS C J (2004), Conjugated linoleic acid: health implications and effects on body composition, *J Am Diet Assoc* **104**, 963–968, quiz 1032.

205 WANG Y and JONES P J (2004), Dietary conjugated linoleic acid and body composition, *Am J Clin Nutr* **79**, 1153S–1158S.

206 WANG Y W and JONES P J (2004), Conjugated linoleic acid and obesity control: efficacy and mechanisms, *Int J Obes Relat Metab Disord* **28**, 941–955.

207 TERPSTRA A H (2004), Effect of conjugated linoleic acid on body composition and plasma lipids in humans: an overview of the literature, *Am J Clin Nutr* **79**, 352–361.

208 GAULLIER J M, HALSE J, HOYE K, KRISTIANSEN K, FAGERTUN H, VIK H and GUDMUNDSEN O (2004), Conjugated linoleic acid supplementation for 1 y reduces body fat mass in healthy overweight humans, *Am J Clin Nutr* **79**, 1118–1125.

209 GAULLIER J M, HALSE J, HOYE K, KRISTIANSEN K, FAGERTUN H, VIK H and GUDMUNDSEN O (2005), Supplementation with conjugated linoleic acid for 24 months is well tolerated by and reduces body fat mass in healthy, overweight humans, *J Nutr* **135**, 778–784.

210 KAMPHUIS M M, LEJEUNE M P, SARIS W H and WESTERTERP-PLANTENGA M S (2003), The effect of conjugated linoleic acid supplementation after weight loss on body weight regain, body composition, and resting metabolic rate in overweight subjects, *Int J Obes Relat Metab Disord* **27**, 840–847.

211 RISERUS U, SMEDMAN A, BASU S and VESSBY B (2004), Metabolic effects of conjugated linoleic acid in humans: the Swedish experience, *Am J Clin Nutr* **79**, 1146S–1148S.

212 WHIGHAM L D, O'SHEA M, MOHEDE I C, WALASKI H P and ATKINSON R L (2004), Safety profile of conjugated linoleic acid in a 12-month trial in obese humans, *Food Chem Toxicol* **42**, 1701–1709.

213 VINCENT J B (2003), The potential value and toxicity of chromium picolinate as a nutritional supplement, weight loss agent and muscle development agent, *Sports Med* **33**, 213–230.

214 PITTLER M H, STEVINSON C and ERNST E (2003), Chromium picolinate for reducing body weight: meta-analysis of randomized trials, *Int J Obes Relat Metab Disord* **27**, 522–529.

215 KLEEFSTRA N, HOUWELING S T, JANSMAN F G, GROENIER K H, GANS R O, MEYBOOM-DE JONG B, BAKKER S J and BILO H J (2006), Chromium treatment has no effect in patients with poorly controlled, insulin-treated type 2 diabetes in an obese Western population: a randomized, double-blind, placebo-controlled trial, *Diabetes Care* **29**, 521–525.

216 NISSEN S, SHARP R, RAY M, RATHMACHER J A, RICE D, FULLER JR J C, CONNELLY A S and ABUMRAD N (1996), Effect of leucine metabolite beta-hydroxy-beta-methylbutyrate on muscle metabolism during resistance-exercise training, *J Appl Physiol* **81**, 2095–2104.

217 KNITTER A E, PANTON L, RATHMACHER J A, PETERSEN A and SHARP R (2000), Effects of beta-hydroxy-beta-methylbutyrate on muscle damage after a prolonged run, *J Appl Physiol* **89**, 1340–1344.

218 TOKISH J M, KOCHER M S and HAWKINS R J (2004), Ergogenic aids: a review of basic science, performance, side effects, and status in sports, *Am J Sports Med* **32** 1543–1553.

219 KARLIC H and LOHNINGER A (2004), Supplementation of L-carnitine in athletes: does it make sense? *Nutrition* **20**, 709–715.

220 BARNETT C, COSTILL D L, VUKOVICH M D, COLE K J, GOODPASTER B H, TRAPPE S W and FINK W J (1994), Effect of L-carnitine supplementation on muscle and blood carnitine content and lactate accumulation during high-intensity sprint cycling, *Int J Sport Nutr* **4**, 280–288.

221 VILLANI R G, GANNON J, SELF M and RICH P A (2000), l-Carnitine supplementation combined with aerobic training does not promote weight loss in moderately obese women, *Int J Sport Nutr Exerc Metab* **10**, 199–207.

222 HAHN A, STROHLE A and WOLTERS M (2003), [Dietary supplements and functional

food for weight reduction – expectations and reality], *MMW Fortschr Med* **145**, 40–45.
223 BRAY G A (2003), Low-carbohydrate diets and realities of weight loss, *JAMA* **289**, 1853–1855.
224 BELL S J and GOODRICK G K (2002), A functional food product for the management of weight, *Crit Rev Food Sci Nutr* **42**, 163–178.

# 5

# Food ingredients implicated in obesity: sugars and sweeteners

**G. H. Anderson, T. Akhavan and R. Mendelson, University of Toronto, Canada**

## 5.1 Introduction

The prevalence of obesity has increased dramatically in the past 35 years and has been associated with increased metabolic diseases including type 2 diabetes, coronary heart disease, hypertension, osteoarthritis and respiratory complications, all of which impose enormous costs on the health care system (Kopelman, 2000).

The etiology of obesity is multifactoral and the underlying reasons for the rapid increase in prevalence have remained unclear. Increased energy intake, decreased physical activity, large numbers of fast-food outlets, large portion sizes and/or increased availability of sweeteners and sugars (especially high-fructose corn syrup, HFCS) have each been proposed as factors contributing to this rise. Among all of the possible contributing factors, sugars and sweeteners have received considerable attention for several reasons. The increased prevalence of obesity has occurred concurrently with the increased availability of caloric (Elliott *et al.*, 2002) and alternative sweeteners (Bright, 1999), the increased replacement of sugar (sucrose) with HFCS (Bray *et al.*, 2004) in foods and beverages and increased consumption of caloric and non-caloric sweetened beverages (Bray *et al.*, 2004; Popkin *et al.*, 2006).

Although many attempts have been made to identify the role of sugars and alternative sweeteners in obesity, direct evidence for cause and effect remains elusive. Food disappearance data and food consumption surveys as well as prospective and intervention studies continuously report a unique role for sugars, especially in beverages, in excessive energy intake and obesity. However many methodological issues arise from these studies (Pereira, 2006). Furthermore, experimental studies and knowledge of the effects of sugars on food intake regulatory mechanisms fail to support a biological mechanism that explains these associations. High-intensity sweeteners have been available for 50 years as substitutes for sugars, but in spite of their increased usage obesity continues to increase. Therefore, it appears that high-intensity sweeteners and sugars in diets are markers of a lifestyle and dietary pattern that contributes to excess energy intake.

The objective of this chapter is to examine the role of caloric and alternative sweeteners in either promoting or preventing overweight and obesity.

## 5.2 Definition of sugars and alternative sweeteners

Carbohydrates are the main source of energy, making up 40–80% of the individual's total energy intake (Anderson *et al.*, 1998). According to the degree of polymerization, carbohydrates are divided into three principal groups, namely sugars, oligosaccharides and polysaccharides (Anderson *et al.*, 1998).

### 5.2.1 Sugars (caloric sweeteners)

Sugars are classified into three groups: monosaccharides, disaccharides, and trisaccharides. The simplest molecules of sugars are the monosaccharides, which include galactose, fructose and glucose, the only monosaccharides absorbed by humans. Disaccharides (including lactose, maltose and sucrose) and trisaccharides (including raffinose, found in cottonseed and sugar beets), are derived from the union of monosaccharides. All of these sugars provide approximately 4 cal/g.

Household 'sugar', or 'table sugar', is extracted mainly from sugar cane or beet. This sugar is a disaccharide composed of 50% glucose and 50% fructose linked by $\alpha$-1,4 glycosidic bonds (Pancoast and Junk, 1980). Glucose, also known as dextrose or corn syrup, is produced from corn starch. Fructose is the sweetest of the simple sugars and is found as the monosaccharide, along with glucose and sucrose, in fruits and vegetables (Park and Yetley, 1993). It is generally present in honey and fruits and vegetables in similar amounts to glucose with the exception that it is found in much higher quantities than glucose in apples and pears. Sucrose is found in smaller quantities (NDL, 2006).

HFCS is a nutritive liquid sweetener containing the monosaccharides fructose and glucose, in varying proportions. The most common forms of HFCS are HFCS 55% and 42%. HFCS 55% is composed of 55% fructose and 45% glucose and is primarily used in sweetened soft drinks. In contrast, HFCS 42% is composed of 42% fructose and 58% glucose and is primarily used in solid foods such as jams, jellies, baked goods, canned goods and dairy products (Hanover and White, 1993).

### 5.2.2 Alternative sweeteners (non-nutritive sweeteners)

The hedonic value of sugars due to their sweetness can be provided in foods and beverages by artificial sweeteners (non-caloric sweeteners) or polyols (low-caloric sweeteners), alternatively called sugar substitutes, sugar replacers or alternative sweeteners.

High-intensity sweeteners provide sweeteness with negligible calories, although the sensation of their sweetness is often different from that of sugar. Saccharine, the oldest artificial sweetener is 300 times as sweet as sucrose. Currently, five of the high-intensity sweeteners have been approved by the US Food and Drug Administration (FDA) and include acesulfame-K, aspartame, sucralose, saccharin and neotame which are 200, 180, 600, 300 and 8000 times sweetener than sugar, respectively (FDA, 2006). Two other artificial sweeteners, alitame and cyclamate (2000 and 30 times sweeter than sugar, respectively), have been used in foods in Europe but not in the United States (CCC, 2006).

Another group of sweeteners provides sweetness with reduced calories. These are the sugar alcohols, identified as sugar replacers or polyols. Sugar alcohols – including mannitol, sorbitol, xylitol, erythritol and lactitol, which, respectively, provide 1.6, 2.6, 2.4, 0.2 and 2.1 kcal/g – are hydrogenated forms of carbohydrate where the ketone group has been reduced at the primary and secondary hydroxyl group (Zumbe *et al.*, 2001; ADA, 2004). Although they have the same bulk and texture as sucrose, they are less sweet and provide fewer calories than sugars. Additionally, they can be used to mask the detectable aftertaste of some artificial sweeteners; therefore, they are often used with high-intensity sweeteners (ADA, 2004).

## 5.3 Sugars and alternative sweeteners: role in obesity

### 5.3.1 Sugars

*Availability of sugars*

The increased prevalence of obesity over the past 35 years has occurred concurrently with an increased availability of added sugars in the food supply (Elliott *et al.*, 2002). Food disappearance data, as an indicator of trends in food consumption, have shown a 30% increase in the availability of sugars in the United States from 1971 to 1997 (Elliott *et al.*, 2002). Thus, it has been suggested that increased consumption of sugars (Ludwig *et al.*, 2001) and the increased availability of HFCS (Bray *et al.*, 2004) have contributed to excess energy intake and obesity.

However, the roles of both increased availability of sugars in the national food supply and of HFCS as an independent contributor to the current epidemic of obesity are uncertain for several reasons. First, although the availability of sugars has increased over the last three decades, it has not increased disproportionately to other components of the food supply. Increases in per capita availability have been seen for most food commodities (Harnack *et al.*, 2000). For instance, US food supply data indicate an increased per capita availability of poultry (84%), fats and oils (47%), dairy products – specifically milks (423%) and yogurts (111%), fruit (28%), vegetables (72%) and even energy (15%) (Harnack *et al.*, 2000). More recent data show that sugar availability has decreased from 151.3 lb (68.7 kg)/capita/year in 1999 to 141.0 lb (64 kg) in 2004 (USDA, 2005) while per capita energy content of the food supply continues to increase.

Secondly, disappearance data are reported as the amount of food available per capita for potential consumption rather than the amount of food eaten. It is estimated that approximately 30% is wasted or spoiled rather than eaten (Harnack *et al.*, 2000). Thus, food disappearance data overestimate actual consumption and do not necessarily predict the food consumed by individuals. Furthermore, an association observed between variables on a group level does not necessarily represent an association that exists at an individual level.

*Dietary associations*

Associations between the intake of sugars and rising rates of obesity have been derived primarily from epidemiological studies (Colditz *et al.*, 1990; Giammattei *et al.*, 2003). The epidemiological evidence for a relationship between obesity and the consumption of sweeteners is inconsistent. Associations detected by these surveys may be the result of differences in the methods used to collect dietary information rather than a reflection of actual food and nutrient intake. For example, self-reported dietary information used in epidemiological studies presents an opportunity for bias in the results because of under-reporting of foods, especially among overweight individuals.

Several studies have shown a positive association between sugars intake and body weight (Colditz *et al.*, 1990; Giammattei *et al.*, 2003), but others have found an inverse association (Bolton-Smith and Woodward, 1994; Hill and Prentice, 1995). A cross-sectional study in middle-aged men and women ($n = 11\,626$) found a negative association between the prevalence of overweight and obesity and the consumption of sugars (Bolton-Smith and Woodward, 1994). Similarly, a survey of youths aged 10–16 years from 34 countries in 2001–2002 found that the frequency of consumption of sweet foods and beverages was lower in overweight youths than in normal-weight youths; in addition, overweight status was not associated with the intake of soft drinks (Janssen *et al.*, 2005).

*Replacement of sucrose with HFCS*

The United States per capita sugars disappearance data for sugars show that sucrose has declined from 80% of total caloric sweeteners available in 1970 to 40% in 1997; in contrast, HFCS has increased from constituting nearly 0% of total caloric sweeteners in 1970 to a level of 40% in 1997 (Elliott *et al.*, 2002). As a result of these changes in the food supply, total fructose availability (from both sucrose and HFCS) has increased, by 26% (from 64 g/day in 1970 to 81 g/day in 1997). Based on the composition of HFCS, it is unlikely that the ratio of fructose and glucose consumed from sugars has increased over the past two decades (Elliott *et al.*, 2002).

HFCS has replaced sucrose in food and beverage applications over the last 30 years in the United States for two main reasons. First, HFCS is the preferred sweetener of many food and beverage manufacturers because of its characteristics, including higher stability and better crystallization control compared with sucrose. In addition, the sweetness of HFCS is set at 120 compared with 100 for sucrose; therefore, less HFCS is required in some food and beverage applications to achieve the same sweetness as sugar. Furthermore, in many countries HFCS has a price advantage over sucrose (Vuilleumier, 1993). In the United States, the price of HFCS has been well below the price of raw sugar and, since 1985, the use of sucrose in foods, especially in soft drinks, has been reduced by 50% and it has been replaced by HFCS (Putnam and Allshouse, 1999).

Because HFCS has replaced sucrose in many foods and beverages, it has been hypothesized that HFCS has led to the current increased prevalence of obesity (Bray *et al.*, 2004). The rationale for this hypothesis is also based on the metabolism of fructose. Fructose, compared with a similar amount of glucose or sucrose, induces a smaller postprandial blood glucose response, and consequently lower concentrations of the two mediating satiety hormones: insulin and leptin (Crapo *et al.*, 1980; Horowitz *et al.*, 1996; Lee and Wolever, 1998). Moreover, in contrast to glucose, fructose enters muscle and other cells via a GLUT-5 transporter that is not insulin dependent. Without this transporter in pancreatic β cells and in the brain, fructose entry into these tissues is limited. Since fructose is not transported into the brain, it is suggested that fructose can not provide 'satiety' signals to the brain (Bray *et al.*, 2004). In addition, fructose can rapidly enter glycerol pathways to substitute for fatty acid synthesis in the liver. Therefore, when large quantities of fructose are consumed, it can promote lipogenesis (Elliott *et al.*, 2002).

Two reports provide support for the hypothesis that a high-fructose diet results in involuntary increases in energy intake, lipogenesis and storage. A 2-day consumption of a diet containing 30% of daily total energy as fructose from beverages resulted in lowered 24-h plasma insulin and leptin concentrations and increased fasting and postprandial triglycerides when compared with a diet containing 30% of energy from glucose beverages in 12 healthy women (Teff *et al.*, 2004). The high-fructose diet provided 17% of energy as fructose, and the high-glucose diet was nearly devoid of fructose. Because insulin and leptin act as key signals to the central nervous system for the long-term regulation of energy balance, decreased circulating insulin due to excess fructose consumption, may lead to increased caloric intake and ultimately contribute to weight gain and obesity (Teff *et al.*, 2004).

In another longer-term study, 24 healthy adults consumed two isoenergetic diets with additions of either fructose or glucose. In the fructose diet, 17% of total energy was contributed by fructose whereas in the glucose diet only 3% of total energy was contributed by fructose. After 6 weeks, decreased glucose and insulin concentrations – as well as increased fasting, postprandial and daylong plasma triacyglycerol concentrations – were reported after the fructose diet for the 12 men, but not for the women (Bantle *et al.*, 2000).

While the results of both of these studies are consistent with the metabolic action of fructose, the diets were formulated to have concentrations of fructose well above those consumed in a typical human diet. The average dietary energy intake in the United States provides only 9% of calories from fructose (Gibney *et al.*, 1995). Furthermore, blood glucose and insulin responses after 400 kcal meals containing 35 g of sugars were similar when sucrose and HFCS meals were provided, but were significantly higher for fructose meals (Akgun and Ertel, 1985). Thus, studies of the effects of fructose in high amounts and in isolation are unlikely to cast much light on the proposed effects of replacing sucrose with HFCS.

Because there are no published studies investigating the effect of different types of HFCS, not as part of the food, compared with sucrose in the literature, well-designed studies are required to compare the effect of HFCS (55% and 42%) with other sugars. More importantly, although the prevalence of obesity has continually increased, the availability of HFCS in the US food supply has not changed from 1997 (60.4 lb (27.5 kg)/capita/year) to 2004 (59.2 lb (26.9 kg)/capita/year) (USDA, 2005).

*Sugars and short-term food intake*

It has been proposed that energy from sugars and sugars-sweetened drinks, due to the inability of physiological regulatory mechanisms to recognize this form of calories, leads to increased total energy intake (Bray *et al.*, 2004), and the development of overweight and obesity especially in children and young adults (Canty and Chan, 1991; Ludwig *et al.*, 2001; Wylie-Rosett *et al.*, 2004).

A number of factors influence short-term food intake and satiety after preloads of sugars: the form (liquid *versus* solid), energy density, taste and palatability of the preload; the dose of sugars in the preload; the time interval between the preload and the subsequent meal; characteristics of the subjects, e.g. body mass index (BMI), gender, activity level and the subject's knowledge about the treatments. However, if studies designed to test the effect of sugars on satiety and short-term food intake consider the quantity of sugars based on the time interval between the preload and the test meal, they report remarkably precise compensation in the subsequent test meal for the energy consumed in the sweetened preload (Anderson and Woodend, 2003a).

Experimental studies have consistently shown that sugars suppress short-term food intake in children (Birch and Fisher, 1997; Birch *et al.*, 1989) and in adults (Woodend and Anderson, 2001; Anderson *et al.*, 2002; Anderson and Woodend, 2003), and the magnitude of this effect is inversely related to the glycemic response that the sugars elicit (Anderson *et al.*, 2002; Anderson and Woodend, 2003b).

#### Sucrose (sugar)

The effect of a sucrose solution on satiety and subsequent food intake depends on both the dose and the time interval between the preload and the test meal. The majority of the literature indicates that approximately 50g sucrose in solution, the quantity in one and one-half soft drinks, consistently reduces food intake at 60min in young adults (Anderson, 1995; Anderson and Woodend, 2003a). However, in one study, 25g sucrose in 300ml also suppressed food intake (Woodend and Anderson, 2001). For larger amounts of sucrose (135g) in solution, 12 healthy males had a strong feeling of fullness and reduced food intake after 3 h when compared with water (Lavin *et al.*, 2002a).

Timing of the test meal in relation to the dose of sugar in solution is an important factor affecting the food intake outcome. This is illustrated by the failure of 50–60g sucrose to suppress food intake of 9- to 10-year-old children when the meal was given 90min later (Anderson *et al.*, 1989). Similarly, sucrose drinks (Rolls *et al.*, 1990) or desserts (Rolls *et al.*, 1988) (150–200kcal) given either shortly before or with lunch resulted in an increased cumulative energy intake (energy from the preloads plus the test meal energy) compared with the non-caloric sweetened drinks or desserts. The results can be explained because the energy from the sucrose drink or dessert may have been below the threshold needed to suppress food intake or the time interval between treatment and test meal may have been insufficient to enhance satiety.

#### Glucose

In young men, a preload of glucose as either 75g (Anderson *et al.*, 2002) or 50g (Rogers *et al.*, 1988) in drinks or 50g in yogurt (Rogers and Blundell, 1989) reduced food intake 1 h later with almost full compensation for the energy in the preloads. Similarly, 75g glucose in solution significantly suppressed food intake in young men; at a test meal given 120min later, greater compensation (about 60%) was seen compared with the amylose solution (which had a caloric compensation of 15%) and the water control (Walters, 2002).

#### Fructose

Several studies have reported that fructose (when consumed alone in a beverage) decreases short-term food intake and enhances satiety (Spitzer and Rodin, 1987; Rodin, 1990). These studies indicated that consumption of a drink with 50g fructose suppressed energy intake to a greater extent than glucose at test meals given 38min (Rodin, 1990) to 2.25h later (Spitzer and

Rodin, 1987; Rodin *et al.*, 1988; Rodin, 1991). These results are not consistent with known mechanisms of satiety because glucose results in much higher blood concentrations of both insulin and glucose, known satiety signals (Lee and Wolever, 1998). It is more likely that the reduced food intake can be accounted for by absorption characteristics and gastrointestinal effects of fructose.

The rate of absorption of fructose from the small intestine is slower than that of glucose. This is partly due to the differences in the absorption process between the two monosaccharides. Glucose is absorbed by an active sodium glucose co-transporter protein, GLUT-1 and GLUT-2 insulin-dependent transporters, from the intestine. Fructose is absorbed at a slower rate from the lower part of duodenum and jejunum by the brush-border membrane transporter 5, GLUT-5, which is insulin independent (Riby *et al.*, 1993). The capacity for fructose absorption in humans is not clear (Holdsworth and Dawson, 1965). Early studies suggest that fructose absorption is quite efficient, although it is less efficient than glucose or sucrose (Riby *et al.*, 1993). Thus, the prolonged contact time with receptors in the luminal intestinal wall would be expected to result in the stimulation of satiety signals and release of hormones from enteroendocrine cells (Read *et al.*, 1994) (Lavin *et al.*, 1998). However, when fructose is consumed as the sole carbohydrate source, it is incompletely absorbed and, as a result, produces a hyperosmolar environment in the large intestine (Ravich *et al.*, 1983). A high concentration of solute within the gut lumen draws fluid into the intestine which can produce feelings of malaise, stomach ache or diarrhea (Ravich *et al.*, 1983), resulting in decreased food intake.

Addition of glucose or starch to the oral dose of fructose reduces the frequency and severity of gastrointestinal symptoms, because it facilitates a more rapid and complete absorption of fructose (Riby *et al.*, 1993). When taken with a glucose source there is no advantage of fructose over glucose on food intake suppression. Equicaloric cereal preloads containing additions of fructose (30 g) or glucose (33.5 g) equally reduced energy intake in meals taken either 30 or 120 min later (Stewart *et al.*, 1997). Similarly, no differences in food intake were observed between 50 g fructose and 50 g glucose at 2.25 h when preloads were given in a mixed-nutrient meal containing starch (Rodin, 1991).

### High-fructose corn syrup (HFCS)

Currently, there are no published studies in the peer-reviewed literature in which HFCS has been compared with sucrose for its effects on short-term food intake. However in a preliminary report, HFCS (55% fructose) and sucrose solutions resulted in similar blood glucose, insulin responses, subjective appetite and food intake 80 min later (Akhavan, 2006).

Although it is clear that sugars in solutions suppress food intake, compensation for the calories is highly variable dependent on the study designs. Birch *et al.* (1989) reported accurate caloric compensation (on average

120%) in 24 young children (aged 2–5 years) during test meals given at 0, 30 or 60 min after a sucrose drink (90 kcal). Similarly in adults, average compensation at a test meal 1 h later for the energy in three preloads of 25, 50 and 75 g sucrose was 70% compared with a sweet control (sucralose) (Woodend and Anderson, 2001). While compensation is not precise, it is no less variable than that observed after other carbohydrate sources (Anderson *et al.*, 2002). However the source of the variability remains to be explored but may merit further examination to help identify those most at risk of poor caloric compensation for previously ingested food and beverages (Cecil *et al.*, 2005).

*Sweetened beverage consumption, food intake and obesity*

Associations between increased intake of sugars-sweetened beverages, more specifically soft drinks, and the increased prevalence of obesity have been found in several epidemiological prospective and interventional studies in both children and adults. However the focus on regular soft drinks as a major contributor to obesity over the past 20 years seems to be based on an overestimate of their role. Because of the strong association between childhood and adult obesity and the rapidly rising prevalence of obesity among children, there have been several reports in the past decade of studies focused on children but it is difficult to derive from these studies a straightforward conclusion of cause and effect.

Sweetened beverage consumption has increased among children and adolescents in the United States over the last two decades (Harnack *et al.*, 1999; Ludwig *et al.*, 2001). Data from the US Department of Agriculture (USDA) also indicate that 56–85% of children consume at least one soft drink daily at school (Gleason and Suitor, 2001) and 20% of this group consume four or more servings daily (12 oz, 375 ml). On average, each caloric soft drink contains 40 g of sugars (150 kcal per serving) (AAPC, 2004).

An analysis of data collected as part of the 1994 Continuing Survey of Food Intakes by Individuals, for 1810 children aged 2–18 years in the United States found that school children who did not consume soft drinks had a mean energy intake of 1830 kcal/day compared with 2018 kcal/day for school children who consumed an average of 9 oz (280 ml) or more of soft drinks per day (Harnack *et al.*, 1999). This comparison suggests that children who drink one regular carbonated drink a day have an average of 10% more total energy intake than non-consumers but the energy differences were not reflected in body weights (Harnack *et al.*, 1999). A prospective study on 548 school children over a 19-month period reported a positive association between the consumption of caloric-sweetened beverages and obesity (Ludwig *et al.*, 2001). As acknowledged by the authors, this was an observational study and, again, cause and effect could not be determined (Ludwig *et al.*, 2001). In addition, while this was a 19-month study, dietary intake was obtained only at two points, once at baseline and once at the end, and consisted of a self-reported youth food-frequency questionnaire. Similarly, higher consumption of sweetened drinks [>12 oz (375 ml)/day] for a period of 4–8 weeks by 30 children aged 6–13 years resulted in no detectable difference in weight gain compared with children who consumed <12 oz (375 ml)/day despite the higher total energy intake (Mrdjenovic and Levitsky, 2003).

In a cluster randomized controlled trial of 1 year duration on 644 children, aged 7–11 years, the percentage of overweight and obese children decreased in the intervention group who decreased their consumption of carbonated drinks by 0.6 glasses (average glass size 250 ml) compared with the control group who increased their consumption by 0.2 glasses (James *et al.*, 2004). However, the change in BMI did not differ between the two groups. The design of this study had several limitations, some of which were acknowledged by the authors, for example, the use of only 3-day drink diaries at baseline and at the end of the trial, and the low return rate of drink diaries at both time points. In addition, the most important bias ignored by the authors is that the four educational sessions were assigned only to the intervention group in order to inform them about healthier lifestyles and to promote the drinking of water. Therefore, it is not clear whether the decreased percentage of overweight children in the intervention group was mediated by lower consumption of sugars-sweetened beverages or by modifications to other aspects of the diet and activity levels.

In another intervention study, 103 adolescents, between ages of 13 to 18 years, who regularly consumed sugars-sweetened beverages, were divided into intervention and control groups and the beverages were delivered to the participant's home (Ebbeling *et al.*, 2006). Sugar-sweetened beverage consumption was completely displaced by non-caloric beverage consumption in the intervention group and was unchanged in the control group for 25 weeks. Decreased consumption of caloric-sweetened drinks was expected to reduce body weights, but BMI changes in the two groups were not significantly different. Nonetheless, some children with a high BMI at baseline reduced body weight on this intervention, raising the possibility that an intervention to decrease sugar-sweetened beverage consumption and BMI among adolescents who are obese would assist in reducing energy intake. However, this study does not explain the etiology of their obesity.

Associations between sugars-sweetened beverages and body weight have also been observed in adults. A 4-year prospective cohort analysis of 51 603 women suggests an association between soft drinks and weight gain (Schulze *et al.*, 2004). Women who increased their soft drink consumption from one or fewer drinks per week to one or more drinks per day had a higher weight gain compared with those who had stable consumption patterns (Schulze *et al.*, 2004). However, it is important to note that women who maintained a high level of sweetened soft drink intake over time had changes in body weight and BMI that were similar to those who maintained either a low intake or substantially reduced their intake. Additionally, women with higher intakes of soft drinks tended to engage in less physical activity, smoke more and have higher total energy intake. Thus there were major lifestyle differences between the two groups of women, differences that may have been much greater determinants of their obesity than their soft-drink intake.

*Caloric beverages and obesity*

From the above, it is clear that soft drinks have been implicated in the etiology of obesity. Regular soft drink availability has increased by only 20% from 31 gal in 1985 to 36.5 gal/capita/year in 2004, and this availability decreased from 39.7 in 1999 to 36.5 gal/capita/year in 2004 (USDA, 2005). However, the relationship between intake of other caloric beverages and the increased prevalence of obesity is unclear. The question of whether sugar-sweetened beverages are a unique source of excessive energy intake needs to be answered. The data available suggest that there is little difference among beverages and that all can contribute to excess energy intakes.

Longitudinal changes have recently been reported in the consumption of six types of beverages (milk, diet and regular soda, fruit juice, fruit-flavored drinks and coffee/tea) and their relationship with BMI based on 3-day food diaries from 2371 girls aged 9–10 years (Striegel-Moore *et al.*, 2006). Consumption of milk decreased, while consumption of soda increased over the 10 years of the study. However, all types of beverages contributed to increased caloric intake. Although the only statistical association found with increased BMI was with soda consumption, this would be expected because soda was overwhelmingly the most frequently consumed beverage. The association between BMI and total caloric beverage consumption or caloric beverages excluding soft drinks was not reported.

The time of consumption of beverages in relation to a meal may be a greater determinant of their effect on excess energy intake than their composition. Orange juice, regular cola, low-fat milk (1%) and sparkling water (control) resulted in similar food intakes in 2 h 15 min later in 32 adult volunteers. All three caloric beverages were isocaloric (1036 kJ, 248 kcal) and equally reduced hunger ratings and desire to eat and increased fullness ratings, compared with sparkling water (Almiron-Roig and Drewnowski, 2003). The similar effect of beverages on food intake is not surprising because of the time interval between the preload and the lunch meal. When the time interval between the cola preload (1254 kJ, 300 kcal, 300 ml) and the test meal was reduced to 20 min, food intake was suppressed more than when the food intake was measured at 2 h (Almiron-Roig *et al.*, 2004). When equicaloric amounts of orange juice, regular cola and 1%-fat milk beverages (360 ml) were consumed at mealtime, they had no effect on food intake and consequently resulted in higher energy intake at the test meal compared with water or diet coke consumption (Della Valle *et al.*, 2005).

Further investigation is needed to explain why caloric beverages consumed shortly before the test meal suppress food intake, while caloric beverages consumed at the test meal fail to do so. It seems that intake of caloric beverages at the test meal is too late to stimulate satiety and food intake regulatory mechanisms to suppress energy intake, but this may be because the beverages satisfy thirst. Cola, orange juice and milk satisfied thirst equally well (Almiron-Roig and Drewnowski, 2003). Possibly thirst leads to greater energy intake in these circumstances, and overrides the ability of food intake control mechanisms to respond in the short term. The interaction between thirst and hunger in determining excess energy intake requires investigation.

*Sugars: liquid versus solids and food intake*

Energy compensation at a test meal following a liquid preload has been proposed to be less than after a solid preload (Matthes, 1996; DiMeglio and Mattes, 2000; Bray *et al.*, 2004). In contrast a more recent review came to the conclusion that the evidence for solid foods being more likely to suppress food intake compared with liquids is inconsistent and the time interval between the beverage preload and test meal is crucial (Almiron-Roig *et al.*, 2003). However, only one study reported in the two reviews (Matthes 1996; Almiron-Roig *et al.*, 2003) addressed the question of differences in the effects of solid *versus* liquid sugars on satiety and food intake.

Two studies have been interpreted to show that sugars-containing beverages lead to higher cumulative energy intake than when the sugars are consumed in solid form (DiMeglio and Mattes, 2000; Lavin *et al.*, 2002b). In the first study, the effect of added sugars (450 kcal/day) in a liquid (soda) or solid form (jellybeans) was examined over two separate 4-week periods. Soda preload consumption increased energy intake, consequently resulting in higher body weight gain and BMI compared with the solid form. Energy compensation at a subsequent test meal was quite precise when the preload was given as solid food (jellybeans), but not when given as a liquid (soda) (DiMeglio and Mattes, 2000). However, the energy densities of the two treatments were different; the liquid treatment (soda) had lower energy density than the jellybeans. In addition, the pattern of consumption of the preloads was different in this study. Subjects were free to consume the treatments whenever they wanted. Because the jellybeans were predominantly consumed between meals as a snack, while the sodas were mostly consumed with meals, the time of consumption rather than the form of the sugar may have been a greater determinant of the outcomes. Logically, the time of consumption should have been controlled. In addition, one might expect better adherence to consumption of the liquid compared with the solid form.

The second study demonstrated a significant reduction in subsequent food intake (3 h later) after consumption of sucrose-containing pastilles (solid food) compared with an isocaloric (251 kJ, 60 kcal) sucrose-containing drink (liquid) or water in ten male and ten female subjects (Lavin *et al.*, 2002b). Subjects consumed the pastilles over a 10-min period, but they consumed the sweetened drink or water within 2 min. The authors attribute the greater reduction in food intake following the solid food to the impact of chewing. The liquid sucrose could decrease pancreatic exocrine and endocrine responses, and promote a faster rate of gastric emptying and intestinal absorption, actions that are predicted to provide a more transient satiety signal (Lavin *et al.*, 2002b). It is possible, however, that if the sucrose-containing drink was consumed slowly over the same time as the pastilles, food intake 3 h later would have been the same. In addition, it is a puzzle how such a small energy intake of 251 kJ (60 kcal) would lead to food intake suppression 3 h later. This intake is below the threshold doses found to suppress short-term food intake.

A recent well-designed experiment provided isocaloric preloads (300 kcal) of either regular cola or fat-free raspberry cookies on two occasions to 32 adult volunteers and their food intake was measured either 20 min or 2 h after preloads. The satiety and food intake responses were similar between preload forms, although food intake was suppressed more at 20 min than at 2 h (Almiron-Roig *et al.*, 2004).

However, further research is required to confirm whether there is a difference in the effect of liquid *versus* solid sources of energy on subsequent food intake. It is premature to conclude that solid forms of sugars compared with liquid forms have a more favorable effect on the regulation of energy intake and food intake and energy balance.

### 5.3.2 Alternative sweeteners (non-nutritive sweeteners)

Although the role of alternative sweeteners as substitutes for caloric sweeteners in the prevention and management of obesity has been under examination for many years, uncertainty remains about their benefits.

*Availability of alternative sweeteners*

Due to the growing interest in non-caloric and caloric-reduced beverages and foods, consumption of alternative sweeteners has increased worldwide (WHO, 1998). Currently in the United States, 79% of adults consume low-calorie and sugar-free beverages and foods and two-thirds of the US population consume such products more than twice a week (NCS, 2000). This demand for alternative sweeteners is derived from an assumption that replacement of sugars with alternative sweeteners prevents weight gain.

*Alternative sweeteners and obesity*

As with caloric sweeteners and the purported association with obesity, it is difficult to discern a specific role for high-intensity sweeteners in managing weight gain or assisting in weight loss. Interpretation of associative data based on disappearance data or on epidemiological surveys is particularly difficult because body weight reflects the habitual diet whereas most surveys provide only a snapshot of present intake. Thus, it is not clear if the association of greater usage of high-intensity sweeteners by individuals of high body fatness is because they have changed their dietary habits and are trying to reduce energy intake or because they have accumulated excess energy from other sources even though they habitually consume high-intensity sweeteners.

Based on food disappearance data, it is clear that an increase in the availability of diet beverages and bottled water has occurred concurrently with the increased prevalence of obesity (USDA, 2005). Diet beverages and bottled water availability have increased from 14 to 39 gal/capita/year between 1984 and 2004. In that time, diet carbonated soft drink availability increased almost two-fold to make up 30% of all soft drinks consumed in the United States. Bottle water availability has increased five-fold over the same time. The availability of these beverages now exceeds the availability of caloric soft drinks (36.5 gal/capita/year). The availability of caloric soft drinks has increased by 20% over the same time, milk decreased by 20% from 26.4 to 21.2 gal/capita/year and fruit juices remained fairly consistent at between 8 and 9 gal/capita/year. It would appear that increased availability and consumption of alternatives to sugars-sweetened beverages has done little to solve the obesity epidemic.

Consumption of alternative sweeteners has been associated with both higher body weights (Colditz *et al.*, 1990; Giammattei *et al.*, 2003) and lower body weights (Serra-Majem *et al.*, 1996). An 8-year cohort study in non-smoking women ($n = 31\,940$), aged 30–55 years, found a positive correlation between saccharine consumption and weight gain. However, as acknowledged by the authors, the strongest correlation with weight change was with age, while dietary intakes were only weakly related. (Colditz *et al.*, 1990). In contrast, a survey in Spain of 2450 individuals aged 6–75 years found a negative association between non-caloric sweetener (cyclamate) consumption and BMI (Serra-Majem *et al.*, 1996).

Long-term intervention studies are the preferred design for determining the role of sugars and alternative sweeteners in weight loss and maintenance. However, only a few comparisons have been in the absence of concurrent energy restriction (Blundell and Hill, 1986; Rolls *et al.*, 1990; Canty and Chan, 1991; Black *et al.*, 1993; Lavin *et al.*, 1997). In an early study by Tordoff and colleagues (Tordoff and Alleva, 1990), the diets of 9 women and 21 men were supplemented daily with 1150 g sodas sweetened with aspartame for 3 weeks followed by another 3 weeks with HFCS sodas. Aspartame-sweetened drinks reduced energy intake in both men and women resulting in decreased body weight for men compared with when no soda was consumed. In contrast, HFCS-sweetened soda increased energy intake and body weight in both sexes, although in men the decrease was about one-half that in the women. Sugar intake from the diet was reduced by about 200 kcal/day after consumption of both soda treatments. However, in this study, subjects were required to consume much larger amounts of the beverages compared with their usual diets. It remains unclear, therefore, if simple substitution of diet soft drinks for caloric soft drinks in their usual diet would have had any impact.

In one randomized control trial, two parallel groups of overweight adults consumed either a sucrose-sweetened beverage (2g sucrose/kg body weight), or a high-intensity sweetened beverage (10g sucrose/kg body weight daily) mostly as beverages in an *ad libitum* diet for 10 weeks (Raben *et al.*, 2002).

The artificial-sweeteners beverages contained 54% aspartame, 22% acesulfame K, 23% cyclamate and 1% saccharine. On average, subjects received 815 and 240kcal/day from supplemented-sucrose and artificially sweetened diets, respectively. After 10 weeks, body weight gain was greater after the sucrose beverage by 1.6kg (about 50% of that expected), whereas, the other group lost 1.0kg. These results indicate that artificial sweeteners have the potential to reduce energy intake and promote weight loss compared with sugars (Raben *et al.,* 2002). Nevertheless, the calories from the sucrose drinks were also compensated for at subsequent test meals by 56%. Based on the solutions' extra calories, if subjects had not compensated for the solution's calories, 7.4 and 2.2kg weight gain would have been expected after the sucrose and artificially sweetened diets, respectively (Raben *et al.*, 2002).

The reduced energy intake associated with the consumption of the artificial-sweetener diets led to a change in the distribution of the macronutrient contribution to the energy intake of the diets as predicted earlier by Beaton *et al.* (1992). Individuals in the artificially sweetened diet group reduced the proportion of carbohydrate and consumed higher proportions of fat and protein whereas individuals in the sucrose-supplemented group maintained their carbohydrate consumption. Therefore, the difference in energy intake and weight loss in these two groups may also be explained by the higher percentage of fat and protein in the diets of those who consumed artificially sweetened drinks because proteins suppress short-term energy intake more than carbohydrate (Anderson and Moore, 2004).

*Alternative sweeteners and short-term food intake*

High-intensity sweeteners

Although it seems reasonable to expect that a reduction in energy intake would occur if caloric beverages were replaced by non-caloric beverages in the diet, this expected benefit was hypothesized to be contradicted if the beverage was sweetened. In the 1980s it was proposed that high-intensity beverages stimulate appetite and increase subsequent food intake (Rogers *et al.*, 1988) through their cephalic-phase (Blundell and Hill, 1986) and postingestive effects (Rolls *et al.*, 1990; Anderson, 1995). The initial hypothesis by Blundell and Hill (1986) suggested that sweetness consumption is often linked with calorie intake and when non-caloric sweeteners are consumed they induce metabolic responses that prepare the body for an inflow of calories. When this expectation is not met, these anticipatory changes lead to increased appetite (Blundell and Hill, 1986). While appealing, this hypothesis has not been supported by short-term studies of the effect of consuming a high-intensity sweetened beverage at a defined time before a meal (Black *et al.*, 1991; Canty and Chan, 1991; Black and Anderson, 1994; Lavin *et al.*, 1997).

Several studies have shown that sweet taste without calories contributes to the reduction of hunger and increased feeling of fullness (Birch *et al.*, 1989; Rodin, 1990; Black *et al.*, 1993; Lavin and Read, 1995; Anderson *et al.*, 2002). In a study involving 44 children aged 2–5 years, an aspartame-sweetened beverage produced a significant suppression of food intake 30 min later in comparison with an isovolumetric water control (150 ml), but not compared with the sugar-sweetened drink (200 kcal) (Birch *et al.*, 1989). After consumption of non-caloric sweetened beverages (either aspartame or saccharin), adult subjects responded with reduced hunger ratings intermediate between those after a 20 g sucrose solution and those after a water control (Canty and Chan, 1991). Similarly, in healthy men, a 560-ml soft drink sweetened with aspartame significantly reduced subjective hunger for the first half hour after consumption compared with smaller volumes of the same drinks (Black *et al.*, 1991). Because food intake was measured at 1 h and was not affected by the drink, it remains possible that earlier measurement of food intake, for example at 30 min, would have demonstrated treatment effects. In adults a sucralose-sweetened drink also resulted in lower, although not statistically significant, food intake 1 h later compared with a water control in 15 healthy young men (Woodend and Anderson, 2001).

Overall, short-term study comparisons of the effect of high-intensity sweetened beverages compared with sugars-sweetened beverages on energy balance would support an advantage of energy-free beverages. The most obvious effect of consuming water or a high-intensity sweetened beverage on food intake at a subsequent meal can be seen in the cumulative energy intakes. Cumulative intake is the sum of the energy from the pre-meal beverage and the test meal that follows and is most often less after consuming a calorie-free beverage than after consuming a calorie-containing beverage (Woodend and Anderson, 2001; Akhavan, 2006). This is to be expected because, as noted earlier, compensation at the test meal for previously consumed calories is not precise and tends to underestimate the compensation required.

### Sugar alcohols

As a result of negative perceptions surrounding sugars and the recent demand for low-carbohydrate foods created by the Atkins diet (Atkins, 1998; Liu *et al.*, 2000; Daniels, 2003), interest in the use of sugar alcohols as alternative sweeteners has increased. Previous studies on sugar alcohols showed that ingestion of 25 g lactitol or xylitol caused smaller changes in plasma glucose, insulin and C-peptide concentrations, and a lower thermogenic response, than ingestion of 25 g glucose, with no difference between the two polyols (Natah *et al.*, 1997). Although short-term energy intake was not assessed in this study, the authors suggested that the small change in blood glucose after sugar alcohols may be beneficial for overweight and diabetic patients (Natah *et al.*, 1997). However, the relationship between the glycemic index of food and weight loss has not been established (ADA, 2004), nor has it been shown that sugar alcohols have an advantage over sugars in a weight-loss diet.

However, in the short-term, sugar alcohols may have some advantage. In a recent clinical study, the effects of sugar alcohols and sugar (sucrose) on appetite and short-term food intake were compared in 15 lean subjects. The effects of 200 g yogurt sweetened with one of 25 g sucrose, 25 g xylitol, 25 g polydextrose or 12.5 xylitol + 12.5 polydextrose were assessed by measuring food intake at an *ad libitum* lunch and also subjective appetite. Sugar-alcohol-sweetened yogurts induced a stronger satiating effect and lower cumulative energy intake (energy content of the yogurt preloads plus lunch intake) compared with the sucrose-sweetened yogurt (King *et al.*, 2005).

In summary, several studies suggest that alternative sweeteners reduce cumulative energy intake in short-term controlled experiments. However, the long-term benefits remain uncertain for several reasons. First, the replacement of sugars with alternative sweeteners alters the macronutrient distribution (dietary intake patterns) of the habitual diet by increasing fat and protein intakes (Beaton *et al.*, 1992). Secondly, solid foods containing artificial sweeteners are not necessarily energy reduced. Most sugar-alcohol-sweetened foods are energy dense and have a higher percentage of fat compared with sugars-sweetened foods (ADA, 2004). Thirdly, it is not clear what the motivation is for those who use artificially sweetened foods and how that affects their food choices and energy intakes. Therefore in the long term, increased use of alternative sweeteners in foods may result in greater energy intake (Wolever *et al.*, 2002) and promote weight gain (Lissner *et al.*, 1987; Saris *et al.*, 2000).

## 5.4 Conclusion

As discussed in this chapter, the results of epidemiological intervention studies and short-term clinical studies on sugars and alternative sweeteners are insufficient to identify the role of these sweeteners as independent factors in the etiology of obesity. Associations found in food availability data and epidemiological studies between consumption of sweeteners and obesity perhaps indicate an overall lifestyle with a food supply that simply provides too much of a good thing (Jenkins *et al.*, 2004). A combination of increased energy intake from all sources and decreased physical activity is the most likely explanation for the current increase in obesity.

## 5.5 Implications and recommendations

It seems unlikely that any approach other than expensive, long-term randomized clinical trials will contribute further to the identification of the specific role for sweeteners in the management of body weight and the prevention of obesity. Even so, the difficulty of designing double-blind experiments involving food and beverages is an obvious limitation. Thus, it is virtually impossible to formulate an ideal design that does not result in behavior change in the participating subjects.

Therefore, a more promising but difficult approach to terminating the current rise in overweight and obesity may involve multi-sector cooperation of government, academia and industry – to design comprehensive overweight prevention programs (Koplan *et al.*, 2004; Anon., 2006). These programs need to collaborate in several ways including: educating healthy eating approaches for parents and children; producing healthy foods and beverages; developing an evidence-based approach to dietary guidance and policy formulation. A public health approach that has a singular focus on sugars and sugars-sweetened beverages is unlikely to provide a solution (Dietz, 2006).

## 5.6 Future trends

Although cause and effect for the role of sweeteners in the etiology of obesity has not been established, the perception that it has been is becoming widespread among health professionals and the public. For this reason it is likely that the consumption of traditional sugars-sweetened beverages will decline. They will be replaced by reduced-energy or energy-free beverages, but also by energy-dense beverages based on sugars or fat and sugars (e.g. specialty coffees) aimed at selected audiences. Clearly more choices will be available but it remains to be seen how the consumer will utilize these choices to maintain healthy body weights. Based on the past, it can be predicted that the obesity epidemic has provided the beverage industry with more product opportunities but health professionals will find they have gained little ground from a public health perspective.

On the other hand, specific answers on the role of sweeteners in determining dietary patterns and energy intake will emerge. Researchers will put more effort into the conduct of randomized clinical trials. Clinical studies will put an increasing emphasis on the impact of caloric and non-caloric sweeteners on satiety and food intake regulatory mechanisms in an attempt to identify the role of environment *versus* physiology as determinants of energy imbalances. The role of genetics, especially of taste, as a determinant of the metabolic and behavioral responses to sweeteners and in the determination of energy imbalances will be increasingly emphasized.

## 5.7 References

AAPC (American Academy of Pediatrics Committee on School Health) (2004), 'Soft drinks in schools.' *Pediatrics*, **113** (1 Pt 1), 152–4.

ADA (American Dietetics Association) (2004), ADA Report. 'Position of the American Dietetic Association. Use of nutritive and non-nutritive sweeteners.' *J Am Diet Assoc*, **104**, 255–75.

AKGUN S and ERTEL N H (1985), 'The effects of sucrose, fructose, and high-fructose corn syrup meals on plasma glucose and insulin in non-insulin-dependent diabetic subjects.' *Diabetes Care*, **8** (3), 279–83.

AKHAVAN T (2006), 'The effects of different ratios of fructose to glucose solutions on glycemic, insulin and appetite responses, and short-term food intake.' Department of Nutritional Sciences, University of Toronto, Canada, Thesis.

ALMIRON-ROIG E and DREWNOWSKI A (2003), 'Hunger, thirst, and energy intakes following consumption of caloric beverages.' *Physiol Behav*, **79** (4–5), 767–73.

ALMIRON-ROIG E, CHEN Y and DREWNOWSKI A (2003), 'Liquid calories and the failure of satiety: how good is the evidence?' *Obes Rev*, **4** (4), 201–12.

ALMIRON-ROIG E, FLORES S Y and DREWNOWSKI A (2004), 'No difference in satiety or in subsequent energy intakes between a beverage and a solid food.' *Physiol Behav*, **82** (4), 671–7.

ANDERSON G H (1995), 'Sugars, sweetness and food intake.' *Am J Clin Nutr*, **62**, 195–202.

ANDERSON G H and MOORE S E (2004), 'Dietary proteins in the regulation of food intake and body weight in humans.' *J Nutr*, **134**, 974–9.

ANDERSON G H and WOODEND D (2003a), 'Effect of glycemic carbohydrates on short-term satiety and food intake.' *Nutr Rev*, **61** (5 Pt 2), 17–26.

ANDERSON G H and WOODEND D (2003b), 'Consumption of sugar and the regulation of short-term satiety and food intake.' *Am J Clin Nutr*, **78** (4), 843–9.

ANDERSON G H, SARAVIS S, SCHACHER R, ZLOTKIN S and LEITER L (1989), 'Aspartame: effect on lunch-time food intake, appetite and hedonic response in children.' *Appetite*, **13**, 93–103.

ANDERSON G H, STEWART S and KAPLAN R (1998), 'Carbohydrate behavior and health.' *Bahrain Med Bull*, **20**, 69–76.

ANDERSON G H, CATHERINE N L, WOODEND D M and WOLEVER T M (2002), 'Inverse association between the effect of carbohydrates on blood glucose and subsequent short-term food intake in young men.' *Am J Clin Nutr*, **76** (5), 1023–30.

ANON. (2006), 'Curbing the obesity epidemic.' Editorial. *Lancet*, **367** (9522), 1549.

ATKINS R C (1998), '*Dr. Atkins' New Diet Revolution*.' Avon, New York.

BANTLE J P, RAATZ S K, THOMAS W and GEORGOPOULOS A (2000), 'Effects of dietary fructose on plasma lipids in healthy subjects.' *Am J Clin Nutr*, **72** (5), 1128–34.

BEATON G H, TARASUK V and ANDERSON G H (1992), 'Estimation of possible impact of non-caloric fat and carbohydrate substitutes on macronutrient intake in the human.' *Appetite*, **19**, 87–103.

BIRCH L L and FISHER J O (1997), 'Food intake regulation in children. Fat and sugar substitutes and intake.' *Ann N Y Acad Sci*, **819**, 194–220.

BIRCH L L, MCPHEE L and SULLIVAN S (1989), 'Children's food intake following drinks sweetened with sucrose or aspartame, time course effects.' *Physiol Behav*, **45**, 387–95.

BLACK R M and ANDERSON G H (1994), 'Sweeteners, food intake and selection.' In Eds. Fernstrom J D and Miller G F. *Appetite and Body Weight Regulation: Sugar, Fat and Macronutrient Substitutes*, CRC, Press, Boca Raton, FL, USA, pp. 125–36.

BLACK R M, TANAKA P, LEITER L A and ANDERSON G H (1991), 'Soft drinks with aspartame: effect on subjective hunger, food selection, and food intake of young adult males.' *Physiol Behav*, **49** (4), 803–10.

BLACK R M, LEITER L A and ANDERSON G H (1993), 'Consuming aspartame with and without taste: differential effects on appetite and food intake of young adult males.' *Physiol Behav*, **53** (3), 459–66.

BLUNDELL J E and HILL A J (1986), 'Paradoxical effects of an intense sweetener (aspartame) on appetite.' *Lancet*, **1** (8489), 1092–3.

BOLTON-SMITH C, and WOODWARD M (1994), 'Dietary composition and fat to sugar ratios in relation to obesity.' *Int J Obes Relat Metab Disord*, **18** (12), 820–8.

BRAY G A, NIELSEN S J and POPKIN B M (2004), 'Consumption of high-fructose corn syrup in beverages may play a role in the epidemic of obesity.' *Am J Clin Nutr*, **79** (4), 537–43.

BRIGHT G (1999), 'Low-calorie sweeteners: from molecules to mass markets.' In Ed. Corti A. *Low-calorie Sweeteners Present and Future*, Vol. 85, Krager AG, Basel, Switzerland, pp. 3–8.

CANTY D J and CHAN M M (1991), 'Effects of consumption of caloric vs. noncaloric sweet drinks on indices of hunger and food consumption in normal adults.' *Am J Clin Nutr*, **53**, 1159–64.

CCC (Calorie Control Council) (2006), www.caloriecontrol.org/.

CECIL J E, PALMER C N, WRIEDEN W, MURRIE I, BOLTON-SMITH C, WATT P, WALLIS D J and HETHERINGTON M M (2005), 'Energy intakes of children after preloads: adjustment, not compensation.' *Am J Clin Nutr*, **82** (2), 302–8.

COLDITZ G A, WILLETT W C, STAMPFER M J, LONDON S J, SEGAL M R and SPEIZER F E (1990), 'Patterns of weight change and their relation to diet in a cohort of healthy women' *Am J Clin Nutr*, **51**, 1100–5.

CRAPO P A, REAVEN G and OLEFSKY J (1980), 'Effects of oral fructose in normal, diabetic, and impaired glucose tolerance subjects.' *Diabetes Care*, **3** (5), 575–82.

DANIELS S R (2003), Abnormal weight gain and weight management: are carbohydrates the enemy. *J Pediatr*, **142** (3), 225–7.

DELLA VALLE D M, ROE L S and ROLLS B J (2005), 'Does the consumption of caloric and non-caloric beverages with a meal affect energy intake?' *Appetite*, **44** (2), 187–93.

DIETZ W H (2006), 'Sugar-sweetened beverages, milk intake, and obesity in children and adolescents.' *J Pediatr*, **148** (2), 152–4.

DIMEGLIO D P and MATTES R D (2000), 'Liquid versus solid carbohydrate: effects on food intake and body weight.' *Int J Obes Relat Metab Disord*, **24** (6), 794–800.

EBBELING C B, FELDMAN H A, OSGANIAN S K, CHOMITZ V R, ELLENBOGEN S J and LUDWIG D S (2006), 'Effects of decreasing sugar-sweetened beverage consumption on body weight in adolescents: a randomized, controlled pilot study.' *Pediatrics*, **117** (3), 673–80.

ELLIOTT S S, KEIM N L, STERN J S, TEFF K and HAVEL P J (2002), 'Fructose, weight gain, and the insulin resistance syndrome.' *Am J Clin Nutr*, **76** (5), 911–22.

FDA (Food and Drug Administration) (2006), Food Additive Status List US Department of Health and Human Services, www.cfsan.fda.gov/~dms/opa-appa.html#ftnA; and www.fda.gov/bbs/topics/ANSWERS/2002/ANS01156.html.

GIAMMATTEI J, BLIX G, MARSHAK H H, WOLLITZER A O and PETTITT D J (2003), 'Television watching and soft drink consumption: associations with obesity in 11- to 13-year-old schoolchildren.' *Arch Pediatr Adolesc Med*, **157**, 882–6.

GIBNEY M, SIGMAN-GRANT M, STANTON J L JR and KEAST D R (1995), 'Consumption of sugars.' *Am J Clin Nutr*, **62** (1 Suppl.), 178S–193S, discussion 194S.

GLEASON P and SUITOR C (2001), '*Children's Diets in the Mid-1990s: Dietary Intake and Its Relationship with School Meal Participation.*' US Department of Agriculture, Food and Nutrition Service, Office of Analysis, Nutrition and Evaluation, Alexandria, VA, USA. Accessed February 12. Available at: http://www.fns.usda.gov/oane/menu/published/cnp/files/childiet.pdf.

HANOVER L M and WHITE J S (1993), Manufacturing, composition, and applications of fructose. *Am J Clin Nutr*, **58** (Suppl. 5), 724–732.

HARNACK L, STANG J and STORY M (1999), 'Soft drink consumption among US children and adolescents: nutritional consequences.' *J Am Diet Assoc*, **99** (4), 436–41.

HARNACK L J, JEFFERY R W and BOUTELLE K N (2000), 'Temporal trends in energy intake in the United States an ecologic perspective.' *Am J Clin Nutr*, **71** (6), 1478–84.

HILL J and PRENTICE A (1995), 'Sugar and body weight regulation.' *Am J Clin Nutr*, **62** (Suppl.), 264–274.

HOLDSWORTH C D and DAWSON A M (1965), 'Absorption of fructose in man.' *Proc Soc Exp Biol Med*, **118**, 142–5.

HOROWITZ M, CUNNINGHAM K M, WISHART J M, JONES K L and READ N W (1996), 'The effect of short-term dietary supplementation with glucose on gastric emptying of glucose and fructose and oral glucose tolerance in normal subjects.' *Diabetologia*, **39** (4), 481–6.

JAMES J, THOMAS P, CAVAN D and KERR D (2004), 'Preventing childhood obesity by reducing consumption of carbonated drinks: cluster randomised controlled trial.' *Br Med J*, **328**, 1237.

JANSSEN I, KATZMARZYK P T, BOYCE W F, VEREECKEN C, MULVIHILL C, ROBERTS C, CURRIE C and PICKETT W; Health Behavior in School-Aged Children Obesity Working Group (2005) 'Comparison of overweight and obesity prevalence in school-aged youth from 34 countries and their relationships with physical activity and dietary patterns.' *Obes Rev*, **6** (2), 123–32.

JENKINS D J, KENDALL C W, MARCHIE A and AUGUSTIN L S (2004), Too much sugar, too much carbohydrate, or just too much? *Am J Clin Nutr*, **79** (5), 711–12.

KING N A, CRAIG S A, PEPPER T and BLUNDELL J E (2005), 'Evaluation of the independent and combined effects of xylitol and polydextrose consumed as a snack on hunger and energy intake over 10 day.' *Br J Nutr*, **93** (6), 911–15.

KOPELMAN P G (2000), 'Physiopathology of prolactin secretion in obesity.' *Int J Obes Relat Metab Disord*, **24** (Suppl. 2), S104–8.

KOPLAN J P, LIVERMAN C T and KRAAK V A, Eds.; Committee on Prevention of Obesity in Children and Youth (2004), *Preventing Childhood Obesity: Health in the Balance*, The Institute of Medicine of the National Academies, Washington, USA.

LAVIN J, WITTERT G and ANDREWS J (1998), 'Interaction of insulin, glucagon-like peptide-1, gastric inhibitory polypeptide and appetite in response to intraduodenal carbohydrate.' *Am J Clin Nutr*, **68** (3), 591–8.

LAVIN J H and READ N W (1995), 'The effect on hunger and satiety of slowing the absorption of glucose: relationship with gastric emptying and postprandial blood glucose and insulin responses.' *Appetite*, **25**, 89–96.

LAVIN J H, FRENCH S J and READ N W (1997), 'The effect of sucrose- and aspartame-sweetened drinks on energy intake, hunger and food choice of female, moderately restrained eaters.' *Int J Obes Relat Metab Disord*, **21** (1), 37–42.

LAVIN J H, FRENCH S J and READ N W (2002a), 'Comparison of oral and gastric administration of sucrose and maltose on gastric emptying rate and appetite.' *Int J Obes Relat Metab Disord*, **26** (1), 80–6.

LAVIN J H and FRENCH S J, RUXTON C H and READ N W (2002b), 'An investigation of the role of oro-sensory stimulation in sugar satiety?' *Int J Obes Relat Metab Disord*, **26** (3), 384–8.

LEE B M and WOLEVER T M S (1998), 'Effect of glucose, sucrose and fructose on plasma glucose and insulin responses in normal humans: comparison with white bread.' *Eur J Clin Nutr*, **52** (12), 924–8.

LISSNER L, LEVITSKY D A, STRUPP B J, KALKWARF H J and ROE D A (1987), 'Dietary fat and the regulation of energy intake in human subjects.' *Am J Clin Nutr*, **46** (6), 886–92.

LIU S, WILLETT W C, STAMPFER M J, HU F B, FRANZ M, SAMPSON L, HENNEKENS C H and MANSON J E (2000), A prospective study of dietary glycemic load, carbohydrate intake, and risk of coronary heart disease in US women. *Am J Clin Nutr*, **71** (6), 1455–61.

LUDWIG D S, PETERSON K E and GORTMAKER S L (2001), 'Relation between consumption of sugar-sweetened drinks and childhood obesity: a prospective, observational analysis.' *Lancet*, **357** (9255), 505–8.

MATTHES R D (1996), 'Dietary compensation by humans for supplemental energy provided as ethanol or carbohydrate in fluids.' *Physiol Behav*, **59** (1), 179–87.

MRDJENOVIC G and LEVITSKY D A (2003), 'Nutritional and energetic consequences of sweetened drink consumption in 6- to 13-year-old children.' *Pediatr*, **142** (6), 604–10.

NATAH S S, HUSSIEN K R, TUOMINEN J A and KOIVISTO V A (1997), 'Metabolic response to lactitol and xylitol in healthy men.' *Am J Clin Nutr*, **65** (4), 947–50.

NCS (National Consumer Survey) (2000), Survey conducted by Booth Research Services for the Calorie Control Council, USA.

NDL (Nutrient Data Laboratory) (2006), USDA, Agricultural Research Service, Washington DC, www.nal.usda.gov/fnic/foodcomp/search/.

PANCOAST H M, JUNK W R (1980), *Handbook of Sugars*, 2nd Edn, AVI Publishing Co, Westport, CT, USA, pp. 81–112.

PARK Y K and YETLEY E A (1993), 'Intakes and food sources of fructose in the United States.' *Am J Clin Nutr*, **58** (5 Suppl.), 737S–747S.

PEREIRA M A (2006), 'The possible role of sugar-sweetened beverages in obesity etiology: A review of the evidence.' *Int J Obes*, **30**, S28–S36.

POPKIN B M, ARMSTRONG L E, BRAY G M, CABALLERO B, FREI B and WILLETT W C (2006), 'A new proposed guidance system for beverage consumption in the United States.' *Am J Clin Nutr*, **83** (3), 529–42.

PUTNAM J J and ALLSHOUSE J E (1999), 'Food consumption, prices and expenditures, 1970–97.' US Department of Agriculture Economic Research Service Statistical Bulletin 965, April, US Government Printing Office, Washington, DC.

RABEN A, VASILARAS T H, MOLLER A C and ASTRUP A (2002), 'Sucrose compared with artificial sweeteners: different effects on ad libitum food intake and body weight after 10 wk of supplementation in overweight.' *Am J Clin Nutr*, **76** (4), 721–9.

RAVICH W J, BAYLESS T M and THOMAS M (1983), 'Fructose: incomplete intestinal absorption in humans.' *Gastroenterology*, **84**, 26–9.

READ N, FRENCH S and CUNNINGHAM K (1994), 'The role of the gut in regulating food intake in man.' *Nutr Rev*, **52**, 1–10.

RIBY J E, FUJISAWA T and KRETCHMER N (1993), 'Fructose absorption.' *Am J Clin Nutr*, **58** (Suppl), 748–53.

RODIN J (1990), 'Comparative effects of fructose, aspartame, glucose and water preloads on calorie and macronutrient intake.' *Am J Clin Nutr*, **51**, 428–35.

RODIN J (1991), 'Effects of pure sugar vs. mixed starch fructose loads on food intake.' *Appetite*, **17**, 213–19.

RODIN J, REED D and JAMNER L (1988), 'Metabolic effect of fructose and glucose: implications for food intake.' *Am J Clin Nutr*, **47** (4), 683–9.

ROGERS P J and BLUNDELL J E (1989), 'Separating the actions of sweetness and calories: effects of saccharin and carbohydrates on hunger and food intake in human subjects.' *Physiol Behav*, **45** (6), 1093–9.

ROGERS P J, CARLYLE J A, HILL A J and BLUNDELL J E (1988), 'Uncoupling sweet taste and calories: comparison of the effects of glucose and three intense sweeteners on hunger and food intake.' *Physiol Behav*, **43** (5), 547–52.

ROLLS B J, HETHERINGTON M and LASTER L J (1988), 'Comparison of the effects of aspartame and sucrose on food intake.' *Appetite*, **11**, 62–7.

ROLLS B J, KIM S and FEDOROFF I C (1990), 'Effects of drinks sweetened with sucrose or aspartame on hunger, thirst and food intake in men.' *Physiol Behav*, **48** (1), 19–26.

SARIS W H, ASTRUP A, PRENTICE A M, ZUNFT H J, FORMIGUERA X, VERBOEKET-VAN DE VENNE W P, RABEN A, POPPITT S D, SEPPELT B, JOHNSTON S, VASILARAS T H and KEOGH G F (2000), 'Randomized controlled trial of changes in dietary carbohydrate/fat ratio and simple vs. complex carbohydrates on body weight and blood lipids: the CARMEN study. The Carbohydrate Ratio Management in European National diets.' *Int J Obes Relat Metab Disord*, **24**, 1310–8.

SCHULZE M B, MANSON J E, LUDWIG D S, COLDITZ G A, STAMPFER M J, WILLETT W C and HU F B (2004), 'Sugar-sweetened beverages, weight gain, and incidence of type 2 diabetes in young and middle-aged women.' *JAMA*, **292**, 927–34.

SERRA-MAJEM L, RIBAS L, INGLES C, FUENTES M, LLOVERAS G and SALLERAS L (1996), 'Cyclamate consumption in Catalonia, Spain (1992): relationship with the body mass index' *Food Addit Contam*, **13**, 695–703.

SPITZER L and RODIN J (1987), 'Effects of fructose and glucose preloads on subsequent food intake.' *Appetite*, **8** (2), 135–45.

STEWART S L, BLACK R, WOLEVER T M S and ANDERSON G H (1997), 'The relationship between the glycaemic response to breakfast cereals and subjective appetite and food intake.' *Nutr Res*, **17** (8), 1249–60.

STRIEGEL-MOORE R H, THOMPSON D, AFFENITO S G, FRANKO D L, OBARZANEK E, BARTON B A, SCHREIBER G B, DANIELS S R, SCHMIDT M and CRAWFORD P B (2006), 'Correlates of beverage intake in adolescent girls: The National Heart, Lung, and Blood Institute Growth and Health Study.' *J Pediatr*, **148**, 183–7.

TEFF K L, ELLIOTT S S, TSCHOP M, KIEFFER T J, RADER D, HEIMAN M, TOWNSEND R R, KEIM N L, D'ALESSIO D and HAVEL P J (2004), 'Dietary fructose reduces circulating insulin and leptin, attenuates postprandial suppression of ghrelin, and increases triglycerides in women.' *J Clin Endocrinol Metab*, **89** (6), 2963–72.

TORDOFF M G and ALLEVA A M (1990), 'Effect of drinking soda sweetened with aspartame or high-fructose corn syrup on food intake and body weight.' *Am J Clin Nutr*, **51** (6), 963–9.

USDA (United States Department of Agriculture/Economic Research Service) (2005), Sugar and Sweetener Yearbook series, Tables 50–53, last updated December 21, 2005.

VUILLEUMIER S (1993), 'Worldwide production of high-fructose syrup and crystalline fructose.' *Am J Clin Nutr*, **58** (5 Suppl.), 733S–736S.

WALTERS S J (2002), 'Glycemic response to liquid and Solid carbohydrate preloads fails to predict appetite or food intake two or four h later in young men.' University of Toronto, Toronto, Canada, Masters Thesis.

WHO (World Health Organization) (1998), Report of a WHO consultation on obesity, WHO, Geneva.

WOLEVER T, PIEKARZ A, HOLLANDS M and YOUNKER K (2002), 'Sugar alcohols and diabetes: a review' *Can J Diabetes*, **26**, 356–62.

WOODEND D M and ANDERSON G H (2001), 'Effect of sucrose and safflower oil preloads on short term appetite and food intake of young men.' *Appetite*, **26**, 384–88.

WYLIE-ROSETT J, SEGAL-ISAACSON C J and SEGAL-ISAACSON A (2004), 'Carbohydrates and increases in obesity: does the type of carbohydrate make a difference?' *Obes Res*, **12** (Suppl. 2), 124S–129S.

ZUMBE A, LEE A and STOREY D (2001), 'Polyols in confectionery: the route to sugar-free, reduced sugar and reduced calorie confectionery', *Br J Nutr*, **85**, S31–45.

# Part II

# Ingredients from grains, fruits and vegetables for weight control

# 6

# β-Glucans

**J.-A. Nazare, M. Laville, Centre de Recherche en Nutrition Humaine Rhône Alpes, France, C. G. Biliaderis, A. Lazaridou, Aristotle University, Thessaloniki, Greece, G. Önning, Lund University, Sweden, M. Salmenkallio-Marttila, VTT, Finland and A. Triantafyllou, Ceba Foods, Sweden**

## 6.1 Introduction

Dietary guidance universally recommends diets with higher fibre content for health promotion and disease prevention. This goal is often difficult to achieve. That is why research has to be developed to find sources of fibre that could easily be worked into a normal diet at levels that could allow beneficial effects.

An official definition of dietary fibre was given by the American Association of Cereal Chemists in 2001:

> Dietary fibre is the edible parts of plants or analogous carbohydrates that are resistant to digestion and absorption in the human small intestine with complete or partial fermentation in the large intestine. Dietary fibres include polysaccharides, oligosaccharides, lignin and associated plant substances. Dietary fibres promote beneficial physiological effects including laxation and/or blood cholesterol attenuation, and/or blood glucose attenuation.[1]

Fibres can be separated into two groups according to whether or not they are soluble. β-Glucans are fibres, they are highly viscous, soluble fermentable polysaccharides. They have been shown to have a positive effect on lipid and carbohydrate metabolism, and could therefore be considered as potentially useful ingredients for weight control.

## 6.2 Sources of β-glucans

Six types of β-glucans have been identified in the cell walls of green plants and fungi. Cellulose is a $(1 \rightarrow 4)$-β-glucan, a long linear glucose polymer, with low flexibility and solubility. It is a ubiquitous component of the fibrillar phase of cell walls while it is also found as an extracellular secretion in certain bacteria.[2]

In cereals, cellulose microfibrils appear to be embedded in a matrix of mixed-linkage (1 → 3, 1 → 4)-β-glucan in the walls of aleurone and starchy endosperm cells. Oat (*Avena sativa*) and barley (*Hordeum vulgare*) both contain large amounts of (1 → 3, 1 → 4)-β-glucan, the latter constituting approximately 75% of the walls of their starchy endosperm cells. The β-glucan found in oat and barley is a soluble fibre that is easily fermented in the intestine and that has a high nutritive value. In addition, the endosperm cell walls of other monocots of the grass family *Gramineae* – such as wheat (*Triticum aestivum*), rye (*Secale cereale*) and rice (*Oryza sativa*) – contain small amounts of β-glucans.[3,4]

A range of fluorescent dyes have been studied for their interaction with endosperm cell walls showing that Calcofluor and Congo red can be used as sensitive and specific markers for the detection of β-glucan.[5] Calcofluor binding reveals that the distribution of β-glucan in the kernels of barley is generally even whereas the concentration of β-glucan is particularly high in the subaleurone layer of the oat groat and this may contribute significantly to the water-binding capacity of the bran and to its efficacy as dietary fibre. Hence dry milling and air-sifting techniques have been exploited to manufacture enriched fractions of oats.[6,7] Enrichment methods have also been employed for barley because the grain is to some extent morphologically differentiated.[8,9] Plant breeding has developed oat and barley cultivars with varying contents of β-glucan.[10] Evaluation of groat characteristics and groat composition in 35 genotypes from 9 taxonomic species of *Avena* has revealed a variation in β-glucan from 2.2 to 11.3%.[11]

Barley has traditionally been seen as a food for human consumption. On the other hand, oat has gained extra attention due to a large number of clinical studies that identified oat β-glucan as the component responsible for the significant cholesterol-lowering properties attributed to oats, particularly the decrease of low-density lipoprotein (LDL) cholesterol.[12] Oat β-glucan hydrolysates are furthermore thought to possess a probiotic effect.[13] Higher plants not only contain significant amounts of mixed linkage (1 → 3, 1 → 4)-β-glucan but also (1 → 3)-β-glucan with a single monomer and linkage type. Deposits of (1 → 3)-β-glucans, referred to as callose, occur in the cell walls of plant tissues during their development and are found in specialized cell walls in response to wounding, infection and physiological stress.[14] Certain bacteria secrete extracellularly a polymer of similar structure, namely curdlan.

Microbial β-glucan is a component of cell walls or is secreted by microorganisms in the growing medium, as in the case of lactic acid bacteria that are living and growing on plants, often under harsh conditions, such as *Pediococcus damnosus*.[15] The glucose molecules in these polymers are generally connected with (1 → 3) linkages with varying proportions of (1 → 6)-

linked β-glucosyl residues substituted at intervals along, or as branches of, the (1 → 3) backbone.

Mushroom myco-polysaccharides such as β-glucan lentinan from shiitake *Lentinus edodes* are also comprised of a β-(1 → 3)-D-glucan backbone with β-(1 → 6)-glucan side chains. The content of β-glucan is typically around 0.3 g per 100 g of mushroom on a dry basis whereas its distribution in the soluble fraction of total dietary fibre ranges widely from 17 to 46%. The soluble: insoluble ratio varies depending on the particular mushroom whereas the content of soluble β-glucan is higher in cereals.[16]

Yeast β-D-glucan, also a polyglucose polysaccharide, derived from the cell walls of baker's yeast or *Saccharomyces cerevisiae*, consists of straight-chain and branched polymers. The straight-chain structures are (1 → 3)-β-D-linked glucose polymers and (1 → 6)-β-D-linked glucose polymers. Similarly the homopolysaccharide of glucose produced by *Botryosphaeria rhodina* (laminaran) consists of a (1 → 3)-β-D-linked backbone containing varying degrees of (1 → 6)-β branches.[17] Yeast β-glucan has been demonstrated to have non-specific immune-enhancing effects in *in vitro* and some animal and human studies.[18]

## 6.3 β-Glucan structure and related properties

Mixed-linkage (1 → 3, 1 → 4) linear β-D-glucans (β-glucans) are major components of endosperm cell walls of commercially important cereals, such as oat, barley, rye and wheat. β-Glucans from cereals are linear homopolysaccharides of D-glucopyranosyl residues (Glc*p*) linked via a mixture of β-(1 → 3) and β-(1 → 4) linkages. The structure features the presence of consecutive (1 → 4)-linked β-D-glucose in blocks (i.e. oligomeric cellulose segments) that are separated by single (1 → 3) linkages. Although most of the cellulose segments are trimers and tetramers, longer cellulosic oligosaccharides are also present in the polymeric chains.[19–25] Cereal β-glucans exhibit diversity with respect to their molecular/structural features, such as molecular size, ratio of tri- to tetramers, amount of longer cellulosic oligomers and ratio of β-(1 → 4):β-(1 → 3) linkages. These structural features seem to be important determinants of their physical properties, such as water solubility, viscosity, and gelation properties. The molecular size and fine structural features of β-glucans play an important role in the solubility and chain conformation, or shape and, therefore, in their rheological properties in solution. The chemical features of cereal β-glucans are reflected in their solubility in water and in their extended, flexible chain conformation.[19] The cellulose-like portions of cereal β-glucans might contribute to the stiffness of the molecules in solution.[22] Furthermore, β-glucans containing blocks of adjacent β-(1 → 4) linkages may exhibit a tendency for interchain aggregation (and hence lower solubility) via strong hydrogen bonds along the cellulose-like segments; the β-(1 → 3) linkages break up the regularity of the β-(1 → 4) linkage sequence, making it more soluble and flexible.[26] On the other hand, it has been shown that a higher content of cellotriosyl units might impose some conformational regularity within the β-glucan chain, and consequently a higher degree of organization of these polymers in solution (i.e. lower solubility).[27,28] Suggestions have been made that differences in the amount of cellotriosyl fragments, long cellulosic oligomers, and the ratio of (1 → 4):(1 → 3) linkages, might explain solubility differences among cereal β-glucans in accord with the two previous aggregation mechanisms.[21,29–31]

Rheologically, solutions of cereal β-glucans fall into the category of viscoelastic fluids behaving similarly to the well-characterized random-coil polysaccharides; i.e. a Newtonian region can be observed at low shear rates and a shear thinning flow at high shear rates. However, the preparation of β-glucan solutions, their storage time (i.e. waiting time before analysis) and their thermal history have been proven to affect their rheological behaviour.[32–37] Time-dependent rheological behaviour is revealed by thixotropic loop experiments for cereal β-glucans with certain structural features, implying the formation of intermolecular networks. Moreover, freshly prepared cereal β-glucan solutions exhibit typical random-coil flow behaviour and an increased storage time induces an unusual shear-thinning flow behaviour at low shear rates. This behaviour becomes more pronounced with increasing storage time before the rheological testing. A strong time-dependent behaviour has been observed for mixed-linked (1 → 3, 1 → 4)-β-glucans with low molecular size and high amounts of cellotriose units and/or long cellulose-like oligomers in the polymeric chain. In addition, the departure from the usual flow behaviour was noticed in shorter storage periods for solutions with increasing concentration of β-glucans.[34,35,37]

As expected, an increased molecular weight induces an increase in the viscosity and the shear-thinning properties of β-glucan dispersions at equivalent polysaccharide concentrations.[34,35,37,38] In addition to solution viscosity enhancement on storage, β-glucans have been shown to gel under certain conditions.[34–45] Two different gelation models have been proposed in the literature for mixed-linkage (1 → 3, 1 → 4)-β-glucans. One model involves the side-by-side interactions of cellulose-like segments of more than three contiguous β-(1 → 4)-linked glucosyl units, whereas the other model involves the association of chain segments with consecutive cellotriosyl units linked by β-(1 → 3) bonds.[39] Among cereal β-glucans of equivalent molecular weight, the gelation time decreased and the gelation rate increased in the order of oat, barley and wheat β-glucans – reflecting the order of the molar ratio DP3/DP4 units.[35,39,40,44] (NB, the enzyme lichenase, a (1 → 3, 1 → 4)-β-D-glucan-4-glucanohydrolase, specifically cleaves the (1 → 4)-glycosidic bond of the 3-substituted glucose residues in β-glucans, yielding oligomers with different degrees of polymerization (DP). The major products for the cereal β-glucans are 3-*O*-β-cellobiosyl-D-glucose (DP3) and 3-*O*-β-cellotriosyl-D-glucose (DP4).) Further to the fine structure, the molecular size of the polymer seems to have a strong impact on polysaccharide gelation ability. For samples with similar distribution of cellulose-like fragments the gelation time decreases and the gelation rate increases with decreasing molecular weight, possibly due to the higher mobility of the shorter chains that enhances diffusion and lateral interchain associations.[34,35,37–39,41,46,47] Although a slower gelation process is noted for the high molecular size β-glucans, the gel network structure consists of structural elements (microaggregates) with better organization and/or it involves interchain associations over longer chain segments.[34,35,37]

Variations in the mechanical properties of cereal β-glucan gels have also been revealed by large deformation compression tests. An increase in strength and a decrease in brittleness of the β-glucan gels cured at room temperature were found with increasing concentration, molecular size and DP3/DP4 ratio of the polysaccharide, whereas cereal β-glucans with high molecular size and low amounts of DP3 units promoted the formation of strong cryogels (formed under repeated freezing–thawing cycles) when tested under large deformation protocols, a fact that was attributed to differences in the nature of the network microstructure among samples.[34,35,37,42]

Overall, the structure–physical property relations for cereal β-glucan isolates have been largely explored. Structural features, such as distribution of cellulosic oligomers, ratio of DP3/DP4 units and molecular size of the polysaccharides were proven to be important determinants of their solubility, rheological behaviour in aqueous solution and gelation ability, as well as of the thermal and mechanical properties of hydrogels obtained by interchain associations either at room temperature or via repeated freeze–thaw cycles.

## 6.4 Effects of β-glucans on lipid metabolism

Cardiovascular diseases, such as myocardial infarction (MI), angina and stroke, are major contributors to the global burden of disease. The diseases are caused by the development of atherosclerosis in the blood vessels and one factor that may influence the atherosclerotic process is the dietary fibre content in the diet. The intake of dietary fibre and risk of coronary heart disease were followed for 10 years among women in the Nurses' Health Study.[48] In total, 68782 women were included in the analysis and the age-adjusted relative risk for major cardiovascular events was 0.53 for women in the highest quintile of total dietary fibre intake (median 22.9 g/day) compared with women in the lowest quintile (median 11.5 g/day). Among different sources of dietary fibre, only cereal fibre was strongly associated with a reduced risk of cardiovascular events. Male health professionals have been followed in a similar study.[49] Their food habits were assessed using a 131-item food frequency questionnaire. During 6 years of follow-up there were 511 non-fatal cases of MI and 229 coronary deaths. The age-adjusted relative risk of MI for the top quintile of total dietary fibre intake was 0.64 (median intake 28.9 g/day) compared with men in the lowest quintile (median intake 12.4 g/day). Cereal fibre was most strongly associated with a reduced risk of MI compared with other fibre sources like vegetables and fruits. Thus, the same associations were found for male health professionals as for female health professionals. In the study on female health professionals, an inverse relation between both soluble and insoluble fibre and the risk of cardiovascular diseases and MI was also found, but after multivariate adjustments the associations were no longer significant.[50]

More data on the effect of dietary fibre on cardiovascular diseases have been gained from intervention trials. Over 50 studies have investigated the effect of β-glucans on blood cholesterol levels. Some investigators have also addressed the task to make overall evaluations on the relation between oat β-glucan intake and its cholesterol-lowering effects. A large meta-analysis of oat products and their lowering effects on plasma cholesterol was made by Ripsin *et al.*[51] The included studies presented differences in study designs, oat products, doses of oats and control products, and subjects with different initial cholesterol levels, gender and age; the influence of these parameters was assessed in the meta-analysis. To be included in the meta-analysis, studies had to be controlled and randomized and the control product had to have a low soluble fibre content. Moreover, the trial should also have included a dietary assessment and measurement of body weight. Twelve trials were included in the calculation of the summary effect size.[51] Most of the trials used a parallel design and the length of the treatment phase varied between 18 days and 12 weeks. The summary effect size for change in total cholesterol was –0.13 mmol/l. The initial cholesterol level was highly predictive of the reduction in total cholesterol level while age and gender could not predict the response to oats. The dose–response effect was also evaluated and, after dividing the material into intakes of $<3$ g and $\geq 3$ g of soluble fibre, the interaction was statistically significant. Mälkki[52] also evaluated the dose–response effect of oats. She identified 53 clinical trials, and 37 of them showed significant reductions in blood cholesterol levels after consumption of oat products while in 10 studies no significant effects were detected. The dose–response effect was not very obvious. The Food and Drug Administration (FDA) reviewed 37 oat trials and 17 studies showed a positive effect of oat bran and oat meal on total and LDL cholesterol.[53] The amount of oat bran or oat meal given in the studies ranged from 34 g (2.5 g soluble fibre) to 123 g (10.3 g soluble fibre). Five studies showed equivocal results in reducing serum cholesterol, 4 had too short a study period and 11 showed no effect on serum lipid levels. However, the overall conclusion was that oats could lower serum cholesterol levels, specifically LDL cholesterol, without any significant change in the high-density lipoprotein (HDL) fraction. The FDA thus authorized a health claim stating: 'Diets high in oat bran or oat meal and low in saturated fat and cholesterol may reduce the risk of heart disease.' To be able to use the health claim a product must contain at least 0.75 g β-glucan soluble fibre per serving and the recommended daily intake is 3 g.[53] It is known that the cholesterol-lowering effect is larger in subjects with increased cholesterol levels. Ripsin *et al.*[51] indicated that if the initial cholesterol levels were over 5.9 mmol/l the reduction was larger. The molecular weight of the β-glucans may also be of importance for the cholesterol-lowering effects. In one study an intake of 5.9 g β-glucan from oat bran incorporated into bread and cookies did not have any significant effect on blood lipids while an intake of 5 g β-glucans mixed in orange juice significantly lowered LDL cholesterol compared with a control group.[54] The molecular weight of the β-glucans was lower in the bread compared with the muffins and the preparation mixed with orange juice. However, the molecular weight is probably not the only important factor for the cholesterol-reducing potential. In another trial an oat drink containing β-glucans of rather low molecular weight (peak molecular weight 82 400) was compared with a control drink with low β-glucans content.[55] The intake of oat drink (3.8 g β-glucan/day) resulted in significantly lower cholesterol (6%) and LDL cholesterol (6%) levels compared with the control drink and, thus, the oat drink had the expected quantitative cholesterol-lowering effects as in products containing β-glucans with a higher molecular weight. One explanation for the results could be that the β-glucans were in a soluble form. Önning[56] compared the method for administration of β-glucans in 17 human studies that included hyperlipidaemic subjects. The total cholesterol level at the end of the intervention period in the control group was between 5.9 and 7.4 mmol/l. The change in total cholesterol in the oat group in comparison with the control group varied from 0 to –13% while the change in LDL cholesterol varied from 0 to –16.5%. The studies with the largest reductions incorporated the oats in crisps, hot cereals, muffins and beverages while in the studies with small reductions the oats were given in cold cereals and also in bread. Inclusion of the β-glucans in liquid foods and also using some heat treatment seemed to increase the lipid-lowering effect probably by increasing the solubility of the β-glucans. The fact that the solubility of the β-glucans varies a lot in foods was confirmed in a study by Lia Amundsen *et al.*[57] Products like bread, teacakes, muesli, muffins, macaroni, pasta and apple drinks were supplemented with an oat bran concentrate and the solubility of the β-glucans varied from 22% in pasta to 70% in the apple drink. Thus, the solubility of the β-glucans in the products was rather low (mean value of about 50%) but the daily dose of soluble β-glucans consumed by hypercholesterolaemic subjects (2.7 g) was still high enough to significantly decrease blood cholesterol levels compared with a control diet. The molecular weight and the solubility of the β-glucans used in human studies have seldom been documented and this makes it difficult to compare results from different studies in relation to the doses used.

Several mechanisms have been proposed for the cholesterol-lowering effects of β-glucans. The main hypothesis is that they decrease the intestinal uptake of bile acids. In subjects with ileostomy, intake of oat bran bread lead to an increased excretion of chenodeoxycholic acid and total bile acids in comparison with intake of wheat flour bread.[58] A recent study focused on the effects of oat β-glucans incorporated into a drink on cholesterol absorption (measurement of plant sterols) and cholesterol synthesis (analysis of lathosterol) in humans.[59] Intake of 5 g β-glucan daily led to a significant decrease in serum total and LDL cholesterol levels and, at the same time, the concentration of lathosterol was increased and that of sitosterol was decreased. This indicates that β-glucans reduce cholesterol absorption in the intestine.

Furthermore, β-glucans are fermented in the colon and the short-chain fatty acids produced may influence cholesterol metabolism in the liver. However, only a few human studies exist on this subject and more studies are needed to evaluate this effect. Soluble fibre can also decrease gastric emptying, prolong glucose absorption and increase insulin sensitivity. These changes can also have an effect on lipid metabolism in the liver. In animals the main outcome of the action of fibre is a lowering of hepatic cholesterol pools as a result of more cholesterol being diverted to bile acid synthesis and lower cholesterol delivery to the liver through chylomicron remnants.[60]

## 6.5 Effects of β-glucans on energy and carbohydrate metabolism

β-Glucan has been suspected of influencing glucose metabolism by modulation of glycaemia or insulin response to a meal. It works by slowing the rate of nutrient absorption leading to a smaller increase in glycaemia and insulinaemia whenever nutrients are ingested concomitantly with β-glucans as opposed to without β-glucans.[61] A study by Battilana *et al.*[62] performed in healthy subjects was designed to observe the action of β-glucans on post-prandial metabolism independently of a delayed absorption effect. The absence of any relevant effect in this case led the authors to conclude that the action of β-glucans after a single meal was mainly due to their delaying the rate of carbohydrate absorption. In addition, it is known that β-glucans taken in a meal increase the viscosity of the meal bolus, thereby reducing the rate of absorption and flattening post-prandial glycaemia. In fact, the viscosity of fibres relates positively with the degree of flattening of post-prandial glycaemia.[63–66] In epidemiological studies, the precise type of fibre ingested is seldom reported but could be important to record. Few studies have been published comparing the differential effects of fermentable and non-fermentable fibres on energy intake and metabolism. Howarth *et al.*[67] did not find any differential effects of fermentable fibres versus non-fermentable fibres (taken as a supplement in flavoured water before the meal) on energy intake or changes in body fatness in a population whose body mass index (BMI) ranged from 20 to 34 kg/m$^2$. However, in animal models, fermentable fibres enhanced satiety to a greater extent. Therefore, a greater reduction in energy intake and body fatness over time was expected. A study in which 10 healthy men ingested either a diet with β-glucans or a diet with cellulose failed to produce significantly different effects on plasma glucose and insulin concentrations.[62] In this case, the effects of the specific action of the β-glucans (colic fermentation, production of short-chain fatty acids) did not seem to interfere with carbohydrate metabolism.

The glycaemic index (GI) of the carbohydrate and fibre content can be related since viscous fibres and foods with intact natural cell walls generally have a lower GI.[68] Dietary fibre was shown to account for about 40% of the variance in GI among 18 starchy foods.[69] In fact, epidemiological and intervention studies showed that body weight is positively correlated with GI. Ma *et al.*[68] carried out a study of 572 healthy men, in which BMI was positively associated with GI: a 5-unit increase in GI was significantly associated with a 0.75-unit increase in BMI ($p = 0.01$). Therefore, dietary fibres like β-glucans, which affect food digestion and absorption rate, also affect GI values as a consequence. Jenkins *et al.*[66] found that addition of β-glucans reduces GI (4 units/g) while maintaining palatability.

Some intervention studies have been carried out with specific test products with high β-glucan content to evaluate the glycaemic and insulin responses in healthy and diabetic subjects. It has been shown that 8–10% of β-glucans in cereals can decrease the glycaemia peak by 50%.[70] Juntunen *et al.*[71] showed that the lowered insulin response observed after consumption of different grain products in healthy men was not dependent on the type of cereals. In another study, β-glucan-enriched products consisted of barley-enriched pasta. Healthy men fed barley pasta enriched with β-glucans did not show any difference in glycaemia response but did show a greater insulin response compared with men fed low-fibre-content pasta. This discrepancy between insulin and glycaemia schemes, also found in other studies, indicates a complicated pattern for the effect of fibres on glucose metabolism, which could be modulated by the action of hormones such as cholecystokinin[65] and glucagon-like peptide 1.[71] These intervention studies showed that a high β-glucan content is required to obtain a significant effect on post-prandial glycaemia and insulinaemia in healthy subjects.

The antidiabetic effects of β-glucans have been suspected in response to their actions on energy and glucose metabolism. Longer studies have been designed to observe the beneficial metabolic effects of β-glucans on type 2 diabetes. The risk of developing type 2 diabetes has been shown to be more than twice as high when consuming a diet high in glycaemic load in combination with a low fibre intake.[70,72] Another study has shown that the addition of β-glucan greatly reduced hyperglycaemia but that there was a threshold level for the amount of fibre.[64] In diabetics, β-glucans-enriched diets have also been shown to improve metabolic control with a decrease in haemoglobin A1c (HbA1c).[73,74] However, only a few studies have focused on the specific effects of β-glucans on HbA1c, and no clear and direct correlation has been found to date.[61] Nevertheless, the improved glycaemic control and the reduction of cardiovascular risks (due to lowered blood lipid levels) associated with fibre intake indicate that it could be a recommended part of the diet for subjects with type 2 diabetes.

## 6.6 β-Glucans and weight control

β-Glucans could play a role in body weight regulation through different mechanisms: it increases satiation, decreases the absorption efficiency of the small intestine, regulates glucose and insulin responses, and has beneficial effects on lipid metabolism.

Various epidemiological studies have shown an inverse correlation between fibre intake and body weight, BMI and body fat.[75] In the CARDIA study, a population-based cohort study of the change in cardiovascular risk factors over 10 years, it was shown that dietary fibre was inversely associated with fasting insulin levels (mean difference across quintiles: –5.6 pmol/l, $p = 0.007$ in whites; –9.7 pmol/l in blacks, $p = 0.01$), weight gain (mean difference across quintiles in both populations: –3.65 kg, $p > 0.001$) and other risk factors for cardiovascular diseases in young adults.[76] White men and women consuming diets supposed to be the lowest in GI (high fibre, high fat) had the least weight gain over 10 years compared with those consuming supposedly high-GI diets (low fibre, low fat).

Another epidemiological study carried out on a cohort of 27 802 men demonstrated a reduced risk of weight gain (8 years of observation) associated with increased whole-grain or bran intake.[77] Dietary fibre was inversely related to weight gain independent of whole-grains ($p$ for trend <0.0001). They found that for every 20 g/day increase in dietary fibre, weight gain was reduced by 1.18 kg.

Few intervention studies had been done until 2000 on the effects of fibre on body weight. In fact, the focus was on the use of fibre in enhancing compliance with low-caloric diets designed for weight loss by reducing hunger.[78] Intervention studies performed in healthy, overweight or obese humans led to conflicting results. Some reported no effect on body weight.[66,79] In the study of Nicolosi *et al.*,[79] the subjects had consumed enough energy to maintain their body weight. Some other studies did report an effect of fibre on body weight loss.[80,81] In these last two studies (with demonstrated effects of fibre on body weight loss), fibre supplementation was associated with reduced energy intake and it was not possible to relate the weight loss solely to fibre intake. In addition, no evidence has been shown of an enhanced effect of fibre supplementation compared with caloric restriction alone. It is also interesting to record that a greater suppression of energy intake and a greater weight loss was observed in overweight or obese subjects versus normal-weight subjects: mean energy intake in all studies was reduced to 82% by higher fibre intake in overweight/obese people versus 94% in lean people and body weight loss was 2.4 kg versus 0.8 kg, respectively.[78,82] Fibre supplementation could be considered at the least as a good support for weight loss diets by enhancing satiety. However, more clinical studies are required to determine which kind of fibre and what quantities are suitable for the prevention of weight gain and obesity in different populations.

## 6.7 β-Glucans in the regulation of satiety and acceptance by consumers

A significant number of studies have demonstrated suppressed hunger and greater satiety with fibres that have the viscous-producing property, whereas satiation and gastric fullness may be more closely related to the bulking effects of fibre.[78] The relationship of body weight status and fibre effect on energy intake suggests that obese individuals may be more likely to reduce food intake with dietary fibre inclusion.[78] Dietary fibre plays a role in weight management as a result of its effect on satiety and blood cholesterol.[83] Both soluble and insoluble fibres prolong after-meal satiety, but soluble fibre is more effective. A fibre-rich meal is usually lower in fat and added sugars, is less energy dense and is processed more slowly, which promotes earlier satiety.[83]

The soluble oat β-glucan has been found to have positive effects on health, such as reducing blood cholesterol levels.[49,51] The consumption of a hypocaloric diet containing oats over 6 weeks resulted in a greater decrease in systolic blood pressure, total cholesterol and LDL cholesterol than did a similar diet without oats.[84] Oat β-glucans can also be used in controlling weight. Ingesting oat β-glucans can increase the viscosity of gut contents enhancing the feeling of fullness. Oat β-glucans can lower the rate at which nutrients are absorbed from the small intestine, delay gastric emptying and prolong the feeling of satiety.[65,85,86] The first effect occurs in the stomach, where swelling and water binding by the fibre causes distension that contributes to the feeling of satiety. In the small intestine, fat and protein or amino acids induce release of the gut hormone cholecystokinin, which delays gastric emptying, blunts glycaemic responses and enhances satiety.[87] The effect is believed to be caused by increased viscosity, which increases the contact time of fat and amino acids with receptors. Other dietary fibres and food consistency have been shown to affect the secretion of cholecystokinin.[88,89]

The physiological effects of β-glucans appear to be related to their rheological characteristics. An inverse relationship between the viscosity of oat β-glucans-containing beverages and the levels of both blood glucose and blood insulin has been shown with beverages varying in the dose and molecular weight of oat β-glucan.[63,90] Thus, physiological responses appear to be affected by the concentration and the molecular weight of β-glucans, probably through effects on gut-content viscosity. Owing to its high water-binding capacity β-glucan also affects the structure of food in a similar way to other soluble dietary fibre.[91–94] This in turn could affect the rate of food digestion, especially the susceptibility of the starch component of the food to amylolysis. Thus it is likely that both the viscosity-increasing and structure-modifying properties of β-glucan are involved in the health-promoting effects of β-glucan-rich foods.

The role of dietary fibre in energy intake regulation and weight control is related to the special physical and chemical properties of fibre that promote the feeling of satiation and enhance or prolong the feeling of satiety.[78] Satiation is related to the effects of dietary fibre on structure and energy density of food, whereas the viscosity-increasing effect of soluble fibres may enhance satiety through delayed gastric emptying and subsequent delay in fat absorption. Fat in the intestine stimulates the feeling of satiety whereas diets low in fat and energy are associated with feelings of hunger. In women, incorporation of foods rich in viscous fibres into mixed low-fat meals resulted in suppressed sensation of hunger and enhanced post-meal satiety compared with a low-fat, low-fibre meal of equal energy content and palatability.[78] Plasma cholecystokinin concentrations were elevated and sustained in response to both the low-fat, high-fibre meal and the high-fat, low-fibre meal.[78] Bourden *et al.*[65] have shown a similar cholecystokinin response when viscous fibres were included in a low-fat meal. If inclusion of viscous-type fibres in low-fat diets effectively slows fat absorption and imparts a greater sense of satiety, this would be a promising way to improve compliance with low-fat diets.

Oat β-glucan is already added to some products, mostly cereal products. The mouth feel of oat products is determined by the unbranched polysaccharide, β-glucan, which also significantly influences the flavour release. The special feature of β-glucan is that it forms highly viscous water solutions. The viscosity of food is known to modify the perception of tastes even though the composition of the thickener has been suggested to have a greater effect on the perception of flavours than the viscosity.[95–98] A negative correlation has been reported between the intensities of flavour attributes and the viscosity of oat β-glucan-enriched soups.[99]

Generally, European consumers seem to know current dietary recommendations rather well. However, the reasons for healthy eating may vary for different people. Healthy food can be chosen for many reasons such as to prevent chronic diseases, to improve general well-being, or for ideological or moral reasons. Preventing disease or getting help for a particular health problem are the most frequently cited reasons for healthy eating.[100–102] The potential benefits of healthy eating only affect behaviour if a person feels it is relevant for him-/herself, is motivated and has sufficient knowledge to change his/her behaviour.[103] If the person is motivated, e.g. has a need to pay attention to their blood pressure, then the information concerning the health-benefit effects of a given product may encourage them to try products that promise to affect blood pressure. There are limitations in the use of information when functional foods are marketed to consumers. Health-related claims are not allowed to promise the curing, treating or prevention of diseases. However, the claims can include statements regarding reducing risk of disease and improved state of health.[104] Urala *et al.*[105] found health-related claims to be advantageous for the products used in their study. However, when the strength of the claims was increased by promising stronger and more definite effects for the consumers, it did not automatically increase the perceived benefit of the product.

Factors affecting consumers' willingness to use beverages and ready-to-eat frozen soups containing oat β-glucan have been studied in Finland, France and Sweden.[106] The presence of a health claim (concerning either cholesterol or glucose) significantly increased the perceived benefit and willingness of the consumers to use the soups and beverages before tasting the sample. Although, the perceived benefit of the β-glucan sample with the health claim decreased after tasting, it was rated either higher (in the glucose-claim subgroup) or equal (in the cholesterol-claim subgroup) in perceived benefit after tasting than the sample without β-glucan. Respondents in both the cholesterol-claim subgroup and the glucose-claim subgroup rated samples similarly in different countries. In general, health claims (glucose or cholesterol claims) had a small positive impact on willingness to use beverages and soups containing β-glucan, but the taste of the products strongly affected the willingness to use them.[106] β-glucan affected the mouth feel of both the beverages and soups. Although, β-glucan addition altered the sensory characteristics of both the beverages and soups, liking for soups, benefit perceived and willingness to use the soups were not remarkably lower in β-glucan soups than in soups without β-glucan. Thus, in the first instance the taste of the product must be pleasing taste, and then health effects can give added value to the product.

## 6.8 Use of β-glucans in food products

It is well known that the source (e.g. species), processing treatments (e.g. milling, temperature, pH effects) and interactions with other constituents in the source – and then in a composite food matrix – are likely to influence structural features, concentration and dispersibility–solubility of β-glucans and so modulate their physiological action. β-Glucans enrichment in some products, leading to concentrated products, has increasingly been studied because it allows a larger β-glucan intake per serving with a minimum decrease in palatability and an increase in volume ingested.[66] In most intervention studies, specific concentrated or processed products have been used, whereas commercially available foods are seldom used.[61] Several studies have shown the advantages of enrichment of oat products in achieving physiological effects. In fact, greater beneficial effects are obtained with these enriched products than with products naturally high in β-glucan.[66] Moreover, the use of β-glucan concentrates in processed food such as muesli bars, pasta, and cereal does not drastically reduce the efficacy of reducing post-prandial glycaemia.[66]

The sensory properties of β-glucan, especially its high viscosity, influence the sensory quality of the products. Positive health effects of products may not guarantee that the product is chosen repeatedly if its sensory quality is not adequate. Taste pleasantness has been found to be the most important factor affecting food choice of novel foods and food choices overall.[107–109] Their good viscosity-forming properties make β-glucans potential alternatives as thickening agents in different food applications, e.g. ice creams, sauces and salad dressings.[110] Compared with other thickening agents, oat gum was less viscous than xanthan and guar at 0.5%, but slightly more viscous than locust bean gum at the same concentration.[111] To make the daily consumption of the FDA-recommended four portions of 0.75 g β-glucan feasible, new types of β-glucan-containing foods need to be developed in addition to cereal products where β-glucan is an intrinsic component. One option for these new products is frozen, ready-to-eat foods, as the consumption of these is growing in general.[112] Frozen ready-to-eat soups are one possible product category, where β-glucan could be used as a thickening agent.[99]

β-glucan is suitable for a wide range of food products, because, being a neutral and non-ionic polymer, its viscosity is not affected by pH.[111] As the viscosity of β-glucan reversibly decreases with increased temperature, warm food products would be ideal products for enrichment with β-glucan.[111,113] In warm foods the concentration of β-glucan could be higher than in cold foods because the product would have decreased sensory thickness during eating or drinking as a result of increased temperature. Technologically, more-processed β-glucan preparations are easier to add into foods in amounts sufficient for achieving a physiologically functional amount of β-glucan in a product. However, the relationship between physiological functionality and molecular weight has to be kept in mind.

The effects of different β-glucan preparations on the sensory texture and instrumental viscosity of beverage prototypes and soups have been evaluated.[99,114] The results showed that both the type and concentration of β-glucan are important in determining the characteristics of foods. Different β-glucan preparations gave different viscosities (both sensory and instrumental) in beverages and soups containing the same amount of β-glucan. The effect was dependent on the molecular weight of the soluble fibre. Currently, the focus of the food-related industries is on developing new foods with sufficient β-glucans content, maintained viscosity and good palatability, in order to facilitate long-term intake and effectiveness. The appearance of new products combining health potential and high acceptability is very important and depends, in the case of cereals, on the development of new processing technologies and improved knowledge of fibre distribution in the matrix.[115] In an EU project entitled 'Design of foods with improved functionality and superior health effects using cereal β-glucans (QLK1-2000-00535)', different foods that normally do not contain cereals were enriched with β-glucans and the health effects were documented.

## 6.9 Future trends

β-Glucan has been intensively studied because of its ability to regulate glucose and insulin levels as well as cholesterol and body weight. Cereals rich in β-glucans may thus be useful nutritional tools to better control different metabolic disorders. One problem, however, is that the acceptability of these products – and hence compliance – is too low for many consumers. This could be improved by offering a wider range of foods enriched in β-glucans. Extended work is still needed from research groups to determine the precise molecular pathways of the action of β-glucans on carbohydrate metabolism and to understand the potential interactions with the other components of the food matrix and their consequences. Rather than relying solely on the effects of β-glucan on body composition a wider approach is needed: the combination of increased consumption of dietary fibre with incorporation of low-GI foods, physical activity and a balanced diet, could help in weight control, and obesity and type 2 diabetes management. In parallel, food industries have to integrate all this information in the development of new products with health potential and high palatability.

## 6.10 Acknowledgements

This chapter was written by a consortium involved in the EU project 'Design of foods with improved functionality and superior health effects using cereal β-glucans (QLK1-2000-00535).'

## 6.11 References

1 AACC (American Association of Cereal Chemists) (2001), The definition of dietary fibre, *Cereal Foods World*, **46** (3), 112–126.
2 DELMER D P (1987), Cellulose biosynthesis, *Annu. Rev. Plant Physiol.*, **38**, 258–290.
3 SHIBUYA N and MISAKI A (1978), Polysaccharides and glycoproteins in the rice endosperm cell wall, *Agric. Biol. Chem.*, **42**, 2267–2274.
4 GENC H, ÖZDEMIR M and DEMIRBAS A (2001), Analysis of mixed-linked ($1 \rightarrow 3$, $1 \rightarrow 4$)-β-glucans in cereal grains from Turkey, *Food Chem.*, **73**, 221–224.

5 AUTIO K (2001), Light microscopic investigation on dietary fibre, in *Advanced Dietary Fibre Technology*, Eds McCleary B and Prosky L, Blackwell Publishing Ltd, Ames, Iowa, pp. 25–29.

6 HELLWEG J H, MCKEEHEN J D and DIETSCH M (2005), Methods for preparing oat bran enriched in beta-glucan and oat products prepared therefrom, Patent Application.

7 MALKKI Y, MYLLYMAKI O, TEINILA K and KOPONEN S (2003), Method for preparing an oat product and a foodstuff enriched in the content of beta-glucan, US Patent 6,797,307.

8 FOEHSE K B (1991), Method of dry milling and preparing high soluble fibre barley fraction, US Patent 5,063,078.

9 KIRYLUK J, KAWKA A, GASIOROWSKI H, CHALCARZ A and ANIOLA J (2000), Milling of barley to obtain β-glucan enriched products, *Nahrung*, **44** (4), 238–241.

10 KIANIAN S F, PHILLIPS R L, RINES H W, FULCHER R G, WEBSTER F H and STUTHMAN D D (2000), Quantitative trait loci influencing β-glucan content in oat (*Avena sativa*, 2n = 6x = 42), *Theor. Appl. Genet.*, **101**, 1039–1048.

11 WELCH R W, BROWN J C and LEGGETT J M (2000), Interspecific and intraspecific variation in grain and groat characteristics of wild oat (Avena) species: very high groat (1 → 93, 1 → 4)-β-D-glucan in an *Avena atlantica* genotype, *J. Cereal Sci.*, **31**, 273–279.

12 FDA (Food and Drug Administration) (2006), Food labeling: Health claims; soluble fibre from certain foods and risk for coronary heart disease, Final rule, *Fed. Regist.*, May 22, **71** (98), 29248–29250.

13 JASKARI J, KONTULA P, SITONEN A, JOUSIMIES-SOMER M, MAT-TILA-SANDHOLM T and POUTANEN K (1998), Oat β-glucan and xylan hydrolysates as selective substrates for Bifidobacterium and Lactobacillus strains, *Appl. Microbiol. Biotechnol.*, **49**, 175–181.

14 SHIBUYA N and MINAMI E (2001), Oligosaccharide signalling for defense responses in plant, *Physiol. Molecul. Plant Pathol.*, **59**, 223–233.

15 MÅRTENSSON O, BIÖRKLUND M, LAMBO A, DUENAS-CHASCO M, IRASTORZA A, HOLST O, NORIN E, WELLING G, ÖSTE R and ÖNNING G (2005), Fermented, ropy, oat-based products reduce cholesterol levels and stimulate the bifidobacteria flora in humans, *Nutr. Res.*, **25**, 429–442.

16 MANZI P and PIZZOFERRATO L (2000), Beta-glucans in edible mushrooms, *Food Chemistry*, **68**, 315–318.

17 SELBMANN L, STINGELE F and PETRUCCIOLLI M (2003), Exo-polysaccharide production by filamentous fungi: the example of Botryo-sphaeria rhodina, *Ant. Van Leeuwenh*, **84**, 135–145.

18 BABINEAU T J, HACKFORD A, KENLER A, BISTRIAN B, FORSE R A, FAIRCHILD P G, HEARD S, KEROACK M, CAUSHAJ P and BENOTTI P (1994), A phase II multicenter, double-blind, randomized, placebo-controlled study of three dosages of an immunomodulator (PGG-glucan) in high-risk surgical patients, *Arch. Surg.*, **129**, 1204–1210.

19 WOODWARD J R, FINCHER G B and STONE B A (1983), Water-soluble (1 → 3),(1 → 4)-β-D-glucans from barley (Hordeum vulgare) endosperm. II. Fine structure, *Carbohydr. Polym.*, **3**, 207–225.

20 DAIS P and PERLIN A S (1982), High-field, $^{13}$C-N.M.R. spectroscopy of β-D-glucans, amylopectin, and glycogen, *Carbohydr. Res.*, **100**, 103–116.

21 IZYDORCZYK M S, MACRI L J and MACGREGOR A W (1998), Structure and physicochemical properties of barley non-starch polysaccharides – II. Alkali-extractable β-glucans and arabinoxylans, *Carbohydr. Polym.*, **35**, 259–269.

22 VARUM K M and SMIDSROD O (1988), Partial chemical and physical characterization of (1 → 3),(1 → 4)-β-D-glucans from oat (Avena sativa L.) aleurone, *Carbohydr. Polym.*, **9**, 103–117.

23 WOOD P J, WEISZ J, and BLACKWELL B A (1991), Molecular characterization of cereal β-D-glucans. Structural analysis of oat β-D-glucan and rapid structural evaluation of β-D-glucans from different sources by high-performance liquid chromatography of oligosaccharides released by lichenase, *Cereal Chem.*, **68**, 31–39.
24 WOOD P J, WEISZ J, and BLACKWELL B A (1994), Structural studies of (1 → 3)(1 → 4)-β-D-glucans by $^{13}$C-nuclear magnetic resonance spectroscopy and by rapid analysis of cellulose-like regions using high-performance anion-exchange chromatography of oligosaccharides released by lichenase, *Cereal Chem.*, **71**, 301–307.
25 WOODWARD J R, PHILLIPS D R and FINCHER G B (1988), Water-soluble (1 → 3, 1 → 4)-β-D-glucans from barley (Hordeum vulgare) endosperm. IV. Comparison of 40 °C and 65 °C soluble fractions, *Carbohydr. Polym.*, **8**, 85–97.
26 BULIGA G S, BRANT D A and FINCHER G B (1986), The sequence statistics and solution conformation of a barley (1 → 3, 1 → 4)-β-D-glucan, *Carbohydr. Res.*, **157**, 139–156.
27 IZYDORCZYK M S, MACRI L J and MACGREGOR A W (1998), Structure and physicochemical properties of barley non-starch polysaccharides – I. Water-extractable β-glucans and arabinoxylans, *Carbohydr. Polym.*, **35**, 249–258.
28 IZYDORCZYK M S, JACOBS M and DEXTER J E (2003), Distribution and structural variation of nonstarch polysaccharides in milling fractions of hull-less barley with variable amylose content, *Cereal Chem.*, **80**, 645–653.
29 CUI W, WOOD P J, BLACKWELL B and NIKIFORUK J (2000), Phy-sicochemical properties and structural characterization by two-dimensional NMR spectroscopy of wheat β-D-glucan – comparison with other cereal β-D-glucans, *Carbohydr. Polym.*, **41**, 249–258.
30 IZYDORCZYK M S, BILIADERIS C G, MACRI L J and MACGREGOR A W (1998), Fractionation of oat (1 → 3), (1 → 4)-β-D-glucans and characterization of the fractions, *J. Cereal Sci.*, **27**, 321–325.
31 STORSLEY J M, IZYDORCZYK M S, YOU S, BILIADERIS C G and ROSSNAGEL B (2003), Structure and physicochemical properties of β-glucans and arabinoxylans isolated from hull-less barley, *Food Hydrocoll.*, **17**, 831–844.
32 BOHM N and KULICKE W M (1999), Rheological studies of barley (1 → 3)(1 → 4)-β-D-glucan in concentrated solution: investigation of the visco-elastic flow behaviour in the sol state, *Carbohydr. Res.*, **315**, 293–301.
33 GOMEZ C, NAVARRO A, GARNIER C, HORTA A and CARBONELL J V (1997), Physical and structural properties of barley (1 → 3), (1 → 4)-β-D-glucan. Part III. Formation of aggregates analysed through its viscoelastic and flow behavior, *Carbohydr. Polym.*, **34**, 141–148.
34 LAZARIDOU A, BILIADERIS C G and IZYDORCZYK M S (2003), Molecular size effects on rheological properties of oat β-glucans in solutions and gels, *Food Hydrocoll.*, **17**, 693–712.
35 LAZARIDOU A, BILIADERIS C G, MICHA-SCRETTAS M and STEELE B R (2004), A comparative study on structure–function relations of mixed linkage (1 → 3), (1 → 4) linear β-D-glucans, *Food Hydrocoll.*, **18**, 837–855.
36 TOSH S M, WOOD P J and WANG Q (2003), Gelation characteristics of acid-hydrolyzed oat beta-glucan solutions solubilized at a range of temperatures, *Food Hydrocoll.*, **17**, 523–527.
37 VAIKOUSI H, BILIADERIS C G and IZYDORCZYK M S (2004), Solution flow behavior and gelling properties of water-soluble barley (1 → 3, 1 → 4)-β-glucans varying in molecular size, *J. Cereal Sci.*, **39**, 119–137.
38 SKENDI A, BILIADERIS C G, LAZARIDOU A and IZYDORCZYK M S (2003), Structure and rheological properties of water soluble β-glucans from oat cultivars of Avena sativa and Avena bysantina, *J. Cereal Sci.*, **38**, 15–31.

39 BOHM N and KULICKE W M (1999), Rheological studies of barley (1 → 3)(1 .020 4)-β-D-glucan in concentrated solution: mechanistic and kinetic investigation of the gel formation, *Carbohydr. Res.*, **315**, 302–311.

40 CUI W and WOOD P J (2000), Relationships between structural features, molecular weight and rheological properties of cereal β-D-glucan, in *Hydrocolloids – Part 1 Physical Chemistry and Industrial Applications of Gels, Polysaccharides and Proteins*, Ed. Nishinari K, Elsevier Science B. V, Amsterdam, pp. 159–168.

41 IRAKLI M, BILIADERIS C G, IZYDORCZYK M S and PAPADOYANNIS I N (2004), Isolation, structural features and rheological properties of water-extractable β-glucans from different Greek barley cultivars, *J. Sci. Food Agric.*, **84**, 1170–1178.

42 LAZARIDOU A and BILIADERIS C G (2004), Cryogelation of cereal β-glucans: structure and molecular size effects, *Food Hydrocoll.*, **18**, 933–947.

43 PAPAGEORGIOU M, LAKHDARAB N, LAZARIDOU A, BILIADERIS C G and IZYDORCZYK M S (2005), Water extractable (1 → 3, 1 → 4)-β-D-glucans from barley and oats: An intervarietal study on their structural features and rheological behaviour, *J. Cereal Sci.*, **42**, 213–224.

44 TOSH S M, BRUMMER Y, WOOD P J, WANG Q and WEISZ J (2004), Evaluation of structure in the formation of gels by structurally diverse (1 → 3)(1 → 4)-β-D-glucans from four cereal and one lichen species, *Carbohydr. Polym.*, **57**, 249–259.

45 VAIKOUSI H and BILIADERIS C G (2005), Processing and formulation effects on rheological behavior of barley β-glucan aqueous dispersions, *Food Chem.*, **91**, 505–516.

46 DOUBLIER J L and WOOD P J (1995), Rheological properties of aqueous solutions of (1-3)(1-4)-β-D-glucan from oats (Avena sativa L.). *Cereal Chem.*, **72**, 335–340.

47 TOSH S M, WOOD P J, WANG Q and WEISZ J (2004), Structural characteristics and rheological properties of partially hydrolyzed oat β-glucan: the effects of molecular weight and hydrolysis method, *Carbohydr. Polym.*, **55**, 425–436.

48 WOLK A, MANSON J E, STAMPFER M J, COLDITZ G A, HU F B, SPEIZER F E, HENNEKENS C H and WILLETT W C (1999), Long-term intake of dietary fibre and decreased risk of coronary heart disease among women, *JAMA*, **281** (21), 1998–2004.

49 RIMM E B, ASCHERIO A, GIOVANNUCCI E, SPIEGELMAN D, STAMPFER M J and WILLETT W C (1996), Vegetable, fruit, and cereal fibre intake and risk of coronary heart disease among men, *JAMA*, **275** (6), 447–451.

50 LIU S, BURING J E, SESSO H D, RIMM E B, WILLETT W C and MANSON J E (2002), A prospective study of dietary fibre intake and risk of cardiovascular disease among women, *J. Am. Coll. Cardiol.*, **39** (1), 49–56.

51 RIPSIN C M, KEENAN J M, JACOBS D R, JR, ELMER P J, WELCH R R, VAN HORN L, LIU K, TURNBULL W H, THYE F W, KESTIN M *et al.* (1992), Oat products and lipid lowering. A meta-analysis, *JAMA*, **267** (24), 3317–3325.

52 MÄLKKI Y (2001), Oat fibres: production, composition, physico-chemical properties, physiological effects, safety and food applications, in *Handbook of Dietary Fibre*, Eds Cho S S and Dreher M, Marcel Dekker Inc., New York, pp. 497–517.

53 FDA (Food and Drug Administration) (1996), Food labeling: Health claims; oats and coronary heart disease, *Fed. Regis.*, **61**, 296.

54 KERCKHOFFS D A, HORNSTRA G and MENSINK R P (2003), Cholesterol-lowering effect of beta-glucan from oat bran in mildly hypercholesterolemic subjects

may decrease when beta-glucan is incorporated into bread and cookies, *Am. J. Clin. Nutr.*, **78** (2), 221–227.
55 ONNING G, WALLMARK A, PERSSON M, AKESSON B, ELMSTAHL S and OSTE R (1999), Consumption of oat milk for 5 weeks lowers serum cholesterol and LDL cholesterol in free-living men with moderate hypercholesterolemia, *Ann. Nutr. Metab.*, **43** (5), 301–309.
56 ÖNNING G (2004), Cereal beta-glucans as a functional ingredient to control diabetes and cardiovascular disease, in *Functional Foods, Diet, Cardiovascular Disease and Diabetes*, Woodhead Publishing Ltd, Cambridge, UK.
57 LIA AMUNDSEN Å, HAUGUM B and ANDERSSON H (2003), Changes in serum cholesterol and sterol metabolites after intake of products enriched with an oat bran concentrate within a controlled diet, *Scand. J. Nutr.*, **47**, 68–74.
58 LIA A, HALLMANS G, SANDBERG A S, SUNDBERG B, AMAN P and ANDERSSON H (1995), Oat beta-glucan increases bile acid excretion and a fibre-rich barley fraction increases cholesterol excretion in ileostomy subjects, *Am. J. Clin. Nutr.*, **62** (6), 1245–1251.
59 NAUMANN E, VAN REES A B, ÖNNING G, ÖSTE R, WYDRA M and MENSINK R P (2006), β-Glucan incorporated into a fruit drink reduces serum concentrations of total and LDL cholesterol at least in part by reducing cholesterol absorption, *Am. J. Clin. Nutr.*, **83** (3), 601–605.
60 FERNANDEZ M L (2001), Soluble fibre and nondigestible carbohydrate effects on plasma lipids and cardiovascular risk, *Curr. Opin. Lipidol.*, **12** (1), 35–40.
61 BIORKLUND M (2005), Health effects of foods enriched with beta-glucans from cereals, PhD thesis, Lund University, Lund.
62 BATTILANA P, ORNSTEIN K, MINEHIRA K, SCHWARZ J M, ACHESON K, SCHNEITER P, BURRI J, JEQUIER E and TAPPY L (2001), Mechanisms of action of beta-glucan in postprandial glucose metabolism in healthy men, *Eur. J. Clin. Nutr.*, **55** (5), 327–333.
63 WOOD P J, BRAATEN J T, SCOTT F W, RIEDEL K D, WOLYNETZ M S and COLLINS M W (1994), Effect of dose and modification of viscous properties of oat gum on plasma glucose and insulin following an oral glucose load, *Br. J. Nutr.*, **72** (5), 731–743.
64 TAPPY L, GUGOLZ E and WURSCH P (1996), Effects of breakfast cereals containing various amounts of beta-glucan fibres on plasma glucose and insulin responses in NIDDM subjects, *Diabetes Care*, **19** (8), 831–834.
65 BOURDON I, YOKOYAMA W, DAVIS P, HUDSON C, BACKUS R, RICHTER D, KNUCKLES B and SCHNEEMAN B O (1999), Postprandial lipid, glucose, insulin, and cholecystokinin responses in men fed barley pasta enriched with beta-glucan, *Am. J. Clin. Nutr.*, **69** (1), 55–63.
66 JENKINS A L, JENKINS D J, ZDRAVKOVIC U, WURSCH P and VUKSAN V (2002), Depression of the glycemic index by high levels of beta-glucan fibre in two functional foods tested in type 2 diabetes, *Eur. J. Clin. Nutr.*, **56** (7), 622–628.
67 HOWARTH N C, SALTZMAN E, MCCRORY M A, GREENBERG A S, DWYER J, AUSMAN L, KRAMER D G and ROBERTS S B (2003), Fermentable and nonfermentable fibre supplements did not alter hunger, satiety or body weight in a pilot study of men and women consuming self-selected diets, *J. Nutr.*, **133** (10), 3141–3144.
68 MA Y, OLENDZKI B, CHIRIBOGA D, HEBERT J R, LI Y, LI W, CAMPBELL M, GENDREAU K and OCKENE I S (2005), Association between dietary carbohydrates and body weight, *Am. J. Epidemiol.*, **161** (4), 359–367.
69 TROUT D L, BEHALL K M and OSILESI O (1993), Prediction of glycemic index for starchy foods, *Am. J. Clin. Nutr.*, **58** (6), 873–878.

70 WURSCH P and PI-SUNYER F X (1997), The role of viscous soluble fibre in the metabolic control of diabetes. A review with special emphasis on cereals rich in beta-glucan, *Diabetes Care*, **20** (11), 1774–1780.

71 JUNTUNEN K S, NISKANEN L K, LIUKKONEN K H, POUTANEN K S, HOLST J J and MYKKANEN H M (2002), Postprandial glucose, insulin, and incretin responses to grain products in healthy subjects, *Am. J. Clin. Nutr.*, **75** (2), 254–262.

72 SALMERON J, ASCHERIO A, RIMM E B, COLDITZ G A, SPIEGELMAN D, JENKINS D J, STAMPFER M J, WING A L and WILLETT W C (1997), Dietary fibre, glycemic load, and risk of NIDDM in men, *Diabetes Care*, **20** (4), 545–550.

73 BRAATEN J T, SCOTT F W, WOOD P J, RIEDEL K D, WOLYNETZ M S, BRULE D and COLLINS M W (1994), High beta-glucan oat bran and oat gum reduce post-prandial blood glucose and insulin in subjects with and without type 2 diabetes, *Diabet. Med.*, **11** (3), 312–318.

74 REYNA N Y, CANO C, BERMUDEZ V J, MEDINA M T, SOUKI A J, AMBARD M, NUNEZ M, FERRER M A and INGLETT G E (2003), Sweeteners and beta-glucans improve metabolic and anthropometrics variables in well controlled type 2 diabetic patients, *Am. J. Ther.*, **10** (6), 438–443.

75 SLAVIN J L (2005), Dietary fibre and body weight, *Nutrition*, **21** (3), 411–418.

76 LUDWIG D S, PEREIRA M A, KROENKE C H, HILNER J E, VAN HORN L, SLATTERY M L and JACOBS D R, JR. (1999), Dietary fibre, weight gain, and cardiovascular disease risk factors in young adults, *JAMA*, **282** (16), 1539–1546.

77 KOH-BANERJEE P, FRANZ M, SAMPSON L, LIU S, JACOBS D R, JR, SPIEGELMAN D, WILLETT W and RIMM E (2004), Changes in whole-grain, bran, and cereal fibre consumption in relation to 8-y weight gain among men, *Am. J. Clin. Nutr.*, **80** (5), 1237–1245.

78 BURTON-FREEMAN B (2000), Dietary fibre and energy regulation, *J. Nutr.*, **130** (2S Suppl.), 272S–275S.

79 NICOLOSI R, BELL S J, BISTRIAN B R, GREENBERG I, FORSE R A and BLACKBURN G L (1999), Plasma lipid changes after supplementation with beta-glucan fibre from yeast, *Am. J. Clin. Nutr.*, **70** (2), 208–212.

80 THOMPSON W G, ROSTAD HOLDMAN N, JANZOW D J, SLEZAK J M, MORRIS K L and ZEMEL M B (2005), Effect of energy-reduced diets high in dairy products and fibre on weight loss in obese adults, *Obes. Res.*, **13** (8), 1344–1353.

81 BIRKETVEDT G S, AASETH J, FLORHOLMEN J R and RYTTIG K (2000), Long-term effect of fibre supplement and reduced energy intake on body weight and blood lipids in overweight subjects, *Acta Medica (Hradec Kralove)*, **43** (4), 129–132.

82 HOWARTH N C, SALTZMAN E and ROBERTS S B (2001), Dietary fibre and weight regulation, *Nutr. Rev.*, **59** (5), 129–139.

83 MARLETT J A, MCBURNEY M I and SLAVIN J L (2002), Position of the American Dietetic Association: health implications of dietary fibre, *J. Am. Diet. Assoc.*, **102** (7), 993–1000.

84 SALTZMAN E, DAS S K, LICHTENSTEIN A H, DALLAL G E, CORRALES A, SCHAEFER E J, GREENBERG A S and ROBERTS S B (2001), An oat-containing hypocaloric diet reduces systolic blood pressure and improves lipid profile beyond effects of weight loss in men and women, *J. Nutr.*, **131** (5), 1465–1470.

85 EDWARDS C A, JOHNSON I T and READ N W (1988), Do viscous polysaccharides slow absorption by inhibiting diffusion or convection?, *Eur. J. Clin. Nutr.*, **42** (4), 307–312.

86 LUND E K, GEE J M, BROWN J C, WOOD P J and JOHNSON I T (1989), Effect of oat gum on the physical properties of the gastrointestinal contents and on the uptake of d-galactose and cholesterol by rat small intestine in vitro, *Br. J. Nutr.*, **62** (1), 91–101.

87 HOLT S, BRAND J, SOVENY C and HANSKY J (1992), Relationship of satiety to postprandial glycaemic, insulin and cholecystokinin responses, *Appetite*, **18** (2), 129–141.
88 BOURDON I, OLSON B, BACKUS R, RICHTER B D, DAVIS P A and SCHNEEMAN B O (2001), Beans, as a source of dietary fiber, increase cholecystokinin and apolipoprotein B48 response to test meals in men, *J. Nutr.*, **131** (5), 1485–1490.
89 SANTANGELO A, PERACCHI M, CONTE D, FRAQUELLI M and PORRINI M (1998), Physical state of meal affects gastric emptying, cholecystokinin release and satiety, *Br. J. Nutr.*, **80** (6), 521–527.
90 WOOD P J, BEER M U and BUTLER G (2000), Evaluation of role of concentration and molecular weight of oat beta-glucan in determining effect of viscosity on plasma glucose and insulin following an oral glucose load, *Br. J. Nutr.*, **84** (1), 19–23.
91 BRENNAN C S and CLEARY L J (2005), The potential use of cereal (1 → 3, 1 → 4)-β-D-glucans as fuctional food ingredients, *J. Cereal Chem.*, **42**, 1–13.
92 BRENNAN C S, BLAKE D E, ELLIS P R and SCHOFIELD J D (1996), Effects of guar galactomannan on wheat bread microstructure and on the in vitro and in vivo digestibility of starch in bread, *J. Cereal. Sci.*, **24**, 151–160.
93 SALMENKALLIO-MARTTILA M, ROININEN K, AUTIO K and LÄHTEENMÄKI L (2004), Effects of gluten and transglutaminase on microstructure, sensory characteristics and instrumental texture of oat bread, *Agric. Food Sci.*, **13**, 138–150.
94 SYMONS L J and BRENNAN C S (2004), The influence of (1 → 3) (1 → 4)-β-D-glucan-rich fractions from barley on the physicochemical properties and in vitro reducing sugar release of white wheat breads, *J. Food Sci.*, **69**, C463–467.
95 GODSHALL M A (1988), The role of carbohydrates in flavour development, *Food Technol.*, **11**, 71–78.
96 PAULUS K and HAAS E M (1980), The influence of solvent viscosity on the threshold values of primary tastes, *Chem. Senses*, **5** (Suppl. 1), 23–32.
97 MÄLKKI Y, HEINIÖ R-L and AUTIO K (1993), Influence of oat gum, guar gum and carboxymethyl cellulose on the perception of sweetness and flavour, *Food Hydrocoll.*, **6**, 525–532.
98 PANGBORN R M, TRABUE I and SZCZESNIAK A (1973), Effect of hydrocolloid on oral viscosity and basic taste intensities, *J. Text. Stud.*, **4**, 224–241.
99 LYLY M, SALMENKALLIO-MARTTILA M, SUORTTI T, AUTIO K, POUTANEN K and LÄHTEENMÄKI L (2004), The sensory characteristics and rheological properties of soups containing oat and barley beta-glucan before and after freezing, *Lebensmittel Wiss. Technol.*, **37**, 749–761.
100 RAPPAPORT L, PETERS G, HUFF-CORZINE L and DOWNEY R (1992), Reasons for eating: an exploratory cognitive analysis, *Ecol. Food Nutr.*, **28**, 171–189.
101 GOODE J, BEARDSWORTH A, HASLAM C, KEIL T and SHERRATT E (1995), Dietary dilemmas: nutritional concerns of the 1990s, *Br. Food J.*, **97**, 3–12.
102 ZUNFT H J, FRIEBE D, SEPPELT B, DE GRAAF C, MARGETTS B, SCHMITT A and GIBNEY M J (1997), Perceived benefits of healthy eating among a nationally-representative sample of adults in the European Union, *Eur. J. Clin. Nutr.*, **51** (Suppl. 2), 41–46.
103 MOORMAN C and MATULICH E (1993), A model of consumers' preventive health behaviors: the role of health motivation and health ability, *J. Consumer Res.*, **20**, 208–228.
104 DIPLOCK A T, AGGET P J, ASHWELL M, BORNET F, FERN E B and ROBERFROID M B (1999), Scientific concepts of functional foods in Europe: Consensus Document, *Br. J. Nutr.*, **81**, 1–27.

105 URALA N, ARVOLA A and LÄHTEENMÄKI L (2003), Strength of health-related claims and their perceived advantage, *Int. J. Food Sci. Technol.*, **38**, 815–826.
106 LYLY M, ROININEN K, HONKAPÄÄ K, POUTANEN K and LÄHTEENMÄKI L (2007), Factors influencing consumers' willingness to use beverages and ready-to-eat frozen soups containing oat beta-glucan in Finland, France and Sweden, *Food Qual. Preference*, **18**, 242–255.
107 ARVOLA A, LÄHTEENMÄKI L and TUORILA H (1999), Predicting the intent to purchase unfamiliar and familiar cheeses: the effects of attitudes, expected liking and food neophobia, *Appetite*, **32**, 113–126.
108 STEPTOE A, POLLARD T M and WARDLE J (1995), Development of a measure of the motives underlying the selection of food: the food choice questionnaire, *Appetite*, **25**, 267–284.
109 MARTINS Y and PLINER P (1998), The development of the Food Motivation Scale, *Appetite*, **30** (1), 94.
110 WOOD P J (1986), Oat β-glucan: structure, location and properties, in *Oats: Chemistry and Technology*, Ed. Webster F H, American Association of Cereal Chemists, Inc, Saint Paul, MN, USA, pp. 121–152.
111 DAWKINS N L and NNANNA I A (1995), Studies on oat gum [(1 → 3,1 → 4)-beta-D-glucan]: composition, molecular weight estimation and rheological properties, *Food Hydrocoll.*, **9**, 1–7.
112 DWYER S (1999), Now they're cookin'!, *Prepared Foods*, **168**, 15–16, 18, 22–24, 26.
113 AUTIO K, MYLLYMÄKI O and MÄLKKI Y (1987), Flow properties of solutions of oat β-glucans, *J. Food Sci.*, **52**, 1364–1366.
114 LYLY M, SALMENKALLIO-MARTTILA M, SUORTTI T, AUTIO K, POUTANEN K and LÄHTEENMÄKI L (2003), Influence of oat β-glucan preparations on the perception of mouthfeel and on rheological properties in beverage prototypes, *Cereal Chem.*, **80**, 536–541.
115 CHARALAMPOPOULOS D, WANG R, PANDIELLA S S and WEBB C (2002), Application of cereals and cereal components in functional foods: a review, *Int. J. Food Microbiol.*, **79** (1–2), 131–141.

# 7

# Non-digestible oligosaccharides

**N. M. Delzenne, P. D. Cani, E. Delmée and A. M. Neyrinck, Université catholique de Louvain, Belgium**

## 7.1 Introduction

Dietary fibres (DFs) are typically edible constituents of plants foods (or analogous carbohydrates) that escape digestion in the upper intestine. Definitions of DF now include components that undergo complete or partial fermentation in the large intestine: therefore, components like non-digestible oligosaccharides (NDOs) are now considered DFs (FAO/WHO 1998; DeVries 2003). Several recent reviews report the mechanisms that enable DF to play a role in the control of food intake and weight management, and these are presented in the first part of this chapter. We will place special emphasis on the definition and physiological properties of NDOs, and we will show how those fermentable DFs may act to modulate food intake and appetite, namely by promoting the release of gut peptides.

## 7.2 Dietary fibres and food intake

It was proposed, more than 30 years ago, that DFs act as a physiological obstacle to energy intake by different mechanisms including: (a) displacement of available calories and nutrients from the diet; (b) increasing chewing – which limits intake by promoting saliva and gastric juice resulting in an increased satiety; and (c) decreasing the absorption efficiency of the intestine (Heaton 1973). During *ad libitum* energy intake, a mean loss of weight of about 1.9 kg was found to have occurred after 14 g per day of additional fibre intake, which may have been due to the 10% lower energy intake observed. This effect was more pronounced in obese subjects (Howarth *et al.* 2001). Pereira and Ludwig (2001) report that in most studies, DF intake was associated with beneficial effects on energy intake. Some studies report mixed or no effects on satiety (Pereira & Ludwig 2001). The composition of diet, the type of fibre, the dose, the time of administration, the subject characteristics (healthy or obese), as well as the method of satiety assessment, are confounding parameters rendering the analysis of food intake modulation following DF intake difficult.

The mechanisms by which DF intake modulates food intake and body weight are multiple and are interestingly described in a recent review (Slavin 2005). It is proposed that DF may have an effect on satiation (sensation of fullness during an eating period, leading to the cessation of eating) and/or satiety (sensation of fullness between eating episodes that tends to inhibit the resumption of eating) (Gerstein *et al.* 2004). The effect on satiation may be related to the intrinsic properties of DF-containing foods (such as their lower energy density), prolonged chewing and mastication, or their gelling properties in the stomach. It has been shown that DF forming gels in contact with acids (alginate, guar gum), increases the sensation of fullness, through the distension of the gastric antrum; this may occur without any modification of gastric emptying (Hoad *et al.* 2004). However, delayed gastric emptying may explain *per se* the satiating effect of other DFs (Slavin 2005). Satiation and satiety are under neuronal and hormonal control (Ritter 2004). Recently, progress has been made in the comprehension of the relation between events occurring in the gut, and the central effect of gastro-intestinal peptides involved in the control of food intake (Badman & Flier 2005). This will be discussed later in this chapter.

Various types of DF may be of interest. Maeda *et al.* (2005) demonstrated that the addition of agar in the diet resulted in marked weight loss due to a reduction of food intake, and also improved cholesterol level, glucose and insulin response, and blood pressure. The Framingham Offspring Study reported that the prevalence of metabolic syndrome – defined following the National Cholesterol Education Program criteria – was improved by high cereal fibres intake (contributing to the beneficial effect of whole grain) (McKeown *et al.* 2004).

Knowledge of the biochemical mechanism allowing DF to modulate satiety, glucose or lipid metabolism, and hypertension is essential when proposing key nutritional advice for specific disorders associated with the metabolic syndrome. In this context, the modulation of gastro-intestinal peptides by NDOs, such as fructans, is an interesting area of research, leading to an understanding of how events occurring in the gut participate in the control of food intake, obesity and associated disorders. We propose, before entering into discussion about the relevance of NDOs in the modulation of food intake, to describe current knowledge related to the nutritional properties of NDOs.

## 7.3 Sources and properties of non-digestible oligosaccharides

### 7.3.1 Definition

Following worldwide authorities on chemical nomenclature and terminology (i.e. the International Union of Biochemistry (IUB) and the International Union of Pure and Applied Chemistry (IUPAC), an oligosaccharide is a molecule containing a small number of monosaccharide residues (degree of polymerisation, DP from 2 to 10). NDOs resist hydrolysis and digestion in the human digestive system and are partially or completely fermented by the colonic microbiota in the large intestine.

### 7.3.2 Chemical structure and origin

Several NDOs are considered DFs, itself a broad category. As illustrated in Table 7.1, NDOs may occur naturally in many plants – mainly vegetables, whole grains and fruits (Meyer 2004). Another natural source of NDOs is milk (cow milk galacto-oligosaccharides and human milk oligosaccharides). Moreover, several NDOs – often added in food for their technological properties – may be synthesised from simple or complex carbohydrates. NDOs present in the diet differ from one another in their chemical structure, in other words the number (DP) or the type of hexose moeties (glucosyl-, fructosyl-, galactosyl-, xylosyl-), the position of links between the hexose moeties and their conformation (α- versus β-) (Delzenne 2003). All these characteristics have consequences on the physical properties of NDOs – and therefore on their putative usefulness as food ingredients and their effects and metabolism in the gastro-intestinal tract. Owing to interest in their nutritional properties, biotechnology (enzymatic or thermal processes) has been applied to obtain new types of NDOs either through enzymatic synthesis from simple sugars, or enzymatic hydrolysis from more complex carbohydrates (Murphy 2001). Short-chain fructo-oligosaccharides (FOS), for example, may be obtained by synthesis from saccharose, or through controlled and partial hydrolysis from chicory root inulin (Roberfroid & Slavin 2000).

FOS are often cited as the most important dietary oligosaccharides. They may be of plant origin (garlic, onions, banana, artichoke, chicory root and cereals) (Delzenne 2003). FOS are a linear polydisperse carbohydrate material consisting mainly, if not exclusively, of fructose residues linked by β-2,1 fructosyl-fructose linkages. The generic term for FOS, namely fructans, includes the oligofructose (OFS) (DP 4), high-molecular-weight inulin (Inu) (DP 25) and a Synergy 1 (Syn) consisting of a mix of OFS and Inu (DP 2–60).

Although specific attention is often given to FOS, one must not forget that human milk, remains another 'natural' source that is extremely rich in diverse oligosaccharides. Their presence could explain some of the many health-promoting effects of breast feeding.

**Table 7.1** Dietary NDOs available in food products

| Type of NDO | Natural occurrence | Industrial production process |
|---|---|---|
| Fructo-oligosaccharides | Onions, banana, garlic, Jerusalem artichokes | Synthesis from saccharose<br>Hydrolysis from chicory-root inulin |
| Galacto-oligosaccharides | Cow milk, soybean, legumes | Enzymatic process from lactose |
| Isomalto-oligosaccharides | Miso, soy sauce, sake, honey | Hydrolysis or glycosyl transfer from starch |
| Palatinose or isomaltulose | Honey, cane juice | Produced from sucrose by α-glucosidase reaction of *Protaminobacter rubrum* |
| Theanderose | Sugar, honey | Produced using fungus *Mucor javanicus* |
| Lactulose | — | Synthesis from lactose |
| Lactosucrose, glycosylsucrose | — | Synthesis from saccharose and/or lactose |
| Xylo-oligosaccharides | Wheat bran | Hydrolysis from polyxylans |
| Stacchyose, raffinose | Soybean | — |
| Fibersol-2 | — | Produced by pyrolysis of corn starch |
| Glucomannan | Konjac root | — |
| Cyclodextrin | — | Synthesis from starch |

### 7.3.3 Technological and nutritional properties (including estimated intake)

NDOs are readily water soluble and exhibit some sweetness, which decreases with longer chain length, whereas water binding and gelling properties increase with the number of hexose molecules and reticulation. These properties, together with some interesting physiological effects (low caloric value – close to 1.5 kcal per gram of oligosaccharides, low cariogenicity, prebiotic effect, improvement of mineral absorption, etc.) are used to promote the addition of some NDOs to foodstuffs that normally contain low or no significant amount of such nutrients. Since they are added to foods, quantifying the dietary intake of NDOs in adult humans is difficult. One study, based on the intake of FOS in fruits and vegetable, has estimated the daily intake of inulin-type fructans for a 75-kg person to be 3.2–11.3 g in Western Europe, and 1–4 g in the United States, (van Loo *et al.* 1995). The usual intake of most other NDOs is difficult to assess due to the lack of adequate published data.

### 7.3.4 Effect of non-digestible oligosaccharides in the gastro-intestinal tract

NDOs, once ingested, resist digestion by hydrolytic enzymes secreted or active in the intestine, such as α-glucosidase or maltase/isomaltase. NDOs, which mostly escape the upper digestion, are important sources of energy for bacteria in the caeco-colon, which express enzymes such as β-fructosidase, β-galactosidase, xylanase or any other hydrolases (Bernalier *et al.* 1999). The ingestion of some NDOs may thus lead to the advantageous proliferation of certain types of bacteria, which are generally considered beneficial (e.g. bifidobacteria, lactobacilli) and suppression of more harmful bacteria. Dietary FOS have been demonstrated in many studies in animals and humans to (re)equilibriate the colonic biotope, first defined as the 'prebiotic effect' in 1995 by Gibson and Roberfroid, 1995. In addition, more recently, promising results have been obtained with other NDOs such as galacto-oligosaccharides (GOS) (Delzenne & Williams 2002). The dose and the duration of NDO intake, the place where fermentation mainly occurs (proximal or distal colon) as well as the initial composition of faecal flora, are important factors influencing the extent of the prebiotic effect – namely the increase in bifidobacteria (Rao 2001; Tuohy *et al.* 2001). On the basis of the results of well-designed human studies that have shown significant changes in the composition of human faecal flora, it can be concluded that FOS are prebiotic at a dose of between 5 and 15 g per day. For the GOS, an increase in bifidobacteria and lactobacilli in response to doses ranging from 3 to 10 g per day has been reported. A dose of isomalto-oligosaccharides of 13.5 g per day for 2 weeks significantly increased the number of bifidobacteria in adult and elderly volunteers (Roberfroid 2003).

For soybean oligosaccharides, a dose of 10 g given twice daily for 3 weeks significantly increases the number of bifidobacteria, while slightly decreasing clostridia counts; a dose of 3 g per day increases bifidobacteria, bacteroides and eubacteria. A bifidogenic effect has also been demonstrated in humans after ingestion of lactulose, lactilol and xylo-oligosaccharides (Meyer 2004). A low baseline bifidobacteria count was significantly associated with the bifidogenic response to NDO ingestion (Bouhnik *et al.* 1999, 2004). Recentlys a new quantitative approach for determining *in vitro* prebiotic potential of dietary oligosaccharides has been developed (Vulevic *et al.* 2004). The measure of the prebiotic effect (MPE) includes quantitative changes in the number of bacterial groups, fermentation end products, such as short-chain fatty acids (SCFAs), and substrate assimilation. Although the approach is not meant to define health values, it is formulated to better inform the choice of prebiotic NDOs.

The major products of NDO metabolism are SCFA and gases (hydrogen and carbon dioxide), produced through fermentation by colonic flora. The pattern of fermentation (the proportion of the different short-chain acids (acetate, propionate, butyrate, lactate) produced in the caecum and/or the colon) varies with the nature of the NDO, at least in animals. More butyrate is produced from FOS and lactitol than from raffinose (Nyman 2002). The proportion of SCFA also changes with the duration of the treatment, as was well illustrated by the study of Le Blay *et al.* (1999) performed with FOS. The SCFA are absorbed into the bloodstream of the host. Butyrate is absorbed and used by colonocytes as the preferred fuel, whereas the other SCFA are transferred to various organs – primarily the liver – where they enter different metabolic pathways. Interesting methods have been developed to determine SCFA turn-over in animals and human subjects, using stable isotopes (Pouteau *et al.* 2003).

SCFA have an important effect in the intestinal tract. It is largely accepted that butyrate exerts an essential role in maintaining the metabolism, and the proliferation/differentiation of different epithelial cell types. SCFA, and mostly butyrate, are often evoked to explain the role of NDO in gut immunity, or cell turn-over.

## 7.4 Effect of non-digestible oligosaccharides on glucose and lipid metabolism: a phenomenon linked to a decrease in food intake

### 7.4.1 Non-digestible oligosaccharides and lipid/glucose metabolism in animal studies

Most data published to date relate to experimental studies performed in animals. NDOs are able to modulate hepatic lipid metabolism in rats or hamsters, with consequences on either triglyceride accumulation in the liver, and/or serum lipids. In non-obese rats and/or hamsters fed a high-carbohydrate diet, a decrease in hepatic and serum triglycerides is observed when inulin-type FOS are added to the diet at concentrations from 2.5 to 10% for several weeks (from 2 to 12 weeks) (Delzenne & Williams 2002). In animals, reduced triglyceridaemia is often linked to a decrease in *de novo* lipogenesis in hepatic, but not in adipose, tissue, cells. A decrease in the expression of key hepatic lipogenic enzymes, reflected by a decrease in fatty acid synthase mRNA, seems to be involved in the lower lipogenic capacity after inulin-type FOG supplementation, as also shown with resistant starch (Delzenne *et al.* 2002). In rats fed a lipid-rich diet containing 10% FOS, a decrease in triglyceridaemia also occurs without any protective effect on hepatic triglyceride accumulation and lipogenesis, suggesting a possible peripheral mode of action (Kok *et al.* 1998b). By contrast, in obese Zucker rats, dietary supplementation with FOS lessens hepatic steatosis, with no effect on post-prandial triglyceridaemia when added in the standard diet (Daubioul *et al.* 2000). This effect is likely to result mainly from reduced availability of non-esterified fatty acids coming from adipose tissue, since fat mass and body weight are decreased by the treatment. The protection against steatosis is strongly dependent on fermentation pattern (Daubioul *et al.* 2002). The high proportion of propionate produced in the caecum, which reaches the liver through the portal vein, is, at least in animals, a key event explaining a lower hepatic triglyceride synthesis upon NDO feeding (Morand *et al.* 1993; Delzenne *et al.* 2002; M. Lasa, June 2002, unpublished results).

Rats fed with NDOs (OFS), also exhibit lower fat mass development, as shown in several models (Daubioul *et al.* 2002; Delzenne *et al.* 2005). The epididymal, inguinal and visceral adipose tissue fat mass are lowered by 30% to 40% in OFS-fed rats as compared with controls (Cani *et al.* 2004).

The effects of NDOs on glucose homeostasis have been less well studied. An improvement of glucose/insulin ratio has been observed in rats receiving FOS with a high-fructose diet (Busserolles *et al.* 2003).

We have recently reported that OFS improves glycaemia and plasma insulin, both in the post-prandial state and after an oral glucose load in streptozotocin-treated diabetic rats (STZ). Moreover, treatment with OFS improves pancreatic insulin and β-cell mass (Cani *et al.* 2005a). This 'anti-diabetic' effect of NDOs is partly linked to a decrease in food intake due to the treatment, but is merely due to the promotion of incretins production (see 7.6.2). In diabetes prone-BB rats, which are characterised by a default in the production of gut peptides, no effect of OFS was shown (Perrin *et al.* 2003)

In most studies showing the interesting effects of NDOs on lipid or glucose metabolism, and fat mass development, the animals supplemented with NDOs exhibited a lower energy intake, suggesting that NDOs have a satietogenic effect. How does this take place? Is it really one of the important metabolic effects of NDOs? The second part of the chapter will be devoted to these questions.

## 7.5 Non-digestible oligosaccharides, food intake and weight control: a key role for gastro-intestinal peptides

### 7.5.1 Involvement in the regulation of food intake: from theory to experimental data

Endocrine L-cells are distributed all along the intestinal tract, but are mostly present in the caeco-colon, where fermentation of NDO occurs (Orskov *et al.* 1989). Endocrine cells present in the intestinal mucosa secrete peptides involved in the regulation of food intake, and/or pancreatic functions, the latter being called incretins [glucagon-like peptide-1 (GLP-1) and gastric inhibitory peptide (GIP)]. Among those peptides, GLP-1, peptide YY (PYY) and oxyntomodulin have recently been proposed as important modulators of appetite, through their peripheral effect (vagal nerve) and/or by acting directly on the arcuate nucleus (Druce *et al.* 2004; Wynne *et al.* 2005). GLP-1 is also involved in the regulation of pancreatic secretion of insulin, and in the differentiation and maturation of β-cells (Brubaker & Drucker 2004). Other gastro-intestinal peptides are implicated in the regulation of body weight and food intake such as ghrelin, a gastric orexigenic-derived hormone (Cowley *et al.* 2003).

Interestingly, we had previously observed that OFS feeding led to an increase in total cecal GLP-1 and jejunum GIP concentrations in rats (Kok *et al.* 1998a). Therefore, we postulated that the modulation of gut peptides could involve a key hormone mediating the effect of OFS – and other NDOs – on food intake, and glucose/lipid metabolism. The mechanism and relevance of endogenous modulation of the production of gut peptides by DF is poorly documented, but several experimental data suggest that those peptides could constitute a link between the outcome of fermentation in the lower part of the gut and systemic consequences of 'colonic food' intake.

Reduction of food/energy intake has been observed in several rat models (lean rats or mice, obese Zucker fa/fa rats, high-fat-diet-induced obese mice) in which inulin-type fructans fibres, extensively fermented in the caeco-colon, were added to the diet. The decrease in food/energy intake was not observed when fructans were substituted by non-fermentable DF (microcrystalline cellulose) (Daubioul *et al.* 2002).

*What we knew at the beginning?*

1 The peptides involved are produced in the gut (GIP, ghrelin), or in the lower part of the gut (PYY, GLP-1), where NDOs – including inulin-type fructans – are largely fermented.
2 The products of such a fermentation in the gut – namely SCFAs – are known to increase the expression of proglucagon mRNA (precursor of GLP-1) in the intestinal tissue (Cherbut *et al.* 1998; Tappenden *et al.* 1998; Drozdowski *et al.* 2002).

3 Some fermentable DFs are able to increase proglucagon mRNA expression when given in high doses in the diet of dogs or rats (Reimer & McBurney 1996; Massimino *et al.* 1998).

We report here experiments devoted to: (a) analysing the putative modulation of portal plasma GLP-1 and PYY and peripheral ghrelin concentrations in rats fed three types of fructans, differing in preferential site and extent of fermentation; and (b) identifying the major intestinal site of proglucagon mRNA expression and GLP-1 synthesis after feeding with fructans.

*Are non-digestible oligosaccharides able to modulate gastro-intestinal peptides involved in appetite and body weight regulation?*

We first compared the influence of inulin-type fructans having different DPs – namely OFS, OFS-enriched inulin (Syn) and high-molecular-weight inulin (Inu) – on daily energy intake, and GLP-1 and PYY production. It is important to note that the differences among inulin-type fructans are not only the DP but also the preferential site of fermentation: OFS being fermented in the caecum and the proximal colon, Inu in the distal colon and Syn throughout the colon. The concentration of these peptides, and of the corresponding mRNA precursors, was measured in various segments of the intestinal tract in male Wistar rats that had been given fructans at a dose of 10% (w/w) for 3 weeks. All measurements were performed 8 h after removal of the diet.

We confirm that inulin-type fructans, when added in the diet, significantly reduce energy intake in rats. The short-chain inulin-type fructans (OFS/Syn) significantly increase the concentration of GLP-1 in the proximal colon and, to a lesser extent, in the medial colon (OFS only) (Cani *et al.* 2004). The portal concentration of both GLP-1 and PYY peptides was increased after OFS treatment (Table 7.2). This is quite interesting since it means an increase flux of those peptides towards the hepato-portal system, where vagal 'sensors' act as a potential signal to the hypothalamic centres that control food intake (Schwartz *et al.* 2000; Holst & Deacon 2005; Wynne *et al.* 2005). The portal GLP-1 increase was correlated to the level of proglucagon mRNA in the proximal colon ($R = 0.62$, $P < 0.001$, Pearson's correlation) (Cani *et al.* 2004). Surprisingly, there was no modification of PYY protein or mRNA in the different intestinal segments, thus suggesting that the effect of OFS was linked to a specific effect on proglucagon gene expression in L-cells as previously suggested (Anini *et al.* 1999). Moreover, the co-localisation of PYY and GLP-1 has been reported for only 15% of the colonic L-cells (Aponte *et al.* 1988; Nilsson *et al.* 1991). Interestingly, even though there is no modification of peptides concentration per gram of caecal tissue, the enlargement of the organ was responsible for an increase in the total caecal pool of both GLP-1 and PYY.

**Table 7.2** Portal vein plasma GLP-1 (7–36) amide and PYY (3–36) amide, and cava vein plasma acylated ghrelin concentrations of rats fed a control diet (CT) or a diet supplemented with OFS, OFS-enriched inulin (Syn) or high-molecular-weight inulin (Inu). Values are means ± S.E.M., $n = 6$ per group. Statistical analysis has been performed through one-way ANOVA followed by Tukey's test separately for each peptide. Mean values with unlike superscript letters are significantly different, $P < 0.05$ (Adapted from Cani *et al.,* 2004, and Delzenne *et al.,* 2005)

| | Portal vein | | Cava vein, acylated ghrelin (pM) |
|---|---|---|---|
| | GLP-1$^{(7\text{–}36)\text{ amide}}$ (pM) | PYY$^{(3\text{–}36)\text{ amide}}$ (pM) | |
| CT | $7.8 \pm 0.7^{a}$ | $9.9 \pm 1.9^{a}$ | $131.7 \pm 7.4^{a}$ |
| OFS | $11.4 \pm 1.2^{b}$ | $19.7 \pm 2.4^{b}$ | $91 \pm 7.2^{b}$ |
| Syn | $10.5 \pm 1.7^{b}$ | $12.9 \pm 2.6^{a}$ | $87.2 \pm 12.6^{b}$ |
| Inu | $8.4 \pm 1.3^{a}$ | $11.2 \pm 3.2^{a}$ | $102.6 \pm 12^{ab}$ |

We have shown that the plasma GLP-1 increase in the portal vein was positively correlated to an increase in the number of cells producing GLP-1 in the proximal colon (P. D. Cani, submitted to Br J. Nutr 2006, personal communication). An increase in intestinal proglucagon mRNA concentration has already been shown in rodents or dogs who received fermentable DF (Reimer *et al.* 1997; Massimino *et al.* 1998; Nian *et al.* 2002). In mice, this was accompanied by a higher GLP-1 incremental area under the curve after a glucose load (Nian *et al.* 2002). None of these studies reported an effect on food intake, body weight gain or insulin sensitivity.

A recent study has suggested that plasma GLP-1 might also influence the production of ghrelin (Lippl *et al.* 2004). Ghrelin stimulates feeding behaviour, lowers energy expenditure and drives body weight increase due to a change in fuel partitioning. Acylated ghrelin concentration increases during food deprivation and rapidly falls during meals (Kojima *et al.* 1999; Tschop *et al.* 2000). Ghrelin could constitute a potential relay of the effects of OFS on satiety because plasma GLP-1 and ghrelin concentrations are inversely correlated after glucose ingestion, and GLP-1 reduces ghrelin secretion (Djurhuus *et al.* 2002; Lippl *et al.* 2004). As shown in Table 7.2, the plasma acylated ghrelin level is almost 30% lower in rats fed short-chain fructans. This suggests that a lower ghrelin production can also contribute to a decrease in appetite during fasting, linked to the presence of NDO in the diet.

In conclusion, we may assess that short-chain fructans, which are fermented in the caecum and the proximal colon, are effective NDOs able to increase proglucagon mRNA and portal and intestinal GLP-1 concentrations, and to decrease peripheral plasma acylated ghrelin, at least in animal models. Due to the results of these experiments, we have chosen to investigate further the effects of OFS, as DF, on the modulatation of gut peptides.

### 7.5.2 Putative modulation of gastro-intestinal peptides by non-digestible oligosaccharides in a high-fat-diet induced hyperphagia model in rats

The role of dietary fat as a key nutrient influencing the energy balance has been a topic of interest for researchers and for those concerned with public health in general. Many epidemiological studies, and experimental data obtained in animals, have characterised the response to high-fat feeding in humans and rodents (Bray & Popkin 1998, 1999; West & York 1998). A high-fat diet produces a consistent and significant increase in body fat content, which is dependent on both the amount of fat in the diet and the duration of feeding. Hyperphagia might be one important mechanism by which high-fat diets promote obesity, since fat is less satiating than carbohydrate (Ramirez & Friedman 1990; Lucas *et al.* 1998; Lucas & Sclafani 1999); it has thus been suggested that fat may lead to passive diet overconsumption (Blundell *et al.* 1996; Blundell & Macdiarmid 1997a,b). The model of high-fat-diet induced hyperphagia is known to be associated with an inhibition of ghrelin. Since ghrelin is inhibited, it is unable to counteract hyperphagia (Lee *et al.* 2002). The reduction in plasma ghrelin levels with the high-fat diet is in accordance with results reported in an article that shows decreased circulating ghrelin levels in obese humans (Tschop *et al.* 2001). The authors of the human study suggest that the reduced plasma ghrelin levels reflect an adaptation to the excessive caloric intake in obese subjects.

Only a small amount of data is available concerning the potential modulation of high-fat-diet induced hyperphagia by DFs or NDOs (Sullivan *et al.* 1978; Ramirez & Friedman 1990). The presence of OFS in a high-fat diet as compared with a high-fat diet alone increases proglucagon mRNA in the proximal colon, with consequences on GLP-1 concentrations. This model has no effect, however, on PYY and ghrelin levels (Cani *et al.* 2005b). OFS also reduces dipeptidyl peptidase IV (DPPIV) activity by about 30%. Thus, a lower DPPIV activity due to OFS may contribute, together with the higher intestinal production, to the promotion of GLP-1 production and of its biological activity in the portal vein. In fact, we know neither the origin of soluble portal DPPIV nor by which mechanisms OFS reduces DPPIV activity (Cani *et al.* 2005b). Thus, because of the protective effect of OFS against high-fat-diet induced body weight gain, hyperphagia and fat mass development, despite the lack of effect of OFS on PYY and ghrelin levels, we postulate that the modulation of GLP-1 synthesis and secretion could be linked to the beneficial effects of OFS.

## 7.6 The role of glucagon-like peptide-1 in the improvement of food intake, fat development and diabetic state by non-digestible oligosaccharides

### 7.6.1 Non-digestible oligosaccharides and glucose/insulin homeostasis: lessons from animal models

GLP-1, besides its effect on food intake, is considered a key peptide in the control of glucose tolerance, and glucose-dependent insulin release by pancreatic β-cells (Meier & Nauck 2005). Moreover, it is also responsible for increased β-cell neogenesis in streptozotocin-treated newborn rats – a model of diabetes – thus allowing a partial recuperation of pancreatic function with age (Tourrel *et al.* 2001). We reported that OFS improves glycaemia and plasma insulin, both in the post-prandial state and after an oral glucose load in streptozotocin-treated diabetic rats (STZ). Moreover, the treatment with OFS allows an improvement of pancreatic insulin and β-cell mass. Endogenous GLP-1 production was increased in STZ-OFS rats as compared with other groups (Cani *et al.* 2005a). This GLP-1 overproduction might be part of the protective effect of dietary fructans. Such a mechanism has been proposed to explain the effectiveness of guar gum in improving hyperglycaemia in hyperphagic diabetic rats (Cameron-Smith *et al.* 1997). We may not exclude the fact that the satietogenic effect of OFS could be involved in the improvement of glucose and pancreatic function. By investigating the putative effect of food restriction alone, we have drawn two conclusions: (a) the higher GLP-1 synthesis in STZ-control rats is clearly linked to hyperphagia, since it is avoided by a drastic caloric restriction; (b) the beneficial effect of OFS is not due to food restriction only, since the improvement in glucose tolerance and pancreatic β-cell mass is observed in STZ-OFS rats and not in food-restricted rats.

In another model (mice fed a high-fat diet), we have also shown that OFS improves hepatic insulin sensitivity and increases plasma insulin; these effects of OFS could also be due to a permanent intestinally released GLP-1, promoting perhaps in part progressive insulin sensitivity associated with reduced weight gain.

### 7.6.2 Is glucagon-like peptide-1 a key hormone involved in the oligofructose effects?

The physiological importance of GLP-1 action can be studied using GLP-1R antagonists or GLP-1R–/– mice. The infusion of the peptide exendin (9–39) (Ex-9) in rats, mice, baboons and humans, increases fasting glycaemia and glycaemic excursions after a glucose load, in association with reduced levels of circulating insulin (D'Alessio *et al.* 1996; Schirra *et al.* 1998; Meeran *et al.* 1999; Burcelin *et al.* 2001). Other studies have shown that injection of Ex-9 increases food intake and weight gain in healthy animals (Meeran *et al.* 1999), consistent with a role for endogenous GLP-1 in the control of body weight. The importance of GLP-1 for the regulation of energy metabolism has also been illustrated by the analysis of mice with genetic disruption of the GLP-1R gene, GLP-1R–/– mice (Scrocchi *et al.* 1998). By using both models of: (a) transient disruption of GLP-1R action by infusing Ex-9 in wild-type mice or (b) genetic elimination of GLP-1R action in GLP-1R–/– mice, we have shown that 4 weeks of OFS treatment during high-fat feeding reduces the development of hyperglycaemia, glucose intolerance and body weight gain in mice, whereas Ex-9 abolishes all the OFS effects (Cani *et al.* 2005c). The importance of intact GLP-1R signalling mechanisms for the anti-diabetic actions of OFS were further illustrated in experiments wherein OFS treatment of GLP-1R–/– mice was not able to reduce the high-fat-induced body weight gain and control food intake.

The issue of peripheral versus intraportal GLP-1 delivery is likely to be important since previous studies have demonstrated that GLP-1R–/– mice or wild-type mice with Ex-9 infused into the portal vein have impaired hepatoportal glucose sensor function and reduced insulin secretory capacity (Burcelin *et al.* 2001). We propose that the production of GLP-1 in the proximal colon of OFS-fed mice is a key event explaining the metabolic effect of this NDO, since the decrease in food intake, in fat mass and in glycemia classically observed after OFS treatment is abolished in GLP-1R–/– mice or in EX-9-infused mice (Cani *et al.* 2006a). In addition to the therapeutic effect of GLP-1 through its direct pancreatic effect on insulin or glucagon secretion, the anti-hyperglycaemic effect of OFS could also be attributed to the extra-pancreatic indirect actions of GLP-1 on hepatoportal neural mechanisms. Other authors have recently debated the GLP-1 levels that need to be reached to achieve metabolic effects (Holst & Deacon 2005). The extensive degradation of GLP-1 that occurs before it enters the systemic circulation has led to the suggestion that GLP-1 exerts numerous actions either locally in the gut or in the hepatic portal bed. Once released, but before it comes into contact with endothelial DPPIV, GLP-1 may interact with afferent sensory nerve fibres arising from the nodose ganglion, which send afferent impulses to the nucleus of the solitary tract and onwards to the hypothalamus which may be efferent transmitted to the pancreas (Nishizawa *et al.* 2000; Nakagawa *et al.* 2004). Thus, under physiological conditions, the neural pathway may be more important than the endocrine route for GLP-1-stimulated insulin secretion. This supports the relevance of our observations, showing a higher GLP-1 content in the proximal colon segment of NDO-treated mice or rats.

## 7.7 Relevance of non-digestible oligosaccharide effects in human studies

Three questions are raised at the end of this experimental work:

1 Is OFS able to increase GLP-1 production in humans?
2 Is OFS able to promote satiety in healthy humans and/or in obese/type 2 diabetic patients?

3 Is OFS able to improve insulin sensitivity in obese/type 2 diabetic patients?

Question 1 has been partly answered by the work of Piche *et al.* (2003). They found that OFS feeding (20 g per day) increased plasma GLP-1 in one interventional study performed in patients presenting gastric reflux. This result was not studied in relation to food intake and satiety (Piche *et al.* 2003). The authors suggested that it is important to take into account the 'kinetics' of fermentation – assessed by hydrogen breath test – when assessing the influence of fermented nutrients on circulating gut peptides. The increase in hydrogen expired (marker of fermentation), correlates with the modulation of plasma GLP-1 level, which could explain the link between intestinal fermentation and gut peptide secretion.

Studies intending to provide an answer to question 2 have produced inconclusive results. Reported effects of NDOs on circulating blood lipids in humans are variable. Both positive and negative outcomes were obtained from a small number of well-designed human studies, devoted to analysing the effect of dietary supplementation with FOS (doses from 8 to 20 g per day) exhibiting prebiotic properties (Delzenne & Williams 2002). Studies have been conducted in both normo- and moderately hyperlipidaemic subjects. The effect of FOS supplementation on lipogenesis has been shown in human volunteers: hepatic triglyceride synthesis is lowered by this NDO, as previously shown in rats (Diraison *et al.* 2003). In patients with non-alcoholic steatohepatitis, FOS supplementation lead to a decrease in serum activity of aminotransferases, suggesting an improvement of hepatic alterations in those patients (Daubioul *et al.* 2005). Studies performed with other NDOs are scarce.

We have recently assessed the relevance of OFS feeding (16 g per day, for 2 weeks) on satiety, hunger and energy intake in a single-blinded, cross-over, placebo-controlled design, pilot study in humans. Interestingly, we found that OFS promotes satiety following breakfast and dinner, and reduces hunger and prospective food consumption after the dinner. During OFS feeding, breakfast, lunch and total energy intake were reduced moderately (by about 5–10%) but were significantly lower than those observed during the placebo period (Cani *et al.* 2006b). Thus, on the basis of these results, it is reasonable to suggest a role for OFS in enhancing satiety and reducing energy intake in humans consuming a diet *ad libitum*. Moreover, Archer *et al.* (2004) have recently demonstrated that fermentable fructans, added to food as a fat replacer, were able to induce a lower energy intake during a test day, despite having no effect on satiety at breakfast, suggesting, as mentioned by the authors, a late post-absorptive satiety trigger related to the complete fermentation of this fibre (Archer *et al.* 2004). The influence of DF on GLP-1 release has been only poorly studied. An increase in the post-prandial response of GLP-1 was observed after ingestion of β-glucan-rich rye bread by healthy subjects (Juntunen *et al.*

2002). The administration of guar gum (together with galactose) promoted the increase in GLP-1 in women (but not in men), and this was related to a significant increase in satiety (Adam & Westerterp-Plantenga 2005). Concerning the type of fibres, following results mostly obtained in animals, it is generally admitted that fermentable fibres might enhance satiety to a larger extent than non-fermentable DFs, resulting in greater reductions in energy intake. However, in a pilot study comparing both fermentable (pectin, β-glucan) and non-fermentable DF (methylcellulose) added as supplement (about 27 g per day) in human volunteers for a 3 week period, methylcellulose was shown to be more satiating than the fermentable fibres (Howarth *et al.* 2003). These last observations suggest that the place (proximal or distal colon) and the pattern of fermentation (in terms of SCFA production) of fermentable fibre, including NDOs, are important, but this remains speculative.

Taken together, these results suggest a role for some NDOs in promoting a moderate negative energy balance in humans consuming a diet *ad libitum*.

## 7.8 Conclusions and future trends

As illustrated in this chapter, NDOs could exert interesting effects on food intake and obesity-associated disorders, by a mechanism that may be different from those classically attributed to most DFs (gastric emptying, bulking effects, etc.). As shown for OFS, NDO feeding could modulate several gastro-intestinal peptides (GLP-1, PYY, ghrelin), GLP-1 being a key hormone involved in OFS effects on food intake, fat mass development and glucose homeostasis. No data are available to support a role for GLP-1 in the modulation of lipid metabolism by NDOs.

The extension of these observations to other NDOs is needed. After all, we may not generalise the OFS effect to all the fermentable NDOs, since, for example, high-molecular-weight inulin does not significantly increase GLP-1 production. Nevertheless, a very recent study observed similar effects to those observed in our studies, Gee and Johnson (2005) demonstrated that feeding rats with lactitol (a fermentable carbohydrate) lowers food intake, body weight gain and increases plasma GLP-1 and PYY. The authors did not study the putative modulation of intestinal peptide content. This last study suggests that other dietary fermentable fibres are putative candidates for the promotion of endogenous gut peptide production.

The results of our experiments encourage further study of the putative targeting of gut peptides by 'colonic nutrients' in humans. A sufficient amount of NDOs must be eaten if one wants to target the colon. Data reporting the amount of NDOs eaten by humans in a standard diet are rare, as are data reporting the dose required to promote the release of satietogenic peptides. Some positive effects have been obtained by adding

NDOs, such as OFS, in the diet at a specific dose (about 15 g per day). Studies of the combined effect of NDOs and other DFs in the control of weight – acting by different mechanisms – should also be useful in establishing the relevance of NDOs in the nutritional control of obesity. This would finally enable the development of a nutritional approach to improving insulin sensitivity, satiety and control of body weight gain in obese and type 2 diabetes patients. Further human studies are clearly necessary to prove the relevance of the animal data available at the present time.

## 7.9 References

ADAM T C and WESTERTERP-PLANTENGA M S (2005), Nutrient-stimulated GLP-1 release in normal-weight men and women. *Horm. Metab. Res.*, **37**, 111–117.

ANINI Y, FU-CHENG X, CUBER J C, KERVRAN A, CHARIOT J and ROZ C (1999), Comparison of the postprandial release of peptide YY and proglucagon-derived peptides in the rat. *Pflugers Arch.*, **438**, 299–306.

APONTE G W, TAYLOR I L and SOLL A H (1988), Primary culture of PYY cells from canine colon. *Am. J. Physiol.*, **254**, G829–G836.

ARCHER B J, JOHNSON S K, DEVEREUX H M and BAXTER A L (2004), Effect of fat replacement by inulin or lupin-kernel fibre on sausage patty acceptability, post-meal perceptions of satiety and food intake in men. *Br. J. Nutr.*, **91**, 591–599.

BADMAN M K and FLIER J S (2005), The gut and energy balance: visceral allies in the obesity wars. *Science*, **307**, 1909–1914.

BERNALIER B, DORÉ J and DURAND M (1999), Colonic microbiota, nutrition and health. In *Biochemistry of Fermentation*, ed. GR Gibson and MB Roberfroid, pp. 37–53. The Netherlands: Kluwer Academic Publishers.

BLUNDELL J E and MACDIARMID J I (1997a), Fat as a risk factor for overconsumption: satiation, satiety, and patterns of eating. *J. Am. Diet. Assoc.*, **97**, S63–S69.

BLUNDELL J E and MACDIARMID J I (1997b), Passive overconsumption. Fat intake and short-term energy balance. *Ann. N. Y. Acad. Sci.*, **827**, 392–407.

BLUNDELL J E, LAWTON C L, COTTON J R and MACDIARMID J I (1996), Control of human appetite: implications for the intake of dietary fat. *Annu. Rev. Nutr.*, **16**, 285–319.

BOUHNIK Y, RASKINE L, SIMONEAU G, VICAUT E, NEUT C, FLOURIE B, BROUNS F and BORNET F R (2004), The capacity of nondigestible carbohydrates to stimulate fecal bifidobacteria in healthy humans: a double-blind, randomized, placebo-controlled, parallel-group, dose-response relation study. *Am. J. Clin. Nutr.*, **80**, 1658–1664.

BOUHNIK Y, VAHEDI K, ACHOUR L, ATTAR A, SALFATI J, POCHART P, MARTEAU P, FLOURIE B, BORNET F and RAMBAUD J C (1999), Short-chain fructo-oligosaccharide administration dose-dependently increases fecal bifidobacteria in healthy humans. *J. Nutr.*, **129**, 113–116.

BRAY G A and POPKIN B M (1998), Dietary fat intake does affect obesity! *Am. J. Clin. Nutr.*, **68**, 1157–1173.

BRAY G A and POPKIN B M (1999), Dietary fat affects obesity rate. *Am. J. Clin. Nutr.*, **70**, 572–573.

BRUBAKER P L and DRUCKER D J (2004), Minireview: Glucagon-like peptides regulate cell proliferation and apoptosis in the pancreas, gut, and central nervous system. *Endocrinology*, **145**, 2653–2659.

BURCELIN R, DA COSTA A, DRUCKER D and THORENS B (2001), Glucose competence of the hepatoportal vein sensor requires the presence of an activated glucagon-like peptide-1 receptor. *Diabetes*, **50**, 1720–1728.

BUSSEROLLES J, GUEUX E, ROCK E, DEMIGNE C, MAZUR A and RAYSSIGUIER Y (2003), Oligofructose protects against the hypertriglyceridemic and pro-oxidative effects of a high fructose diet in rats. *J. Nutr.*, **133**, 1903–1908.

CAMERON-SMITH D, HABITO R, BARNETT M and COLLIER G R (1997), Dietary guar gum improves insulin sensitivity in streptozotocin-induced diabetic rats. *J. Nutr.*, **127**, 359–364.

CANI P D, DAUBIOUL C A, REUSENS B, REMACLE C, CATILLON G and DELZENNE N M (2005a), Involvement of endogenous glucagon-like peptide-1(7–36) amide on glycaemia-lowering effect of oligofructose in streptozotocin-treated rats. *J. Endocrinol.*, **185**, 457–465.

CANI P D, DEWEVER C and DELZENNE N M (2004), Inulin-type fructans modulate gastrointestinal peptides involved in appetite regulation (glucagon-like peptide-1 and ghrelin) in rats. *Br. J. Nutr.*, **92**, 521–526.

CANI P D, KNAUF C, IGLESIAS M A, DRUCKER D J, DELZENNE N M and BURCELIN R (2006a), Imrovement of glucose tolerance and hepatic insulin sensitivity by oligofructose requires a functional GLP-1 receptor. *Diabetes*, **55**, 1484–1490.

CANI P D, NEYRINCK A M, MATON N and DELZENNE N M (2005b), Oligofructose promotes satiety in rats fed a high-fat diet: involvement of glucagon-like peptide-1. *Obes. Res.*, **13**, 1000–1007.

CANI P D (2005c), Modulation of gastro-intestinal peptides involved in the regulation of body weight, food intake and glucose metabolism by dietary fructans: from experimental data to human health. PhD Thesis Université catholique de Louvain Belgium.

CANI P D, JOLY E I, HORSMANS Y and DELZENNE N M (2006b), Oligofructose promotes satiety in healthy humans: a pilot study. *Eur. J. Clin. Nutr.*, **60**, 567–572.

CHERBUT C, FERRIER L, ROZE C, ANINI Y, BLOTTIERE H, LECANNU G and GALMICHE J P (1998), Short-chain fatty acids modify colonic motility through nerves and polypeptide YY release in the rat. *Am. J. Physiol*, **275**, G1415–G1422.

COWLEY M A, SMITH R G, DIANO S, TSCHOP M, PRONCHUK N, GROVE K L, STRASBURGER C J, BIDLINGMAIER M, ESTERMAN M, HEIMAN M L, GARCIA-SEGURA L M, NILLNI E A, MENDEZ P, LOW M J, SOTONYI P, FRIEDMAN J M, LIU H, PINTO S, COLMERS W F, CONE R D and HORVATH T L (2003), The distribution and mechanism of action of ghrelin in the CNS demonstrates a novel hypothalamic circuit regulating energy homeostasis. *Neuron*, **37**, 649–661.

D'ALESSIO D A, VOGEL R, PRIGEON R, LASCHANSKY E, KOERKER D, ENG J and ENSINCK J W (1996), Elimination of the action of glucagon-like peptide 1 causes an impairment of glucose tolerance after nutrient ingestion by healthy baboons. *J. Clin. Invest*, **97**, 133–138.

DAUBIOUL C, ROUSSEAU N, DEMEURE R, GALLEZ B, TAPER H, DECLERCK B and DELZENNE N (2002), Dietary fructans, but not cellulose, decrease triglyceride accumulation in the liver of obese Zucker fa/fa rats. *J. Nutr.*, **132**, 967–973.

DAUBIOUL C A, HORSMANS Y, LAMBERT P, DANSE E and DELZENNE N M (2005), Effects of oligofructose on glucose and lipid metabolism in patients with nonalcoholic steatohepatitis: results of a pilot study. *Eur. J. Clin. Nutr.*, **59**, 723–726.

DAUBIOUL C A, TAPER H S, DE WISPELAERE L D and DELZENNE N M (2000), Dietary oligofructose lessens hepatic steatosis, but does not prevent hypertriglyceridemia in obese zucker rats. *J. Nutr.*, **130**, 1314–1319.

DELZENNE N M (2003), Oligosaccharides: state of the art. *Proc. Nutr. Soc.*, **62**, 177–182.

DELZENNE N M and WILLIAMS C M (2002), Prebiotics and lipid metabolism. *Curr. Opin. Lipidol.*, **13**, 61–67.

DELZENNE N M, CANI P D, DAUBIOUL C and NEYRINCK A M (2005), Impact of inulin and oligofructose on gastrointestinal peptides. *Br. J. Nutr.*, **93** (Suppl 1), S157–S161.

DELZENNE N M, DAUBIOUL C, NEYRINCK A, LASA M and TAPER H S (2002), Inulin and oligofructose modulate lipid metabolism in animals: review of biochemical events and future prospects. *Br. J. Nutr.*, **87** (Suppl 2), S255–S259.

DEVRIES J W (2003), On defining dietary fibre. *Proc. Nutr. Soc.*, **62**, 37–43.

DIRAISON F, MOULIN P and BEYLOT M (2003), Contribution of hepatic de novo lipogenesis and reesterification of plasma non esterified fatty acids to plasma triglyceride synthesis during non-alcoholic fatty liver disease. *Diabetes Metab.*, **29**, 478–485.

DJURHUUS C B, HANSEN T K, GRAVHOLT C, ORSKOV L, HOSODA H, KANGAWA K, JORGENSEN J O, HOLST J J and SCHMITZ O (2002), Circulating levels of ghrelin and GLP-1 are inversely related during glucose ingestion. *Horm. Metab. Res.*, **34**, 411–413.

DROZDOWSKI L A, DIXON W T, MCBURNEY M I and THOMSON A B (2002), Short-chain fatty acids and total parenteral nutrition affect intestinal gene expression. *JPEN J. Parenter. Enteral Nutr.*, **26**, 145–150.

DRUCE M R, SMALL C J and BLOOM S R (2004), Minireview: Gut peptides regulating satiety. *Endocrinology*, **145**, 2660–2665.

FAO/WHO (1998), Carbohydrates in human nutrition. Report of a Joint FAO/WHO Expert Consultation. *FAO Food Nutr. Pap.*, **66**, 1–140.

GEE J M and JOHNSON I T (2005), Dietary lactitol fermentation increases circulating peptide YY and glucagon-like peptide-1 in rats and humans. *Nutrition*, **21**, 1036–1043.

GERSTEIN D E, WOODWARD-LOPEZ G, EVANS A E, KELSEY K and DREWNOWSKI A (2004), Clarifying concepts about macronutrients' effects on satiation and satiety. *J. Am. Diet. Assoc.*, **104**, 1151–1153.

GIBSON G and ROBERFROID M (1995), Dietary modulation of the human colonic microbiota; introducing the concept of prebiotics. *J. Nutr.*, **125**, 1401–1412.

HEATON K W (1973), Food fibre as an obstacle to energy intake. *Lancet*, **2**, 1418–1421.

HOAD C L, RAYMENT P, SPILLER R C, MARCIANI L, ALONSO B C, TRAYNOR C, MELA D J, PETERS H P and GOWLAND P A (2004), In vivo imaging of intragastric gelation and its effect on satiety in humans. *J. Nutr.*, **134**, 2293–2300.

HOLST J J and DEACON C F (2005), Glucagon-like peptide-1 mediates the therapeutic actions of DPP-IV inhibitors. *Diabetologia*, **48**, 612–615.

HOWARTH N C, SALTZMAN E, MCCRORY M A, GREENBERG A S, DWYER J, AUSMAN L, KRAMER D G and ROBERTS S B (2003), Fermentable and nonfermentable fiber supplements did not alter hunger, satiety or body weight in a pilot study of men and women consuming self-selected diets. *J. Nutr.*, **133**, 3141–3144.

HOWARTH N C, SALTZMAN E and ROBERTS S B (2001), Dietary fiber and weight regulation. *Nutr. Rev.*, **59**, 129–139.

JUNTUNEN K S, NISKANEN L K, LIUKKONEN K H, POUTANEN K S, HOLST J J and MYKKANEN H M (2002), Postprandial glucose, insulin, and incretin responses to grain products in healthy subjects. *Am. J. Clin. Nutr.*, **75**, 254–262.

KOJIMA M, HOSODA H, DATE Y, NAKAZATO M, MATSUO H and KANGAWA K (1999), Ghrelin is a growth-hormone-releasing acylated peptide from stomach. *Nature*, **402**, 656–660.

KOK N N, MORGAN L M, WILLIAMS C M, ROBERFROID M B, THISSEN J P and DELZENNE N M (1998a), Insulin, glucagon-like peptide 1, glucose-dependent insulinotropic polypeptide and insulin-like growth factor I as putative mediators of the hypolipidemic effect of oligofructose in rats. *J. Nutr.*, **128**, 1099–1103.

KOK N N, TAPER H S and DELZENNE N M (1998b), Oligofructose modulates lipid metabolism alterations induced by a fat-rich diet in rats. *J. Appl. Toxicol.*, **18**, 47–53.

LE BLAY G, MICHEL C, BLOTTIERE H M and CHERBUT C (1999), Prolonged intake of fructo-oligosaccharides induces a short-term elevation of lactic acid-producing bacteria and a persistent increase in cecal butyrate in rats. *J. Nutr.*, **129**, 2231–2235.

LEE H M, WANG G, ENGLANDER E W, KOJIMA M and GREELEY G H, JR (2002), Ghrelin, a new gastrointestinal endocrine peptide that stimulates insulin secretion: enteric distribution, ontogeny, influence of endocrine, and dietary manipulations. *Endocrinology*, **143**, 185–190.

LIPPL F, KIRCHER F, ERDMANN J, ALLESCHER H D and SCHUSDZIARRA V (2004), Effect of GIP, GLP-1, insulin and gastrin on ghrelin release in the isolated rat stomach. *Regul. Pept.*, **119**, 93–98.

LUCAS F, ACKROFF K and SCLAFANI A (1998), High-fat diet preference and overeating mediated by postingestive factors in rats. *Am. J. Physiol.*, **275**, R1511–R1522.

LUCAS F and SCLAFANI A (1999), Differential reinforcing and satiating effects of intragastric fat and carbohydrate infusions in rats. *Physiol. Behav.*, **66**, 381–388.

MAEDA H, YAMAMOTO R, HIRAO K and TOCHIKUBO O (2005), Effects of agar (kanten) diet on obese patients with impaired glucose tolerance and type 2 diabetes. *Diabetes Obes. Metab*, **7**, 40–46.

MASSIMINO S P, MCBURNEY M I, FIELD C J, THOMSON A B, KEELAN M, HAYEK M G and SUNVOLD G D (1998), Fermentable dietary fiber increases GLP-1 secretion and improves glucose homeostasis despite increased intestinal glucose transport capacity in healthy dogs. *J. Nutr.*, **128**, 1786–1793.

MCKEOWN N M, MEIGS J B, LIU S, SALTZMAN E, WILSON P W and JACQUES P F (2004), Carbohydrate nutrition, insulin resistance, and the prevalence of the metabolic syndrome in the Framingham Offspring Cohort. *Diabetes Care*, **27**, 538–546.

MEERAN K, O'SHEA D, EDWARDS C M, TURTON M D, HEATH M M, GUNN I, ABUSNANA S, ROSSI M, SMALL C J, GOLDSTONE A P, TAYLOR G M, SUNTER D, STEERE J, CHOI S J, GHATEI M A and BLOOM S R (1999), Repeated intracerebroventricular administration of glucagon-like peptide-1-(7–36) amide or exendin-(9–39) alters body weight in the rat. *Endocrinology*, **140**, 244–250.

MEIER J J and NAUCK M A (2005), Glucagon-like peptide 1 (GLP-1) in biology and pathology. *Diabetes Metab. Res. Rev.*, **21**, 91–117.

MEYER P D (2004), Nondigestible oligosaccharides as dietary fiber. *J. AOAC Int.*, **87**, 718–726.

MORAND C, REMESY C and DEMIGNE C (1993), Fatty acids are potent modulators of lactate utilization in isolated hepatocytes from fed rats. *Am. J. Physiol.*, **264**, E816–E823.

MURPHY O (2001), Non-polyol low-digestible carbohydrates: food applications and functional benefits. *Br. J. Nutr.*, **85**, S47–S53.

NAKAGAWA A, SATAKE H, NAKABAYASHI H, NISHIZAWA M, FURUYA K, NAKANO S, KIGOSHI T, NAKAYAMA K and UCHIDA K (2004), Receptor gene expression of glucagon-like peptide-1, but not glucose-dependent insulinotropic polypeptide, in rat nodose ganglion cells. *Auton. Neurosci.*, **110**, 36–43.

NIAN M, GU J, IRWIN D M and DRUCKER D J (2002), Human glucagon gene promoter sequences regulating tissue-specific versus nutrient-regulated gene expression. *Am. J. Physiol. Regul. Integr. Comp. Physiol.*, **282**, R173–R183.

NILSSON O, BILCHIK A J, GOLDENRING J R, BALLANTYNE G H, ADRIAN T E and MODLIN I M (1991), Distribution and immunocytochemical colocalization of peptide YY and enteroglucagon in endocrine cells of the rabbit colon. *Endocrinology*, **129**, 139–148.

NISHIZAWA M, NAKABAYASHI H, KAWAI K, ITO T, KAWAKAMI S, NAKAGAWA A, NIIJIMA A and UCHIDA K (2000), The hepatic vagal reception of intraportal GLP-1 is via receptor different from the pancreatic GLP-1 receptor. *J. Auton. Nerv. Syst.*, **80**, 14–21.

NYMAN M (2002), Fermentation and bulking capacity of indigestible carbohydrates: the case of inulin and oligofructose. *Br. J. Nutr.*, **87**, S163–S168.

ORSKOV C, BERSANI M, JOHNSEN A H, HOJRUP P and HOLST J J (1989), Complete sequences of glucagon-like peptide-1 from human and pig small intestine. *J. Biol. Chem.*, **264**, 12826–12829.

PEREIRA M A and LUDWIG D S (2001), Dietary fiber and body-weight regulation. Observations and mechanisms. *Pediatr. Clin. North Am.*, **48**, 969–980.

PERRIN I V, MARCHESINI M, ROCHAT F C, SCHIFFRIN E J and SCHILTER B (2003), Oligofructose does not affect the development of Type 1 diabetes mellitus induced by dietary proteins in the diabetes-prone BB rat model. *Diabetes Nutr. Metab.*, **16**, 94–101.

PICHE T, DES VARANNES S B, SACHER-HUVELIN S, HOLST J J, CUBER J C and GALMICHE J P (2003), Colonic fermentation influences lower esophageal sphincter function in gastroesophageal reflux disease. *Gastroenterology*, **124**, 894–902.

POUTEAU E, NGUYEN P, BALLEVRE O and KREMPF M (2003), Production rates and metabolism of short-chain fatty acids in the colon and whole body using stable isotopes. *Proc. Nutr. Soc.*, **62**, 87–93.

RAMIREZ I and FRIEDMAN M I (1990), Dietary hyperphagia in rats: role of fat, carbohydrate, and energy content. *Physiol. Behav.*, **47**, 1157–1163.

RAO V A (2001), The prebiotic properties of oligofructose at low intake levels. *Nutr. Res.*, **21**, 843–848.

REIMER R A and MCBURNEY M I (1996), Dietary fiber modulates intestinal proglucagon messenger ribonucleic acid and postprandial secretion of glucagon-like peptide-1 and insulin in rats. *Endocrinology*, **137**, 3948–3956.

REIMER R A, THOMSON A B, RAJOTTE R V, BASU T K, OORAIKUL B and MCBURNEY M I (1997), A physiological level of rhubarb fiber increases proglucagon gene expression and modulates intestinal glucose uptake in rats. *J. Nutr.*, **127**, 1923–1928.

RITTER R C (2004), Gastrointestinal mechanisms of satiation for food. *Physiol. Behav.*, **81**, 249–273.

ROBERFROID M (2003), Probiotics and prebiotics: why should the medical community pay attention? *Drug Discov. Today*, **8**, 1107–1108.

ROBERFROID M and SLAVIN J (2000), Nondigestible oligosaccharides. *Crit. Rev. Food Sci. Nutr.*, **40**, 461–480.

SCHIRRA J, STURM K, LEICHT P, ARNOLD R, GOKE B and KATSCHINSKI M (1998), Exendin(9–39)amide is an antagonist of glucagon-like peptide-1(7–36)amide in humans. *J. Clin. Invest*, **101**, 1421–1430.

SCHWARTZ M W, WOODS S C, PORTE D, JR, SEELEY R J and BASKIN D G (2000), Central nervous system control of food intake. *Nature*, **404**, 661–671.

SCROCCHI L A, MARSHALL B A, COOK S M, BRUBAKER P L and DRUCKER D J (1998), Identification of glucagon-like peptide 1 (GLP-1) actions essential for glucose homeostasis in mice with disruption of GLP-1 receptor signaling. *Diabetes*, **47**, 632–639.

SLAVIN J L (2005), Dietary fiber and body weight. *Nutrition*, **21**, 411–418.

SULLIVAN A C, TRISCARI J and COMAI K (1978), Caloric compensatory responses to diets containing either nonabsorbable carbohydrate or lipid by obese and lean Zucker rats. *Am. J. Clin. Nutr.*, **31**, S261–S266.

TAPPENDEN K A, DROZDOWSKI L A, THOMSON A B and MCBURNEY M I (1998), Short-chain fatty acid-supplemented total parenteral nutrition alters intestinal structure, glucose transporter 2 (GLUT2) mRNA and protein, and proglucagon mRNA abundance in normal rats. *Am. J. Clin. Nutr.*, **68**, 118–125.

TOURREL C, BAILBE D, MEILE M J, KERGOAT M, PORTHA B (2001), Glucagon-like peptide 1 and exendin 4 stimulate b-cells neogenesis in streptozotocin treated new born rats resulting in persistently improved glucose homeostasis at adult age. *Diabetes*, **50**, 1562–1570.

TSCHOP M, SMILEY D L and HEIMAN M L (2000), Ghrelin induces adiposity in rodents. *Nature*, **407**, 908–913.

TSCHOP M, WEYER C, TATARANNI P A, DEVANARAYAN V, RAVUSSIN E and HEIMAN M L (2001), Circulating ghrelin levels are decreased in human obesity. *Diabetes*, **50**, 707–709.

TUOHY K M, FINLAY R K, WYNNE A G and GIBSON G R (2001), A human volunteer study on the prebiotic effects of HP-inulin – Faecal bacteria enumerated using fluorescent in situ hybridisation (FISH). *Anaerobe*, **7**, 113–118.

VAN LOO J, COUSSEMENT P, DE LEENHEER L, HOEBREGS H and SMITS G (1995), On the presence of inulin and oligofructose as natural ingredients in the western diet. *Crit. Rev. Food Sci. Nutr.*, **35**, 525–552.

VULEVIC J, RASTALL R A and GIBSON G R (2004), Developing a quantitative approach for determining the in vitro prebiotic potential of dietary oligosaccharides. *FEMS Microbiol. Lett.*, **236**, 153–159.

WEST D B and YORK B (1998), Dietary fat, genetic predisposition, and obesity: lessons from animal models. *Am. J. Clin. Nutr.*, **67**, 505S–512S.

WYNNE K, STANLEY S, MCGOWAN B and BLOOM S (2005), Appetite control. *J. Endocrinol.*, **184**, 291–318.

# 8

# Resistant starch

**A. M. Birkett, National Starch Food Innovation, USA and I. L. Brown, University of Colorado Health Sciences Center, Denver, Colorado, USA**

## 8.1 Introduction

Starch is usually a major component in both the composition and energy value of the foods that we eat. Therefore understanding the contribution that starches make to energy metabolism is an important consideration in both the choice of foods and in the selection of specific ingredients to assist with targeting weight management regimes. The modernization of the Western diet has seen significant changes in the amount and type of starch consumed with increasing amounts being readily digestible. In this sense, type refers not only to the source, but also the nutritional fate of the starch. Traditional starch-rich foods are often relegated to a low dietary status as being merely caloric fillers, and starch ingredients are mostly used by food formulators for their texturizing and viscosifying attributes. However, the potential dietary importance of starchy foods and the variety of starch sub-types that they contain has now elevated the level of interest in this component of the diet and identified opportunities to selectively augment foods with specific starch sub-types.

Starch is the preferred method of storing the carbohydrate glucose in insoluble form in most higher plants, including cereals such as corn, rice and wheat. Starch exists in many forms depending on the plant species and this is reflected in variations in such parameters as granule morphology, thermic properties and nutritional effects. Until the early 1980s it was thought that starch, particularly when cooked, was fully digested within the small intestine and absorbed into the body as glucose. Excreted starch was attributed to malabsorption. Since that time, some starches have been identified that resist normal digestion in humans and animals. These so-called 'resistant starches' (RSs) pass through the small intestine to the large bowel where they are fermented by the resident colonic microflora. Early research focused on the effects of RS consumption in the large bowel and identified an important role for RSs in helping to promote digestive health. Recently, clinical research has suggested a role for dietary RS with respect to energy metabolism and weight management.

Starchy foods have a traditional place in diets globally, although the type and amount of starchy foods consumed does vary with cultural preference. In Western countries usually less starch is consumed (i.e. 73–156 g/day in the UK, USA and Australia) than in countries that consume traditional non-Western diets (i.e. 215–371 g/day in India and China) (Cassidy *et al.*, 1994). Much of the starch that is found in foods in Western diets is readily digested and incorporated into highly processed and refined foods such as bread, pizza and breakfast cereals. Processed foods present an opportunity for food formulators to incorporate starch-based ingredients that have been selected for their specific and simultaneous contribution to both nutritional quality and food performance. For this reason RS ingredients offer enormous potential as functional food ingredients.

### 8.1.1 Relevance of resistant starch to weight management

RS appears to play two roles with respect to weight management. Firstly there is a reduction in the digestible energy available from the RS compared with a readily digestible starch. The presence of RS in foods reduces their caloric density. Recently, research has demonstrated a second role for RS in energy metabolism and metabolic control. The lower glucose and insulin impact of RS causes changes in lipid metabolism that favor lower levels of lipid production and storage. In addition, RS is fermented within the large bowel by the indigenous colonic bacteria producing an important range of compounds called short-chain fatty acids (SCFAs). The amount and type of SCFA produced are proposed to affect carbohydrate and lipid metabolism in the body, particularly in the liver, muscle and adipose tissue. The known effects of RS in relation to weight management are listed in Table 8.1. Each of these aspects will be discussed later in this chapter.

## 8.2 Background

### 8.2.1 Definition of resistant starch

From a nutritional perspective, starches can be classified according to their digestive fate in the gastrointestinal tract. Starches can be fully digestible in the small intestine (either rapidly digested or slowly digested) or indigestible (resistant). Depending upon food consumption practices and individual gastrointestinal processes, it is possible that some digestible starch may

**Table 8.1** Known effects of RS on parameters relevant to weight management

| |
|---|
| Resistant to digestion – does not contribute to available glucose |
| Decreased caloric contribution compared with digestible starch |
| Decreased macronutrient utilization |
| Decreased body fat accumulation |
| Decreased adipocyte volume |
| Increased lipid oxidation at the expense of carbohydrate oxidation |
| Decreased lipid production (lipogenesis) |
| Increased insulin sensitivity |
| Decreased glucose response |
| Decreased insulin response |
| Possible contribution to satiety |

actually pass through the small intestine undigested and contribute to the amount of RS.

Following the discovery that some starch resisted digestion, RS became the subject of widespread attention by a collaborative group of European researchers between 1990 and 1994, known collectively as EURESTA – European FLAIR-Concerted Action on the 'Physiological implication of the consumption of resistant starch in man'. It involved 36 groups from 10 countries, and was organized into the following four areas: (1) definition and analysis of RS; (2) RS production and technological impact; (3) physiological effects of RS, principally as they relate to the upper and lower gastrointestinal tract; and (4) the energy contribution of RS (Brown *et al.*, 2001). Although an officially recognized method to quantify RS did not emerge from this extensive program, it did provide a significant base for subsequent RS research.

The EURESTA group proposed a definition for RS, namely: 'Resistant starch is the sum of starch and products of starch degradation not absorbed in the small intestine of healthy individuals' (Asp, 1992). Although this is not a current regulatory definition, it has become widely accepted. The definition proposed by EURESTA is a physiological and not a chemical definition. As a consequence any measurement of RS must reflect how much starch is digested and what occurs to starch in the body. RS is comprised of many chemically and physically distinct starch and starch-derived materials.

RS is best measured *in vivo* in humans as the starch excreted at the terminal ileum of ileostomate subjects, as this directly accounts for individual variation in the gastrointestinal tract management of starches. However, this remains an estimate because ileostomates are not intact healthy individuals. The *in vitro* quantification of the RS content of foods and ingredients employs enzyme-based methods that simulate the gastrointestinal tract, such as that recommended by the Association of Official Analytical Chemists (AOAC) which make reference to RS, dietary fiber and resistant maltodextrins.

Definitions of dietary fiber have recently been expanded by several groups to recognize a larger range of dietary components that demonstrate appropriate and defined physiological behaviors. RS has been considered a part of dietary fiber according to the definitions proposed by the Institute of Medicine of the National Academies in the USA (IOM, 2002) and the American Association of Cereal Chemists (AACC, 2001) according to the specific physiological effects described. The Codex Alimentarius Commission (FAO/WHO, 2005) has also proposed a definition for dietary fiber that lists physiological effects, and if approved would also recognize RS.

Dietary fiber represents a broad range of compounds, based on structure and chemistry, and each component of dietary fiber should be individually assessed for its role in the formulation of foods. RS has it own unique profile of physiological and food engineering benefits that often recommend its use when compared with other fibers. Typically RS can be used to increase the dietary fiber of foods with minimal changes to their appearance or organoleptic properties.

### 8.2.2 Starch composition and arrangement

Starch is a heterogeneous group when considering structure and conformation, and so too is RS. In order to select appropriate RSs for food development, a basic understanding of starch chemistry is useful. All RSs share one basic similarity – they are all glucose-based polymers. Starch is largely composed of two glucose polymers, either the straight chain (amylose) or the highly branched chain (amylopectin) (see Fig. 8.1). The chain type is dictated by the type of linkages between the glucose monomers – i.e. amylose contains essentially $\alpha$-1→4 linkages and amylopectin contains both $\alpha$-1→4 and $\alpha$-1→6 linkages which facilitate chain branching.

Both starch polymers can theoretically be enzymatically digested within the small intestine. However starches with elevated levels of amylose tend to have higher inherent resistance to amylolysis, particularly in their granular form. The most researched and commercially used form of RS is obtained from high-amylose maize or corn and it is this material that has been used in experiments to investigate the potential impact of RS in weight management regimes.

The digestibility of amylose and amylopectin differs because their polymeric configuration and granule conformation confer a range of physical properties (Table 8.2). These include chain length, molecular weight, melting temperature and three-dimensional structure (e.g. helicity and crystallinity). In corn, the polymeric configuration also determines the properties of the starch on cooking. For example, when heat and moisture are applied simultaneously (as in normal cooking procedures), the amylopectin-rich or waxy maize starch loses its granular definition and undergoes gelatinization. In either the granular or gelatinized state, the waxy corn starch is readily

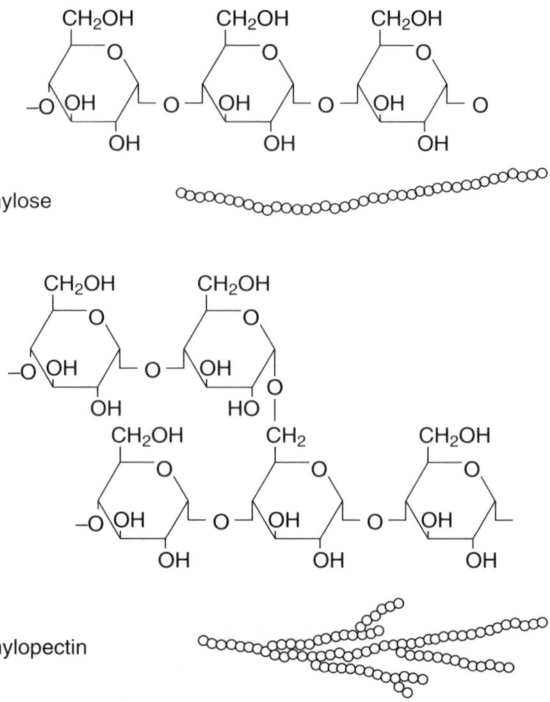


**Fig. 8.1** Polymeric configurations of starch.

**Table 8.2** Relative characteristics of amylose and amylopectin

| Property | Amylose | Amylopectin |
|---|---|---|
| Polymeric arrangement | Linear | Branched |
| Linkage type | $\alpha$-1 → 4 | $\alpha$-1 → 4 and $\alpha$-1 → 6 |
| Degree of polymerization | Smaller | Larger |
| Molecular weight | Smaller | Larger |
| Melting temperature | Higher | Lower |
| Ultrastructure | Higher helicity | Lower helicity |
| Tendency to retrograde | Faster | Slower |
| Degree of resistance | Higher | Lower |

digested by amylases (Brown *et al.*, 2003). In contrast, high-amylose corn starch, as a result of its granule structure and conformation, resists gelatinization during most normal food processing conditions, such as in the baking of bread, and contributes RS and dietary fiber to the food.

Other properties of starch are also known to contribute to their resistance. In nature, starch polymers are localized into granules. Granular morphology and surface properties differ between starch sources, and can affect enzyme interaction and hence the degree and rate of amylolysis. Many of these differences are lost upon cooking, when most starch granules typically gelatinize. One exception is high-amylose corn starch, which retains its granularity under most normal cooking conditions.

### 8.2.3 Starch digestion and absorption

*Fate of digestible starch*

Most of the starch present in the diet is cooked and gelatinized. As such, most dietary starch is easily digested, accounting for approximately 95% of that consumed (Cassidy *et al.*, 1994). Various diet, food processing and physiological factors are known to affect starch digestion, and these are listed in Table 8.3. Starch is digested/hydrolyzed enzymically and sequentially within the upper gastrointestinal tract (Gray, 1992, 2003; Levin, 1994). In the mouth some starch is digested to maltose via salivary amylase. In the small intestine, starch is initially digested in the lumen via pancreatic amylase to smaller compounds that include maltose, maltotriose and branched limit dextrins. Two more enzymes produced by the brush border (sucrase-isomaltase and glucoamylase) further hydrolyze the starch products to glucose which is actively absorbed through the enterocyte membrane. Most dietary starch is absorbed as glucose to participate in energy metabolism in the body.

**Table 8.3** Food and physiological factors affecting the rate and extent of starch digestion

| Category | Detail |
|---|---|
| Food behavior | Type of starchy food eaten |
| | Amount of starchy food eaten |
| | Customs of food preparation and consumption |
| Nature of the starch eaten | Amylose content |
| | Granularity |
| | Conformation |
| Food processing | Loss of cellular and native plant structure |
| | Processing conditions |
| | Extent of gelatinization |
| | Particle size |
| | Other food components – antinutrients, viscous fiber, fat |
| Physiology | Health status |
| | Individual physiological differences |
| | Extent of chewing |
| | Gastric emptying |
| | Viscosity |
| | Gastrointestinal transit time |
| | Enzyme inhibition |

*Fate of resistant starch*
RS is not digested, hydrolyzed or absorbed and so it does not contribute to plasma glucose levels. Instead RS passes into the large bowel where it contributes metabolic energy through bacterially fermented and absorbed SCFAs.

The large bowel is intensely populated with bacteria, with several hundred species present at about $10^{11}$–$10^{12}$ CFU/g dry weight (Cummings and Macfarlane, 1991). These bacteria have a key role in salvaging undigested energy from food residues via metabolic pathways that generate SCFAs – such as acetate, propionate and butyrate. Some of the salvaged energy is utilized by the bacteria for growth but approximately 95% of the SCFAs are absorbed (Cummings and Macfarlane, 1991) and provide energy to the body. For example butyrate is the primary energy source for colonocytes and acetate is mainly used by muscle tissue (Salminen *et al.*, 1998). SCFAs provide approximately 5–10% of our daily energy intake (Cummings, 1996).

Some of the RS is not fermented. The amount will depend on the type of RS, how much RS has been consumed, the composition of the colonic microflora, the digestive transit time and the health status of the individual. As much as 22% of RS can be excreted unfermented from the body (Phillips *et al.*, 1995).

### 8.2.4 Types of resistant starch

As previously indicated, there are different types of RS. This is analogous to dietary fiber, for which there are many different types and sources. Fibers exhibit a broad range of physiological effects and so do RSs. Four classes of RS have been described (Table 8.4) (Brown *et al.*, 1995). Three are found

**Table 8.4** Types of RS (from Brown *et al.*, 1995)

| Type of starch | Example of occurrence | Probable digestion in the small intestine |
|---|---|---|
| Rapidly digestible starch | Freshly cooked starchy food | Rapid |
| Slowly digestible starch | Most raw cereals | Slow, but complete |
| Resistant starch | | |
| RS1: physically inaccessible | Partly milled grains and seeds | Resistant |
| RS2: resistant granules | Raw potato, green banana, some legumes, and high amylose corn starch | Resistant |
| RS3: retrograded starch | Cooked and cooled potato, bread and cornflakes | Resistant |
| RS4: chemically modified starch | Starch ethers, esters and cross-bonded | Resistant |

in nature or are formed as part of normal cooking procedures while the fourth class can be produced using chemical modification methods that are approved for use in foods. Commercial sources of RS-rich ingredients are available for increasing the RS and/or dietary fiber content of foods and these will be described later. RS ingredients from all four classes of RS are available commercially.

- Resistant starch type 1 (RS1). This type of starch is resistant because the starch is physically trapped within the food matrix. Enzymes are physically inhibited from reaching the starch. Milling or grinding foods can release the starch, making it accessible and more digestible.
- Resistant starch type 2 (RS2). This type of starch is naturally resistant because of the nature of the starch granule. RS2 occurs in foods where the starch is eaten raw (e.g. unripe bananas) or where the granules do not gelatinize during cooking (e.g. high-amylose corn starch).
- Resistant starch type 3 (RS3). This type of starch occurs when gelatinized starch is cooked and cooled. It can occur naturally during normal food processing (e.g. cooked and cooled potatoes) or can occur during the manufacture of RS-rich ingredients.
- Resistant starch type 4 (RS4). This type of starch is prepared by the introduction of chemical bonds to the starch polymer that interfere with the action of the digestive amylases. The inhibition is dependent upon the type and extent of the bonding. Chemistries that inhibit amylolysis can include dextrinization, etherification, esterification and oxidation, and cross-linking with difunctional reagents, and can markedly affect the food engineering functionality contributed by the RS to the food, e.g. solubility and process tolerance.

### 8.2.5 Sources of resistant starch

RS is a natural part of our diet but the quantity of RS consumed in foods can vary depending on the amount and type of starch present, how the food was processed, how it was stored before consumption and how it was ingested. RS can constitute as much as 18% of the dry mass of a food (Englyst *et al.*, 1992). However although some foods are relatively high in RS, these foods are not typically consumed on a large scale, hence the need for RS-enriched foods. RS levels present in some common foods range from as low as 1% of the dry matter in white bread, to 5% in hot boiled potatoes (Table 8.5).

Intakes of RS are estimates only due to a lack of internationally agreed methodologies and limited RS values for commonly consumed foods. There are no national food composition databases that contain an exhaustive list of the RS content of starchy foods. However, irrespective of these sources of variation the estimated levels of RS intakes in Western countries are consistently lower than for traditional and less-processed diets. For example in Western countries RS intakes could range between 3 and 9 g/day (see

**Table 8.5** RS content of common foods (from Englyst *et al.*, 1992)

| Food | Dry matter (%) | RS (g/100g dry matter) |
|---|---|---|
| White bread | 54.5 | 1 |
| Wholemeal bread | 52.0 | 1 |
| Cornflakes | 95.8 | 3 |
| Porridge oats | 90.7 | 2 |
| Ryvita crispbread | 94.3 | 3 |
| Boiled potato (hot) | 22.8 | 5 |
| Boiled potato (cold) | 23.8 | 10 |
| Spaghetti (freshly cooked) | 28.3 | 5 |
| Spaghetti (cooled) | 34.7 | 4 |
| Peas (frozen, boiled 5 min) | 18.3 | 5 |
| Lentils (boiled 20 min, cold) | 28.3 | 9 |
| Haricot beans (boiled 40 min) | 41.4 | 18 |

Table 8.6), with the largest source of RS being from cereals; in contrast, in China estimated RS intakes could reach closer to 20 g/day. Recent research has demonstrated a rationale for increasing RS intakes, particularly for designing foods for weight management. Even though some food processing techniques form RS, e.g. cooking/cooling processes, most RS has been removed from the diet by ingredient and food processing techniques. Commercial RS ingredients are an ideal choice for enriching RS intake in the diet. Currently, RSs from all four classes are commercially available. Each type of RS has different physiological properties, so supporting evidence should be independently evaluated for each individual ingredient. The RS ingredients prepared from high-amylose corn are currently the best characterized, both physiologically and for food functionality, of those commercially available.

## 8.3 Role of resistant starch in weight management

### 8.3.1 Weight management, direct evidence

RS is by its very nature indigestible and so does not contribute directly to plasma blood glucose levels. Therefore, replacing digestible starch with RS is a natural fit for low-glycemic foods and diets. In a 2003 report, the World Health Organization (WHO) reviewed the strength of evidence on various factors that might promote or protect against weight gain and obesity. They assessed the totality of evidence, including randomized controlled trials (highest ranking), associated evidence and expert opinions. This group advised that based on the available evidence there is a 'possible' decreased risk of weight gain and obesity with low-glycemic-index foods.

Few studies have looked at the impact of low-glycemic diets on weight loss or maintenance, by directly measuring body weight or body mass index

**Table 8.6** Estimated consumption of RS worldwide

| Country | Estimated intake (g/day) | Reference |
|---|---|---|
| Australia | 5 female, 5.3 male (36% cereals, 26% vegetables, 22% fruits) | Baghurst *et al.*, 1996 |
| | 3.4–9.4 range | Roberts *et al.*, 2004 |
| | 8 g/10 MJ | Muir *et al.*, 1998 |
| | 8.6 g/10 MJ | Walker *et al.*, 1997 |
| Belgium | 3.99 | Dysseler & Hoffem, 1994 |
| China | 20 g/10 MJ | Muir *et al.*, 1998 |
| Denmark | 3.67 | Dysseler and Hoffem, 1994 |
| England | 3.97 | Dysseler and Hoffem, 1994 |
| Europe, mean | 4.11 | Dysseler and Hoffem, 1994 |
| France | 3.73 | Dysseler and Hoffem, 1994 |
| Germany | 3.75 | Dysseler and Hoffem, 1994 |
| India | 10 | Platel and Shurpalekar, 1994 |
| Italy | 8.5 (7.2 g north-west, 9.2 g south) | Brighenti *et al.*, 1998 |
| Netherlands | 5.29 | Dysseler and Hoffem, 1994 |
| New Zealand | 5.7 | Baghurst *et al.*, 1996 |
| Norway | 3.22 | Dysseler and Hoffem, 1994 |
| Spain | 5.74 | Dysseler and Hoffem, 1994 |
| Sweden | 3.36 | Dysseler and Hoffem, 1994 |
| | 3.2 (1.3 g bread, 1.2 g potatoes) | Elmstahl, 2002 |
| Switzerland | 4.38 | Dysseler and Hoffem, 1994 |
| UK | 2.76 | Tomlin and Read, 1990 |

(BMI). However, those that have generally indicate a positive role for low-glycemic diets. Ebbeling *et al.* (2003) compared low-glycemic-load dietary advice with low-fat dietary advice in a group of young people aged 13–21 years with a BMI greater than the 95th percentile. The authors observed a lower BMI with the low-glycemic group after 12 months (6 month intervention plus 6 month follow-up). This supports observations from a US cohort of adults, where glycemic index but not total carbohydrate intake was positively associated with BMI, indicating a role for carbohydrate type over amount (Ma *et al.*, 2005). In shorter-term studies (6 weeks to 4 months), a comparison of low-glycemic-index with high-glycemic-index or low-fat diets showed lower weight and/or BMI with the low-glycemic-index diet (Slabber *et al.*, 1994; Spieth *et al.*, 2000; Jimenez-Cruz *et al.*, 2003).

Studies such as those mentioned above support a role for low-glycemic foods in weight management. More long-term clinical trials in which RS-enriched foods are included are needed to establish this association with greater certainty, particularly for weight loss. However a wealth of associated supporting evidence exists that indicates a clear role for RS in weight management, particularly when digestible starch in foods is at least partly replaced by RS. This evidence will be discussed here.

### 8.3.2 Weight management, supporting evidence

RS is associated with nutritional, metabolic and physiological changes that make it an attractive ingredient not only for weight management (Table 8.1), but also for other chronic diseases associated with the metabolic syndrome such as dyslipidemia, insulin resistance, type 2 diabetes, hypertension and coronary heart disease (Higgins, 2004). Previously a role for RS was attributed to reduced digestibility, and the impact of lower glucose absorption. More recent research, however, indicates a broader health impact of RS on metabolism, via fermentation of RS to SCFAs in the large bowel. Fermentable carbohydrates have their own unique fermentation profile, in terms of relative type and amount of SCFAs. Hence the metabolic impact of fermentation will differ between RS and other fiber types. The hypothesized interaction between fermentation by-products and target metabolic tissues will evolve as more mechanistic information becomes available.

*Energy value*

Foods containing RSs have a lower caloric density than similar foods with digestible starch because RS does not contribute available glucose to the body, and RS increases energy wastage (excretion). However, contrary to expectation, commercial RSs do contribute some metabolic energy for two reasons in particular.

- Commercial RS ingredients typically contain some digestible starch. That is, there are no commercial ingredients currently available that are 100% RS. The higher the RS contribution to the ingredient, the lower the caloric contribution.
- Most of the SCFAs generated by colonic bacterial fermentation of the RS will be absorbed and made available for further metabolism. All fibers that are fermented in the body will contribute some energy through SCFAs.

Typically the energy contribution of RS ingredients is approximately one-third lower than for digestible starches. Reported values will differ between methodologies and ingredients.

Digestible energy: Digestible energy is typically measured as dietary energy less fecal energy. An RS ingredient would be expected to have lower digestible energy because it is partially indigestible, contributes to fecal bulking and increases excretion of other nutrients. Behall and Howe (1996) from the US Department of Agriculture (USDA) reported that high-amylose corn RS2 had 67% of the partial digestible energy of regular cornstarch, at 11.7 kJ/g. This was supported in rats, with the digestible energy contribution from high-amylose corn RS3 being 62% of that from wheat starch (Aust *et al.*, 2001). These values refer to both the digestible and resistant fractions of the RS ingredient. Although the energy value of the RS fraction alone was calculated to be 8.9–9.2 kJ/g (Mathers, 1992) and was measured as 15 kJ/g for corn or 12 kJ/g for potato (Livesey *et al.*, 1990), this energy generated via fermentation does not contribute significantly to whole-body energy (Cummings, 1996).

RS is known to increase energy wastage (excretion) from the gastrointestinal tract. Rats fed high-amylose corn RS2 and RS3 had increased fecal energy (de Schrijver *et al.*, 1999). The increased energy wastage would be partially contributed by increased excretion of lipids (de Deckere *et al.*, 1995), which was measured when rats were fed high-amylose corn RS2.

Metabolic energy: Lower metabolic energy of raw potato RS2 was shown in humans by Tagliabue *et al.* (1995), with 60% reduction in thermic effect. Results are inconsistent in animal studies, possibly due to differences in physiology, particularly fermentative capacity between species (Andrieux and Sacquet, 1986; de Schrijver *et al.*, 1999).

*Body composition and lipid storage*

Not only BMI, but also body composition and regional differences in lipid deposition are associated with increased risk of chronic disease. Incorporating RS into foods lowers body lipid composition and distribution, principally via reduced lipogenesis (lipid production) and increased lipid oxidation (lipid utilization).

Body composition: The ability of RS to lower body lipid composition has been shown consistently across animal studies, indicating that the value of RS in foods for weight management extends beyond lower digestibility into a metabolic role. RS2 from high-amylose corn and potato causes lower body lipid accumulation (Williamson *et al.*, 1999; Pawlak *et al.*, 2004), and more specifically lower epididymal pad weight in the abdomen following consumption of various sources of RS (de Deckere *et al.*, 1993, 1995; Pawlak *et al.*, 2001; Kishida *et al.*, 2001; Zhou and Kaplan, 1997). Confirmatory studies in humans are underway. RS has also been shown to impact the cellular morphology of adipose tissue, with rats fed mung bean RS2 having smaller adipocyte size (Lerer-Metzger *et al.*, 1996; Kabir *et al.*, 1998b). It has also been demonstrated that the consumption of RS2 from high-amylose corn in rats could not only reduce the body's lipid composition but also increase its muscle mass (Kiriyama, 1996).

Lipid storage and associated metabolism: Selective changes in body lipid storage could be associated with the affect of RS on insulin and hence insulin-regulated pathways, such as glucose utilization and lipid metabolism in adipose tissue. Lipogenesis (lipid production) from glucose conversion was lower in adipocytes for rats fed RS from mung beans (Kabir *et al.*, 1998b). This could be explained by lower expression of GLUT4, the protein responsible for insulin-stimulated glucose uptake, and lower fatty acid synthase activity and expression, the enzyme responsible for the rate-limiting step in lipid synthesis, in the adipose tissue of rats fed high-RS diets (Kabir *et al.*, 1998a).

Morand *et al.* (1994) investigated a role for corn-based RS in hepatic lipid and carbohydrate metabolism, and showed that lipogenesis (lipid production) as well as glycolysis was also lower in hepatic tissue. Gluconeogenesis was favored, which is also antagonistic to lipogenesis. Reduced lipogenic enzyme activities included: glucose-6-P dehydrogenase and malic enzyme, which are known for their role in supplying NADPH; ATP citrate lyase, which provides acetyl coenzyme A (CoA); acetyl CoA carboxylase, the key enzyme of lipogenesis; and fatty acid synthetase. Reduced glycolytic enzyme activities included glucokinase and pyruvate kinase activity; with higher gluconeogenesis activity via the rate-controlling enzyme phosphoenolpyruvate carboxykinase (PEPCK).

In the study by Morand *et al.* (1994), in which most lipogenic enzymes were inhibited, acetyl CoA synthetase activity was not affected by RS. This suggests a role for the SCFA acetate in liver metabolism. Higgins (2004) noted that acetate can inhibit glycogenolysis, further suggesting a mechanistic role for SCFA to spare carbohydrate oxidation, potentially promoting lipid oxidation, thereby reducing lipid storage in response to RS consumption.

Lipid oxidation: Evidence supporting increased lipid oxidation with high-RS diets will be described in detail in the following section.

*Whole-body energy metabolism*

RS has been shown to impact whole-body energy metabolism via at least three measurements:

- lower respiratory quotient (RQ);
- lower diet-induced thermogenesis (DIT);
- lower energy expenditure (EE).

Effects in the short term are probably due to the lower supply of available carbohydrate in RS-rich meals, and the direct effect on carbohydrate and lipid oxidation. In the longer term, effects could be due to a contributory role of SCFAs in metabolic substrate selection.

Respiratory quotient: RQ is a comparative measure of oxidative substrate selection, i.e. carbohydrate oxidation relative to lipid oxidation. When the RQ is lower there is relatively more lipid oxidation. Lower RQ or delta RQ up to 5–6 h after a meal was reported with high-amylose corn based and raw potato based RS2 in two human studies (Tagliabue *et al.*, 1995; Higgins *et al.*, 2004). Over 23–24 h this was supported in rats (Aust *et al.*, 2001), but not in humans (Howe *et al.*, 1996; Achour *et al.*, 1997).

Diet-induced thermogenesis: The calculated difference between postprandial metabolic rate and resting metabolic rate can be used to represent DIT, a 'tax' on dietary metabolism. Tagliabue *et al.* (1995) demonstrated that when raw potato RS2 replaced pregelatinized potato starch, DIT was lower in the first 5 h after meal consumption. This is attributed to the lower availability of starch for digestion and metabolism. This was not supported over a longer 8-h time period in the human study by Achour *et al.* (1997), which also did not observe a change in RQ.

Energy expenditure: The impact of RS on EE is less conclusive than for DIT and RQ, with only one study available to report on each of the absorptive, postprandial and total 24 hours periods following a meal. Tagliabue *et al.* (1995) reported a lower EE in the postprandial period, when raw potato RS2 replaced pregelatinized potato starch in a meal. This is probably due to the lower available starch content of the meal.

Carbohydrate versus lipid oxidation: The choice of substrate for energy metabolism affects RQ and DIT. RQ is lower when the balance of lipid: carbohydrate oxidation shifts towards lipids. Studies with RS have demonstrated a shift towards increased lipid oxidation, which may be important for weight management because reduced rates of lipid oxidation have been linked with greater weight gain (Brand-Miller *et al.*, 2002).

When potato RS2 was fed to humans, glucose oxidation was lower and lipid oxidation higher, associated with a lower RQ (Tagliabue *et al.*, 1995). Increased lipid oxidation relates to both total and meal lipid, as demonstrated by Higgins *et al.* (2004) who observed a 23% increase in meal lipid oxidation with as little as 5.4% RS in a single meal. Studies in animals support an effect of RS on substrate oxidation – high-amylose RS3 lowered RQ by lower carbohydrate oxidation (Aust *et al.*, 2001). Mechanistically these observations are probably related to the effects of RS on cellular metabolism described previously.

*Insulin response and sensitivity*

Insulin sensitivity: Insulin is an important regulatory hormone, contributing to carbohydrate, lipid and protein metabolism. Most importantly, insulin is key for glucose homeostasis, regulating glucose uptake by muscle and adipose tissue. Insulin resistance, defined as a sub-optimal biological response to insulin (Hulman and Falkner, 1994) is a characteristic feature of the metabolic syndrome, and is known to develop as people age. High-amylose corn RS2 enhances insulin sensitivity, assisting the body to handle dietary carbohydrate better (Robertson *et al.*, 2003, 2005). Furthermore, in rats, dietary starch type has an important affect on the development of insulin resistance. Rats fed high-amylose corn RS2 were protected against developing insulin resistance for more than three times as long as for rats fed low-RS starch or glucose – up to 26 weeks versus only 8 weeks (Byrnes *et al.*, 1995; Higgins *et al.*, 1996).

Glucose response: Postprandial glucose and insulin response influence insulin sensitivity (Higgins, 2004). One of the most consistent effects of RS is the ability to lower glucose response, with many groups reporting decreased postprandial response when RS replaces digestible starch in foods (Higgins, 2004). This has been observed in non-diabetics, type 2 diabetics and various animal models. The magnitude of this effect is particularly dependent upon two considerations, namely the RS amount relative to other carbohydrates present in the cooked foods as eaten, and the RS type with higher-amylose starches being more effective.

Behall and Hallfrisch (2002) fed breads made with corn starches varying in amylose content from 30–70%. The higher the amylose content, the greater the RS content, hence the lower the effect on glucose response. Overall, bread made with 70% amylose starch had the greatest impact on the reduction in the postprandial plasma glucose response. Furthermore, Brown *et al.* (1995) demonstrated that the amount of RS ingredient included in the bread relative to other carbohydrates already present is an important consideration for obtaining a measurable impact on glucose response. White bread with 5% replacement of flour with high-amylose corn RS2 had a relative glycemic response of 95 (versus 100 for a commercial bread). Bread with higher flour replacement levels had a more marked response, with 10% and 20% flour replacement reducing the relative glycemic response to 74 and 53 respectively.

Insulin response: Insulin is a regulatory hormone for glucose homeostasis, therefore the lower glucose response observed with high-RS foods, causes a lower blood insulin response. In studies where RS has replaced digestible starch, many have reported a decreased postprandial insulin response (Higgins, 2004). Insulin levels may be predictive of weight gain (Ludwig, 2000). Furthermore, hyperinsulinemia in association with hyperglycemia, could reduce insulin sensitivity via mechanisms such as down-regulation of insulin receptors in muscle tissue and increased plasma free fatty acids (Higgins, 2004). SCFAs may also assist in increasing insulin sensitivity, by lowering free fatty acids (Higgins, 2004).

In the assessment of breads made with starches with increasing amylose content described above (Behall and Hallfrisch, 2002), high-amylose corn RS2 (60–70% amylose) had the greatest impact on insulin response reduction. Furthermore, RS is known to be dependent upon food processing, with high-amylose corn RS2 being more tolerant to normal cooking conditions. Brown *et al.* (2003) compared uncooked and cooked rat diets containing corn starches with 0–85% amylose. While insulin response was lower for uncooked starches with 27–85% amylose, only the 60–85% amylose corn RS2 lowered insulin response following cooking.

*Satiety and related observations*

Short-term studies indicate that low-glycemic versus high-glycemic meals can increase satiety and/or reduce subsequent hunger, as determined by visual analog scales or measurement of subsequent energy intake. After controlling for energy intake, macronutrient content, energy density and palatability, people consumed on average 29% less energy after low-glycemic meals than after high-glycemic meals (Roberts, 2000).

When high-amylose RS2- and RS3-containing meals were fed in two studies, people reported increased satiety (Jenkins *et al.*, 1998), particularly in the postabsorptive period (Achour *et al.*, 1997). Effects of RS on other observations relevant to satiety – such as appetite, fullness and satisfaction – are less consistent. van Amelsvoort and Weststrate (1992) fed subjects meals with high-amylose corn and rice, and reported increased satisfaction and fullness, with reduced hunger and desire to eat. de Roos *et al.* (1995) fed high-amylose corn RS2 and reported reduced appetite for a meal or snack. However, other studies were less supportive of these and other descriptors (Weststrate and van Amelsvoort, 1993; Raben *et al.*, 1994; de Roos *et al.*, 1995).

The lack of consistency for subjective satiety questionnaires is not surprising as many food factors other than RS content contribute to satiety descriptors; these food factors are often not adequately controlled for, thereby making interpretation difficult. More research based on objective measurements, such as satiety hormones, is warranted.

## 8.4 Increasing the resistant starch content of foods

### 8.4.1 Commercial ingredients

The first commercially available RS ingredient was a high-amylose corn RS2 released in Australia in 1993, called Hi-maize™ starch, with a dietary fiber content of 30%. Since then, the number and type of RS ingredients has increased. Today, commercial sources of RS1, RS2, RS3 and RS4 are available. Each RS ingredient will have a unique profile of physiological and technological functionality, and so should be considered accordingly. For example using AOAC total dietary fiber methods, RS ingredients can differ in their dietary fiber contents from >60% for RS2 made from high-amylose corn starch, to 0–30% for RS3 made from tapioca or high-amylose corn starch. RS4 has been prepared using various techniques, for example by acid hydrolysis or dextrinization to produce a soluble material while more recently RS4 chemically modified starches have been prepared from various starch bases using difunctional phosphate reagents. Depending on the country, some of the RS4 materials are considered novel foods that must seek official regulatory approval.

Some properties that differ between commercial RS ingredients include:

- the relative ratio of digestible to indigestible starch – some ingredients are higher in RS (and/or total dietary fiber) than others;
- the methodology that can be used to determine the resistant component – different ingredients will use different methods to quantify the RS and/or dietary fiber content (e.g. AOAC 985.29, 991.43, 2002.02, 2001.03), not all of which are approved by local regulatory bodies;
- whether the RS and/or dietary fiber content of the ingredient is preserved in the food as eaten;
- the physiological outcome – as for other fibers (e.g. soluble versus insoluble), different RS ingredients behave uniquely within the body;
- the level of supporting evidence – more established RS ingredients such as RS2 and RS3 from high-amylose corn have a broad body of scientific evidence available to support their inclusion into functional foods while newer forms of RS may have little or no supporting clinical evidence;
- the contribution of the starch to technological functionality – different RS ingredients have different technological characteristics, which favor certain food applications;
- impact on the organoleptic properties of foods – RSs from various sources will affect sensory dimensions such as taste in different ways.

Most evidence for the health benefits of RS has been demonstrated using high-amylose corn RS2, largely due to its process tolerance and ease of incorporation into foods relative to other sources of RS and dietary fibers. Table 8.7 describes some important digestive health benefits attributed to high-amylose corn RS2.

### 8.4.2 Formulating foods with resistant starch ingredients

RS is found in starchy foods that we eat every day, but the amount present is very small. Ingredients rich in RS can be used to increase the RS content of a wide variety of foods including breads, buns, breakfast cereals, extruded foods, cereal bars, pasta, noodles, biscuits, confectionery, beverages and yogurt. These ingredients can increase the RS content, increase the total dietary fiber content, add physiological benefit and improve food quality.

**Table 8.7** Important digestive health benefits of high-amylose corn RS2 ingredients (modified from Brown *et al.*, 2000, and Brown, 2004)

| General physiological highlight | Specific physiological effect |
|---|---|
| Improved bowel health | Controlled fermentation<br>Cecal bulking, increased fecal weight<br>Increased production of colonic SCFAs<br>Reduced intestinal pH<br>Reduced levels of secondary bile acids and ammonia<br>Cecal bulking, increased fecal weight<br>Reduced symptoms of diarrhea |
| Prebiotic | Selectively utilized by bifidobacteria<br>Promotes growth of beneficial indigenous microbes – lactobacilli and bifidobacteria<br>Promotes probiotic growth and activity<br>Reduced pathogenic bacteria levels<br>Elevated colonic butyrate levels |
| Culture protagonist | Improves yield of probiotic cultures during growth<br>Improves survival of probiotic cultures during processing, in foods, *in vivo* |
| Increased absorption of micronutrients | Calcium |
| Potential for protection against bowel cancer | Increased butyrate production<br>Increased apoptotic index<br>Decreased levels of cytotoxic compounds |
| Synergistic interactions with other dietary components | Protein, probiotics, lipids, fructo-oligosaccharide |
| Tolerance | Tolerated at high levels |

The functional properties of high-amylose corn RS2 relevant to food use are listed in Table 8.8. RS ingredients are incorporated into many commercially available foods. The most successful foods have capitalized on the ability of RS to deliver high-quality fiber-enriched foods, with potential physiological benefits. Selected RS ingredients show good promise for inclusion into the following foods:

- baked goods – due to low water absorptive capacity relative to other fibers, which causes less disruption of crumb structure, improved loaf volume, lighter crumb color and more even color;
- extruded high-fiber breakfast cereals – due to reduced bulk density, improved expansion, extended bowl life and crispiness;
- dairy foods – due to enhanced viability of probiotics during manufacturing.

**Table 8.8** Functional properties of high-amylose corn RS2 ingredients (Brown, 2004)

| |
|---|
| Natural |
| Source of dietary fiber and RS |
| White |
| Fine particle size (average granule size is <10 μm) |
| High gelatinization temperature |
| Low water absorption compared with some other dietary fibers |
| Extrudes well. Excellent film-forming properties |
| Can give low bulk density, high-fiber products |
| Improves coating crispness |
| Improves the bowl life of breakfast cereals |

## 8.5 Sources of further information and advice

There are now some extensive independent reviews available that describe the physiological effects of RS; some of these are listed below.

- British Nutrition Foundation: Nugent A P. Health properties of resistant starch. *Nutrition Bulletin* 2005, **30**:27–54.
- Association of Official Analytical Chemists: *Journal of AOAC International*, Special Guest Editor Section, Eds: B V McCleary and I L Brown, 2004, **87**:682–796.
- Commonwealth Scientific and Industrial Research Organisation: Baghurst P A, Baghurst K I and Record S J. Dietary fibre, non-starch polysaccharides and resistant starch. A review. *Supplement to Food Australia* 1996, **48**:S1–S36.
- Topping D L and Clifton P M. Short-chain fatty acids and human colonic function: roles of resistant starch and nonstarch polysaccharides. *Physiological Reviews* 2001, **81**:1031–1064.
- Bird A R, Brown I L and Topping D L. Starches, resistant starches, the gut microflora and human health. *Current Issues in Intestinal Microbiology* 2000, **1**:25–37.

## 8.6 Future trends

Research over the past 20 years has helped to establish RS as a valuable ingredient for functional food development. Most research has focused on the distinctive digestive health benefits for RS, to position it as a unique component of dietary fiber. However, a role for RS has also been established in the area of energy metabolism, as described in this chapter. In the future new research will emerge to elucidate a mechanistic understanding of this role.

Future functional food development will aim to leverage nutritional attributes of all the components present in the food, i.e. to truly formulate specialty functional foods as opposed to enriching existing foods with functional ingredients. RS is uniquely positioned to support the creation of multi-benefit functional foods, through its cross-sectional benefits and its synergies with other food ingredients such as protein, lipid, fibers and probiotics. Future weight management approaches will be multi-functional to address diverse etiologies, so a multi-benefit ingredient like RS is an ideal ingredient of choice.

Until recently RS ingredients have mostly been insoluble, and so ideally suited for bakery applications. Recent demand for RS as a functional ingredient has grown, so new ingredients will emerge that are suitable for a broader range of applications. As RSs are such a diverse and heterogeneous group of compounds there will undoubtedly emerge new RS ingredients with discrete health-promoting attributes.

## 8.7 Conclusion

Dietary starch in general and RS in particular are being re-assessed for their contribution to health. A wealth of information collected over 20 years of research, from human and animal studies, supports the use of RS ingredients to enrich new and existing foods. Consumer research highlights the importance of food quality as a major determinant of consumer choice. RS is a versatile option for formulating high-quality foods with added physiological benefits for enhancing their marketability. In the area of weight management, RS is an ideal ingredient choice. Favorable caloric, metabolic and hormonal parameters combine to affect not only energy intake but also energy metabolism. Future research will uncover mechanistic rationales for how RS-rich foods contribute, in particular, to improve insulin sensitivity and reduce lipid metabolism and lipid storage.

## 8.8 References

AACC (American Association of Cereal Chemists) (2001), The definition of dietary fiber. *Cereal Foods World*, **46**, 112–126.

ACHOUR L, FLOURIE B, BRIET F, FRANCHISSEUR C, BORNET F, CHAMP M, RAMBAUD J-C and MESSING B (1997), Metabolic effects of digestible and partially indigestible cornstarch: a study in the absorptive and postabsorptive periods in healthy humans. *American Journal of Clinical Nutrition*, **66**, 1151–1159.

ANDRIEUX C and SACQUET E (1986), Effects of amylomaize starch on mineral metabolism in the adult rat: role of the microflora. *Journal of Nutrition*, **116**, 991–998.

ASP N G (1992), Resistant starch. Proceedings from the second plenary meeting of EURESTA: European FLAIR-Concerted Action No. 11 on the physiological implications of the consumption of resistant starch in man. *European Journal of Clinical Nutrition*, **46** (Suppl 2), S1.

AUST L, DONGOWSKI G, FRENZ U, TAUFEL A and NOACK R (2001), Estimation of available energy of dietary fibres by indirect calorimetry in rats. *European Journal of Nutrition*, **40**, 23–29.

BAGHURST P A, BAGHURST K I and RECORD S J (1996), Dietary fibre, non-starch polysaccharides and resistant starch. A review. *Food Australia*, **48** (Suppl.), S1–S36.

BEHALL K M and HALLFRISCH J (2002), Plasma glucose and insulin reduction after consumption of breads varying in amylose content. *European Journal of Clinical Nutrition*, **56**, 913–920.

BEHALL K M and HOWE J C (1996), Resistant starch as energy. *Journal of the American College of Nutrition*, **15**, 248–254.

BIRD A R, BROWN I L and TOPPING D L (2000), Starches, resistant starches, the gut microflora and human health. *Current Issues in Intestinal Microbiology*, **1**, 25–37.

BRAND-MILLER J C, HOLT S H A, PAWLAK D B and MCMILLAN J (2002), Glycemic index and obesity. *American Journal of Clinical Nutrition*, **76** (Suppl.), 281S–285S.

BRIGHENTI F, CASIRAGHI M C and BAGGIO C (1998), Resistant starch in the Italian diet. *British Journal of Nutrition*, **80**, 333–341.

BROWN I L (2004), Applications and uses of resistant starch. *Journal of AOAC International*, **87**, 727–732.

BROWN I, CONWAY P and TOPPING D (2000), The health potential of resistant starches in foods. An Australian perspective. *Scandinavian Journal of Nutrition*, **44**, 53–58.

BROWN I L, MCNAUGHT K J, ANDREWS D and MORITA T. Resistant starch: plant breeding, applications development and commercial use. chapter 34. in *Advanced Dietary Fibre Technology*, Eds: Bv McCleary and L Prosky. Blackwell Science, Oxford, UK. 2001. pp. 401–412.

BROWN I L, MCNAUGHT K J and MOLONEY E (1995), Hi-maize: new directions in starch technology and nutrition. *Food Australia*, **46**, 272–275.

BROWN M A, STORLIEN L H, BROWN I L and HIGGINS J A (2003), Cooking attenuates the ability of high-amylose meals to reduce plasma insulin concentrations in rats. *British Journal of Nutrition*, **90**, 823–827.

BYRNES S E, BRAND MILLER J C and DENYER G S (1995), Amylopectin starch promotes the development of insulin resistance in rats. *Journal of Nutrition*, **125**, 1430–1437.

CASSIDY A, BINGHAM S A and CUMMINGS J H (1994), Starch intake and colorectal cancer risk: an international comparison. *British Journal of Cancer*, **69**, 937–942.

CUMMINGS J H (1996), *The Large Intestine in Nutrition and Disease*. Chapter 9. Danone Chair Monograph. Danone Institute, France.

CUMMINGS J H and MACFARLANE G T (1991), The control and consequences of bacterial fermentation in the human colon. *Journal of Applied Bacteriology*, **70**, 443–459.

DE DECKERE E A M, KLOOTS W J and VAN AMELSVOORT J M M (1993), Resistant starch decreases serum total cholesterol and triacylglycerol concentrations in rats. *Journal of Nutrition*, **123**, 2142–2151.

DE DECKERE E A M, KLOOTS W J and VAN AMELSVOORT J M M (1995), Both raw and retrograded starch decrease serum triacylglycerol concentration and fat accretion in the rat. *British Journal of Nutrition*, **73**, 287–298.

DE ROOS N, HEIJNEN M L, DE GRAAF C, WOESTENENK G and HOBBEL E (1995), Resistant starch has little effect on appetite, food intake and insulin secretion of healthy young men. *European Journal of Clinical Nutrition*, **49**, 532–541.

DE SCHRIJVER R, VANHOOF K and VANDE GINSTE J (1999), Nutrient utilization in rats and pigs fed enzyme resistant starch. *Nutrition Research*, **19**, 1349–1361.

DYSSELER P and HOFFEM D (1994), Estimation of resistant starch intake in Europe. In *Proceedings of the concluding plenary meeting of EURESTA; including the final reports of the working groups. FLAIR Food-Linked Agro-Industrial Research*. Eds: NG Asp, JMM van Amelsvoort and JGAJ Hautvast. pp. 84–86.

EBBELING C B, LEIDIG M M, SINCLAIR K B, HANGEN J P and LUDWIG D S (2003), A reduced-glycemic load diet in the treatment of adolescent obesity. *Archives of Pediatric Adolescent Medicine*, **157**, 773–779.

ELMSTAHL H L (2002), Resistant starch content in a selection of starchy foods on the Swedish market. *European Journal of Clinical Nutrition*, **56**, 500–505.

ENGLYST H N, KINGMAN S M and CUMMINGS J H (1992), Classification and measurement of nutritionally important starch fractions. *European Journal of Clinical Nutrition*, **46** (Suppl 2), S33–S50.

FAO/WHO (Food and Agriculture Organization and the World Health Organization). codex Alimentarius commission, 2005. Report of the 26th session of the codex committee on nutrition and foods for special dietary uses, Bonn, Germany, November 2004.

GRAY G M (1992), Starch digestion and absorption in nonruminants. *Journal of Nutrition*, **122**, 172–177.

GRAY J (2003), *Carbohydrates: Nutritional and Health Aspects*. International Life Sciences Institute, Washington DC, USA.

HIGGINS J A (2004), Resistant starch: metabolic effects and potential health benefits. *Journal of AOAC International*, **87**, 761–768.

HIGGINS J A, BRAND MILLER J C and DENYER G S (1996), Development of insulin resistance in the rat is dependent on the rate of glucose absorption from the diet. *Journal of Nutrition*, **126**, 596–602.

HIGGINS J A, HIGBEE D R, DONAHOO W T, BROWN I L, BELL M L and BESSESEN D H (2004), Resistant starch consumption promotes lipid oxidation. *Nutrition and Metabolism*, **1**, 8–18.

HOWE J C, RUMPLER W V and BEHALL K M (1996), Dietary starch composition and level of energy intake alter nutrient oxidation in 'carbohydrate-sensitive' men. *Journal of Nutrition*, **126**, 2120–2129.

HULMAN S and FALKNER B (1994), The effect of excess dietary sucrose on growth, blood pressure, and metabolism in developing Sprague–Dawley rats. *Pediatric Research*, **36**, 95–101.

IOM (Institute of Medicine of the National Academies). Dietary, functional and total fiber. Chapter 7. In *Dietary Reference Intakes: Energy, Carbohydrates, Fiber, Fat, Fatty Acids, Cholesterol, Protein, and Amino Acids (Macronutrients)*. National Academies Press, Washington DC, USA. 2002.

JENKINS D J A, VUKSAN V, KENDALL C W C, WURSCH P, JEFFCOAT R, WARING S, MEHLING C C, VIDGEN E, AUGUSTIN L S A and WONG E (1998), Physiological effects of resistant starches on fecal bulk, short chain fatty acids, blood lipids and glycemic index. *Journal of the American College of Nutrition*, **17**, 609–616.

JIMINEZ-CRUZ A, BACARDI-GASCON M, TURNBULL W H, ROSALES-GARAY P and SEVERINO-LUGO I (2003), A flexible, low-glycemic index Mexican-style diet in overweight and obese subjects with Type 2 diabetes improves metabolic parameters during a 6-week treatment period. *Diabetes Care*, **26**, 1967–1970.

KABIR M, RIZKALLA S W, QUIGNARD-BOULANGE, GUERRE-MILLO M, BOILLOT J, ARDOUIN B, LUO J and SLAMA G (1998a), A high glycemic index starch diet affects lipid storage-related enzymes in normal and to a lesser extent in diabetic rats. *Journal of Nutrition*, **128**, 1878–1883.

KABIR M, RIZKALLA S W, CHAMP M, LUO J, BOILLOT J, BRUZZO F and SLAMA G (1998b), Dietary amylose-amylopectin starch content affects glucose and lipid metabolism in adipocytes of normal and diabetic rats. *Journal of Nutrition*, **128**, 35–43.

KIRIYAMA S (1996), Physiological function of resistant starch and its use. *Up-to-date Food Processing*, **31** (2), 34–38.

KISHIDA T, NOGAMI H, HIMENO S and EBIHARA K (2001), Heat moisture treatment of high amylose cornstarch increases its resistant starch content but not its physiologic effects in rats. *Journal of Nutrition*, **131**, 2716–2721.

LERER-METZGER M, RIZKALLA S W, LUO J, CHAMP M, KABIR M, BRUZZO F, BORNET F and SLAMA G (1996), Effects of long-term low-glycaemic index starchy food on plasma glucose and lipid concentrations and adipose tissue cellularity in normal and diabetic rats. *British Journal of Nutrition*, **75**, 723–732.

LEVIN R J (1994), Digestion and absorption of carbohydrates – from molecules and membranes to humans. *American Journal of Clinical Nutrition*, **59**, 690S–698S.

LIVESEY G, DAVIES I R, BROWN J C, FAULKS R M and SOUTHON S (1990), Energy balance and energy values of α-amylase (EC 3.2.1.1)-resistant maize and pea (*Pisum sativum*) starches in the rat. *British Journal of Nutrition*, **63**, 467–480.

LUDWIG D S (2000), Dietary glycemic index and obesity. *Journal of Nutrition*, **130**, 280S–283S.

MA Y, OLENDZKI B, CHIRIBOGA D, HEBERT J R, LI Y, LI W, CAMPBELL M, GENDREAU K and OCKENE I S (2005), Association between dietary carbohydrates and body weight. *American Journal of Epidemiology*, **161**, 359–367.

MATHERS J C (1992), Energy value of resistant starch. *European Journal of Clinical Nutrition*, **46** (Suppl 2), S129–S130.

MORAND C, LEVRAT M A, BESSON C, DEMIGNE C and REMESY C (1994), Effects of a diet rich in resistant starch on hepatic lipid metabolism in the rat. *Journal of Nutritional Biochemistry*, **5**, 138–144.

MUIR J G, WALKER K Z, KAIMAKAMIS M A, CAMERON M A, GOVERS M J A P, LU Z X, YOUNG G P and O'DEA K (1998), Modulation of fecal markers relevant to colon cancer risk: a high-starch Chinese diet did not generate expected beneficial changes relative to a Western-type diet. *American Journal of Clinical Nutrition*, **68**, 372–379.

NUGENT A (2005), Health properties of resistant starch. *Nutrition Bulletin*, **30**, 27–54.

PAWLAK D B, BRYSON J M, DENYER G S and BRAND-MILLER J C (2001), High glycemic index starch promotes hypersecretion of insulin and higher body fat in rats without affecting insulin sensitivity. *Journal of Nutrition*, **131**, 99–104.

PAWLAK D B, KUSHNER J A and LUDWIG D S (2004), Effects of dietary glycemic index on adiposity, glucose homoeostasis, and plasma lipids in animals. *Lancet* **364**, 778–785.

PHILLIPS J, MUIR J G, BIRKETT A, LU Z X, JONES G P, O'DEA K and YOUNG, G P (1995), Effect of resistant starch on fecal bulk and fermentation-dependent events in humans. *American Journal of Clinical Nutrition*, **62**, 121–130.

PLATEL K and SHURPALEKAR K S (1994), Resistant starch content of Indian foods. *Plant Foods for Human Nutrition*, **45**, 91–95.

RABEN A, TAGLIABUE A, CHRISTENSEN N J, MADSEN J, HOLST J J and ASTRUP A (1994), Resistant starch: the effect on postprandial glycemia, hormonal response, and satiety. *American Journal of Clinical Nutrition*, **60**, 544–551.

ROBERTS J, JONES G P, RUTISHAUSER I H E, BIRKETT A and GIBBONS C (2004), Resistant starch in the Australian diet. *Nutrition and Dietetics*, **61**, 98–104.

ROBERTS S B (2000), High-glycemic index foods, hunger, and obesity: is there a connection? *Nutrition Reviews*, **58**, 163–169.

ROBERTSON M D, BICKERTON A S, DENNIS A L, VIDAL H and FRAYN K N (2005), Insulin-sensitizing effects of dietary resistant starch and effects on skeletal muscle and adipose tissue metabolism. *American Journal of Clinical Nutrition*, **82**, 559–567.

ROBERTSON M D, CURRIE J M, MORGAN L M, JEWELL D P and FRAYN K N (2003), Prior short-term consumption of resistant starch enhances postprandial insulin sensitivity in healthy subjects. *Diabetologia*, **46**, 659–665.

SALMINEN S, BOULEY C, BOUTRON-RUAULT M C, CUMMINGS J H, FRANCK A, GIBSON G R, ISOLAURI E, MOREAU M C, ROBERFROID M and ROWLAND I (1998), Functional food science and gastrointestinal physiology and function. *British Journal of Nutrition*, **80**, S147–S171.

SLABBER M, BARNARD H C and KUYL J M (1994), Effects of a low-insulin-response, energy-restricted diet on weight loss and plasma insulin concentrations in hyperinsulinemic obese females. *American Journal of Clinical Nutrition*, **60**, 48–53.

SPIETH L E, HARNISH J D, LENDERS S M, RAEZER L B, PEREIRA M A, HANGEN S J and LUDWIG D S (2000), A low-glycemic index diet in the treatment of pediatric obesity. *Archives of Pediatric Adolescent Medicine*, **154**, 947–951.

TAGLIABUE A, RABEN A, HEIJNEN M L, DEURENBERG P, PASQUALI E and ASTRUP A (1995), The effect of raw potato starch on energy expenditure and substrate oxidation. *American Journal of Clinical Nutrition*, **61**, 1070–1075.

TOMLIN J and READ N W (1990), The effect of resistant starch on colon function in humans. *British Journal of Nutrition*, **64**, 589–595.

TOPPING D L and CLIFTON P M (2001), Short-chain fatty acids and human colonic function: roles of resistant starch and nonstarch polysaccharides. *Physiological Reviews*, **81**, 1031–1064.

VAN AMELSVOORT J M M and WESTSTRATE J A (1992), Amylose–amylopectin ratio in a meal affects postprandial variables in male volunteers. *American Journal of Clinical Nutrition*, **55**, 712–718.

WALKER K Z, BIRKETT A, LU Z X, JONES G, O'DEA K and MUIR J G (1997), Development of a simulated Australian diet for adults which may have use as a research tool. *Australian Journal of Nutrition and Dietetics*, **54**, 190–197.

WESTSTRATE J A and VAN AMELSVOORT J M M (1993), Effects of the amylose content of breakfast and lunch on postprandial variables in male volunteers. *American Journal of Clinical Nutrition*, **58**, 180–186.

WILLIAMSON S L H, KARTHEUSER A, COAKER J, KOOSHKGHAZI M D, FODDE R, BURN J and MATHERS J C (1999), Intestinal tumorigenesis in the Apc1638N mouse treated with aspirin and resistant starch for up to 5 months. *Carcinogenesis*, **20**, 805–810.

WHO (World Health Organization). Diet, nutrition and the prevention of chronic diseases. WHO Technical report series 916. Report of a joint FAO/WHO Expert Consultation. WHO, *Geneva*. 2003. p. 63.

ZHOU X and KAPLAN M L (1997), Soluble amylose cornstarch is more digestible than soluble amylopectin potato starch in rats. *Journal of Nutrition*, **127**, 1349–1356.

# 9

# Modified carbohydrates with lower glycemic index

**B. R. Hamaker, G. Zhang and M. Venkatachalam, Purdue University, USA**

## 9.1 Introduction

Glycemic index (GI) relates to the blood glucose profile seen over a period of 2 h after consumption of a starch-based or sugar-containing food. It is measured as the area under the curve for a given amount of available carbohydrate in a test food as compared with a reference food (usually glucose or white bread) (Wolever *et al.*, 1991). GI, as well as glycemic load, which accounts for the amount of such food consumed in relation to the total diet, has been studied and may relate to a number of disease and pre-disease conditions such as diabetes and pre-diabetes, cardiovascular disease, cancer, obesity; it may also relate to energy expenditure and activity level (Ludwig, 2002; Brand-Miller, 2003; Aston, 2006). While some controversy exists in the nutrition and medical communities on nearly all of these relationships, much research has been and continues to be conducted to elucidate the health consequences of GI.

There is a range of GI values in foods. A comprehensive table was recently published by Foster-Powell *et al.* (2002). Starch, being the principal component in most staple foods such as cereals and tubers, is the major food carbohydrate contributing to postprandial glycemia. However, depending on the food source, other carbohydrates can contribute to the glycemic response, such as sucrose, lactose, high-fructose corn syrup, and maltodextrins. For the purposes of this chapter, the discussion of modified carbohydrates with lower GI will focus on starch-based foods and food products.

From a nutritional standpoint, Englyst *et al.* (1992) classified starch into three categories based on digestion times in *in vitro* digestion assays: rapidly digestible starch (RDS) was digested in 20 min, slowly digestible starch (SDS) was digested in between 20 and 120 min, and resistant starch (RS) was undigested at 120 min. Foods with a high proportion of RDS have a high GI value based on a correlative relationship between RDS and GI (Englyst *et al.*, 1996). The rapid increase in blood glucose levels from RDS triggers the secretion of insulin from pancreas beta cells that promotes glucose uptake by muscle and adipose tissues to maintain blood glucose homeostasis; if the increase in postprandial glycemia is pronounced, this usually generates a hypoglycemic episode between 1 and 2 h after consumption of RDS. In contrast, SDS is that portion of starch that is digested slower than RDS, implying that it is digested throughout the small intestine to provide a slow and prolonged release of glucose. Such a moderated and controlled release of glucose may place less stress on the blood glucose regulatory system. Resistant starch is that portion of starch that is not digested in the small intestine. However, it is digested by colonic microflora enzymes and then fermented to produce short-chain fatty acids (acetic, propionic, and butyric) that have been shown to be beneficial to colonic health (Bird *et al.*, 2000). Thus, the nutritional quality of starch-based foods that is attributed to RDS, SDS, and RS depends on the relative amounts of these fractions. A low-GI starch ingredient should contain lower amounts of RDS, and a higher proportion of SDS and RS. The emphasis of this chapter is on methodologies to create SDS and RS.

The opportunity to alter the GI of foods can be viewed from a number of perspectives. The most obvious is the form in which the food is eaten. A simple example would be that white bread made from refined wheat flour is essentially as rapidly digested and absorbed as glucose itself, while the same flour made into pasta is absorbed at a much slower rate. This difference can be attributed to the 'food form', where the former has starch that is readily accessible to digestive enzymes and in the latter it is less accessible due to a combination of a protein matrix effect and the density of the food. Starchy foods will also change in GI depending on food processing conditions (e.g. degree of starch gelatinization related to temperature and water content, degree of shear, cooling rate, and time) and storage (factors related to starch retrogradation) (Björck *et al.*, 2000; Fernandes *et al.*, 2005). There are many such examples and food form is a large factor to be considered when designing low-glycemic products. Starch itself, being composed of the complex molecules of amylose and amylopectin, can be altered structurally to moderate its digestion rate. In this regard, changes to its molecular architecture at various stages of food processing and storage affect its susceptibility to digestive enzymes. Additionally, other non-starch components in the food can lower starch digestion rate by influencing gastric emptying and luminal viscosity, or can inhibit amylases, all of which affect postprandial glycemia. The various approaches to producing carbohydrates with comparably low GI are described below.

## 9.2 Methods of producing carbohydrates with lower glycemic index

Based on the current Dietary Guidelines for Americans 2005 (USDA, 2005), dietary carbohydrates should provide 45–65% of total calories. Dietary carbohydrates, structurally, can be divided into monosaccharides, disaccharides, oligosaccharides, and polysaccharides. α-1,4- and 1,6-linked glucans (such as starch and maltodextrins) are digestible by human enzymes, while dietary fiber – including some oligosaccharides (like inulin) and non-starch polysaccharides (like pectins, hemicelluloses, cellulose) – cannot be digested by the human body. The majority of starches in cooked and processed foods are rapidly digested and produce high postprandial glycemia. Starches that digest slowly result in a moderated glycemic response and may provide extended energy to an individual. A challenge facing researchers in the public and private sectors is to create such slowly digestible starches with low GI as an ingredient for typically high-GI processed foods, or as new food products, or, through genetics, to be naturally present in starchy foods. Some examples and basic theories will be discussed in this section.

Currently available food products with low-GI properties are not well defined. While RDS, SDS, and RS are defined by *in vitro* digestion times, the structural or other component requirements of each starch grouping are not well understood. For example, RDS has no special structural component associated with fast digestion and generally can be viewed as readily accessible to starch-degrading enzymes. RSs, on the other hand, often consist of highly ordered crystallites that are difficult to digest, physically hindered, or chemically modified. The starch structure or other factors leading to SDS, however, are not well understood. The complexity of factors leading to the creation of an 'SDS state', that is the food form wherein starch has a slow digestion property, is shown in Fig. 9.1. Further investigation of the requirements of the SDS state is needed for its better understanding and preparation. This is particularly so because SDS, compared with RS, is more related to the glycemic response as it alone both reduces the initial postprandial glycemic peak and provides extended glucose release over time for perhaps the optimal glycemic response.

## 9.3 Slow-digestion and digestion-resistant characteristics of raw starch

### 9.3.1 Native starches

Native starch naturally exists in the form of starch granules with different shapes, sizes, and surface properties. X-ray diffraction can be used to classify starches into A-, B-, and C- (combination of A and B) types based on the packing of the semicrystalline structures of starch granules. Most cereal

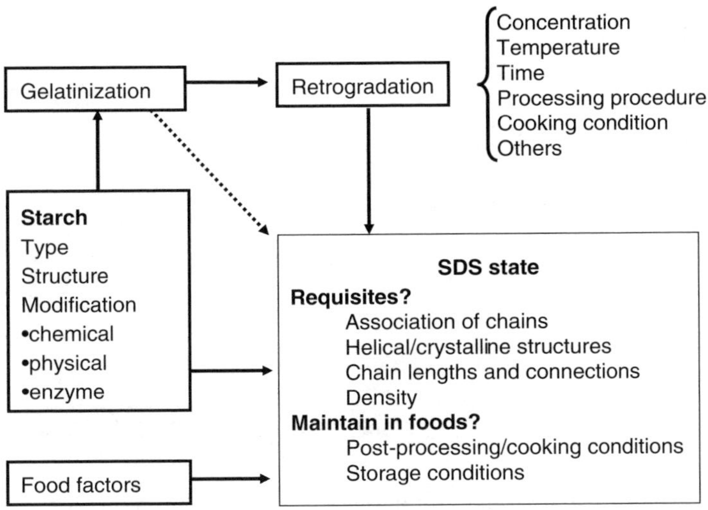


**Fig. 9.1** Factors leading to the SDS state.

starches (maize, wheat, rice) are of the A-type, tuber starches (potato, yam) are B-type, and legume starches (kidney bean, soybean) normally belong to C-type. Some A-type starches (maize, sorghum, millets, and large granules of wheat, rye, and barley at the equatorial groove) have surface pores connected to interior cavities through channels (Fannon *et al.*, 1992). There are no such surface pores in B-type starch granules. This macrostructural difference between native starch granules has importance during digestion as starch-digesting enzymes enter the pores and channels and digest the granules in an inside-out manner. As far as the nutritional quality of starch is concerned, native A-type starches inherently have a high amount of SDS while native B-type starches are essentially resistant (high RS) (Ferguson *et al.*, 2000), based on the *in vitro* Englyst assay (Englyst *et al.*, 1992). In an *in vivo* study, Seal *et al.* (2003) clearly showed the changes in blood glucose levels after consumption of native maize starch (Fig. 9.2), producing a typical profile of SDS. There have been two patents (Axelsen and Smith, 2001; Qi and Tester, 2005) on SDS in which native A-type starches were used as the sole ingredient to prepare medical foods for treatment of glycogen storage disease (GSD1) (Chen *et al.*, 1984) and other diabetic conditions.

Our own investigation of native starch digestion properties shows that A-type native maize starch is a near-ideal SDS source (Zhang *et al.*, 2006a,b). This is because native granules, at any given time point of digestion in the Englyst assay, provide similar RDS, SDS, and RS amounts, and thus continue to provide slow release of glucose over an extended period of time. It is well known that the semicrystalline structure of starch granules is composed of alternating concentric layers of ordered and dense crystalline

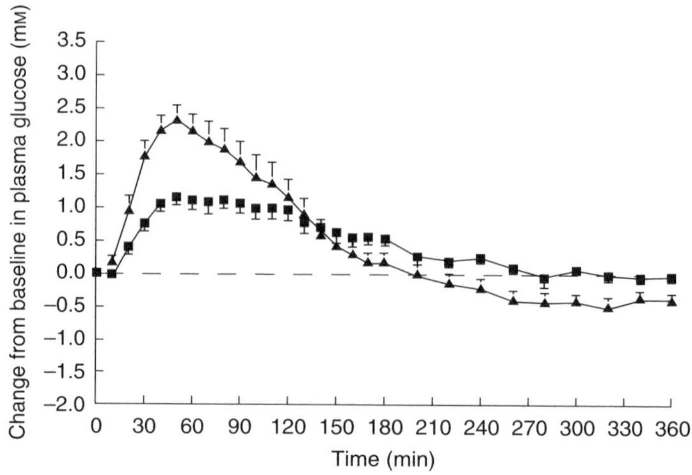


**Fig. 9.2** Change from baseline in plasma glucose concentrations with time after consumption of 50 g rapidly hydrolysed (▲) and 50 g slowly hydrolysed (■) native maize starch for healthy subjects (from Seal *et al.*, 2003).

regions and less ordered amorphous regions (also called amorphous background) from the hilum to the surface of the granules. This is considered a lamellar structure. Based on our investigation (Zhang *et al.*, 2006a), the surface pores and interior channels are the starting points for enzymic digestion, and gradually the amorphous background and dense crystalline regions are evenly digested by enlarging the interior channels through a side-by-side digestion mechanism from the inside of the granule to the outside. This is the mechanism for the slow digestion property of A-type maize starch and could conceivably be replicated in other food materials to create a similar digestion effect. B-type starches have a somewhat similar granular structure with different crystalline and amorphous arrangements, but there are no surface pores or interior cavities. Thus, digestion occurs through pitting from the outside of the starch granules. Additionally, B-type crystallites are somewhat resistant to digestion compared with A-type crystallites (Gérard *et al.*, 2000). Therefore B-type native starch is largely RS (~70%) due to the harder surface and the nature of B-type crystallites.

### 9.3.2 Hydrothermal modification

Hydrothermal modification is one of the physical methods commonly used to modify the functional properties of starch granules while maintaining granular structure. Three parameters are varied in hydrothermal treatment of starch granules: temperature, moisture, and time. Hydrothermal treatments can be divided into two general areas: annealing and heat-moisture treatment. Annealing is usually performed in conditions of excess (>66%) or intermediate water content (40–55% w/w), while heat-moisture treatment is defined for low-moisture conditions (<35% w/w). The temperature range used is generally between the glass transition temperature ($T_g$), the transition point between the glassy and rubbery state of starch, and the gelatinization temperature at which irreversible loss in crystallinity occurs. The time can be varied from hours to a week. Detailed conditions for a variety of starches can be found in the review by Jacobs and Delcour (1998), or determined based on $T_g$ and gelatinization temperature of a specific starch sample.

Hydrothermal treatment results in changes in the crystalline and amorphous regions of starch granules and the interaction between these two regions. It results in an increase in perfection of crystallites, alteration of crystalline packing from B- or C- to A-type, and increased interaction of molecules within amorphous and crystalline regions. As the raw starch granule structure is related to starch digestibility, hydrothermal treatment can be used as a way of changing the slow digestion property of native starch granules resulting in lower GI. Shin *et al.* (2005) reported that hydrothermal treatment of sweet potato converted its C-type structure to A-type, and the SDS of the treated granule increased 200% compared with native starch granules. Owing to the broad range of physicochemical changes caused by hydrothermal treatment, more studies are needed to systematically investigate the effect on the slow digestion property and the related low glycemic response of hydrothermally treated starches.

## 9.4 Starch structural modification

The structure, and perhaps size, of starch molecules can fundamentally affect digestion properties in cooked and processed foods. This can be viewed both from the inherent starch structural properties as well as retrogradation-related structural differences (double helical structures and crystallites) that affect enzyme binding and rate of digestion. Therefore, an understanding of starch structure is critical for the moderation of glycemic response and to design enhanced health value starch ingredients for the food industry. Starch is composed of the essentially linear amylose which consists mostly of α-1,4-linked D-glucopyranosyl units and the highly branched and very large amylopectin (often >1 million glucose units) in which linear α-1,4-linked D-glucopyranosyl chains are joined through α-1,6-linked branches. Starch structural modification therefore can be viewed as a key strategy to achieve SDS. Structural modification of starch molecules can be carried out through genetic, enzymatic, physical, and chemical modifications.

### 9.4.1 Amylose/amylopectin ratio

The amylose/amylopectin ratio is one of the main parameters measured in starch quality evaluation. In a diluted starch solution (<1% w/v) containing both amylose and amylopectin, amylose can be easily digested by α-amylase while amylopectin is slower to be digested due to its branching structure (Park and Rollings, 1994); however, in a concentrated starch system, especially one with a higher ratio of amylose/amylopectin, a firm gel will form and the digestibility will be decreased due to the high amounts of retrograded starch formed by amylose. Much of highly retrograded amylose is classified as RS. Studies have shown that the amylose/amylopectin ratio is an important determinant of starch quality and amylose content is highly correlated with RS content. Thus, foods produced with high-amylose starches generally have low GI value (Miller *et al.*, 1992).

The amount of amylose and amylopectin within starch granules is genetically controlled by the series of enzymes involved in starch biosynthesis. Traditional breeding has been successfully used to produce starches (especially in maize) with a wide range of amylose and amylopectin ratios, such as waxy starches (essentially pure amylopectin) and high-amylose starches (50–70% amylose). Today, the ratio of amylose to amylopectin can be manipulated through modern genetic techniques, such as genetic engineering, to up- or down-regulate genes related to amylose and amylopectin synthesis. Modern techniques such as transposon insertion, site-directed mutagenesis, antisense inactivation, and TILLING (targeting induced local lesions in genomes) of mutagenized populations – as well as producing transgenic lines with the addition of foreign genes – are being used to produce starch mutants with desired properties. High-amylose starch has been an ideal starting material to make heat-stable RS (Brown, 2004) to decrease the postprandial glycemic response of processed foods. Conceivably, novel mutants could cause changes in the molecular weight, amount of amylose, and perhaps its branching structure to produce starches with higher amounts of SDS.

### 9.4.2 Amylopectin fine structure

Amylopectin is the major component, by weight, of normal starch granules (~75%). The cluster model (Fig. 9.3) is the accepted model to describe its fine structure. The branched chains are classified as A chains (no further branching point), B chains (with one or more branching points), and the C chain – the only chain with a reducing end. The fine structure of amylopectin mainly refers to the chain-length distribution, the branching density, internal chain lengths, and cluster repeating distance. The relationship between amylopectin fine structure and starch functionality has been extensively studied. However, its effect on the nutritional quality of starch is not as well investigated. Recent research in our laboratory (G. Zhang and B. R. Hamaker, unpublished data, 2006) shows that both high amounts of short chains (principally the A chains) and high amounts of long chains (intermediate to long B chains) tend to result in more SDS. Shi and Seib (1995) showed that B1 chains having degree of polymerisation (DP) 16–30, are

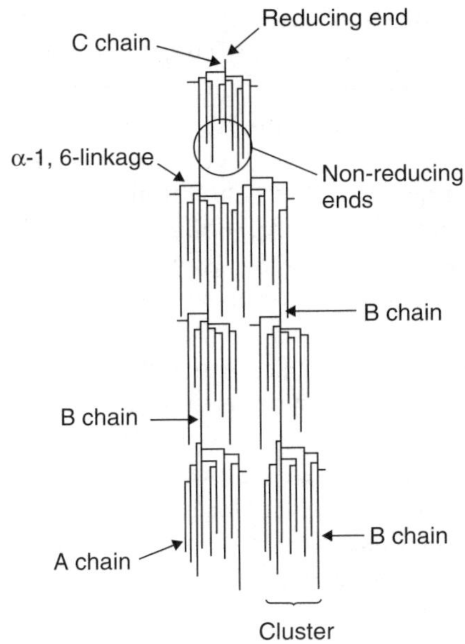


**Fig. 9.3** The cluster model of amylopectin structure including A, B and C chains (Thompson, 2000).

more associated with starch retrogradation and RS content. The amount of amylose appears to have no relationship with SDS. Therefore, the structure of amylopectin may be more critical for SDS, than parameters of amylose.

The fine structure of amylopectin is regulated by soluble starch synthase, branching enzyme isoforms, and debranching enzymes. Variations in activities, or mutations, in these enzymes produce a range of amylopectin with different fine structures. If the relationship between the nutritional quality of starch and amylopectin fine structure is thoroughly understood, genetic engineering or other manipulation methods may be used to produce ideal starches with high-SDS and low-GI properties.

### 9.4.3 Enzyme modification

The molecular structure of amylose and amylopectin is one of the essential intrinsic factors associated with the nutritional quality of starch as described above. Enzyme modification is an alternative way of changing the structure of starch molecules to achieve appropriate digestion or glycemic properties. Theoretically speaking, all of the enzymes involved in starch biosynthesis and degradation can be used to modify starch structure, but in practice only commercially available enzymes are used such as α-amylases, β-amylases, debranching enzymes (isoamylase and pullulanase), transglucosidases, and glycosyltransferases (CGTase). These enzymes decrease the molecular weight of starch molecules, remove outer chains of amylopectin, or add new structures to existing chains. The purpose of using enzyme modification to affect GI is to obtain an optimum structure that will have low GI properties either through an increase in SDS or RS, or both. The approach may be counter to the commonly known enzyme modifications that aim to increase the starch functionality, e.g. texture, gel clarity, and pasting properties. Therefore, definitions of the starch molecular structure needed to produce SDS, as well as RS, are still of critical importance when attempting to improve glycemic properties by enzyme modification.

It has been shown that amylose with DP ~100 rather easily forms RS (Eerlingen *et al.*, 1993) which can be used to decrease the GI of a food, but RS does not, by definition, provide slow-digesting properties. Amylopectin hinders the association of amylose to form RS (Berry, 1986). Starch can be modified using pullulanase or isoamylase and α-amylase to debranch amylopectin and shorten amylose, respectively, so that the RS formation can be increased significantly. Several enzyme-modified RSs have been patented and used commercially [Roquette, France (Nutriose – a new dextrin) and National Starch (Chiu *et al.*, 1994; Shi and Trzasko, 1997)]. Han *et al.* (2006) recently reported a method to produce a starch with RS and some SDS property using α-amylase digestion of partially retrograded normal maize starch. For SDS, partially debranched waxy starch, made using pullulanase, has been used to make SDS (Shin *et al.*, 2004b). In another recent investigation in our laboratory (Z. Ao, G. Zhang and B. R. Hamaker, unpublished data, 2005), a combination of maltogenic α-amylase, β-amylase, and transglucosidase treatment of normal corn starch was used to form starch with an increased proportion of SDS. These studies suggest that the structure of SDSs could be imperfect crystallites, and amylopectin with high branch density or extra long chains might be the structural basis to form an imperfect and entangled structure with substantial density to slow down enzymatic digestion rate.

### 9.4.4 Other physical modifications (retrogradation)

When starch granules are cooked in a food process, the crystalline structure is lost and amylose and amylopectin are dispersed to a certain extent (gelatinization). The extent depends on water content, temperature, time, and degree of shear of the process. To produce low-GI foods in this situation, physical modification (i.e. starch concentration, processing condition, and storage method) can be used to moderate starch digestion properties. Modification of starch gelatinization and retrogradation are the main categories of physical modification used to achieve low-GI benefits in cooked and processed starchy foods.

As described above, native starch (especially A-type) is an ideal SDS, and, if incomplete gelatinization can be achieved through lowering temperature, decreasing water content, or shortening processing time, the nutritional benefits of SDS will be partially retained. However, the organoleptic properties may not be suitable for consumption. This means that improved food processing technologies are needed to impart low glycemic properties. Hydrothermal modifications of the nutritional properties of starch could conceivably also be applied in food processing to achieve a low-glycemic food product.

Extensive research has shown that water content, temperature of storage, and the existence of other ingredients affect starch retrogradation. Most of the RS in food is produced through retrogradation, particularly by amylose retrogradation which occurs very rapidly. Thus, foods produced with high-amylose starch usually have low GI values due to the occurrence of retrogradation. Alternatively, low-GI or controlled glycemic foods can also be made using SDS ingredients. Preliminary data from our laboratory (G. Zhang and B. R. Hamaker, unpublished data, 2005) show that controlled retrogradation can be used to make SDS. Similarly, Shi *et al.* (2003) and Shin *et al.* (2004a) showed that less retrogradation with partially debranched starch ingredients makes it possible to produce SDS. Perhaps SDS, in these cases, is due to the formation of imperfect crystallites.

### 9.4.5 Chemical modification

To improve functionality and create value-added starch-based products, native starches are additionally subjected to various chemical modifications to overcome some of the structural and rheological problems that they inherently have during food processing and storage. These include: loss in viscosity; acid, shear, and/or heat stability; pasting; thickening; syneresis; and retrogradation. Although most chemical treatments have been intended to improve the functionality of the starches in foods, some recent work has focused on such treatments for creating slowly digesting and resistant starches. Many chemical modifications essentially result in the creation of RSs (Wolf *et al.*, 1999). Chemically modified starch derivatives such as citrate starches (Wepner *et al.*, 1999) and cross-linked starches (Woo and Seib, 2002; Shin *et al.*, 2000) have been shown to decrease starch digestion rate depending on the type and degree of modification, extent of gelatinization, and digestion conditions employed. Han and BeMiller (2006) demonstrated high SDS amounts in 2-octen-1-ylsuccinic anhydride esterified waxy starch, and relatively high SDS and RS amounts in cross-linked hydroxypropylated and acetylated waxy starches. However, clinical trials need to be carried out to evaluate the efficacy of such starches in creating low-GI foods.

## 9.5 Influence of other food components

The presence of other major and minor food components, besides starch, has also been shown to influence the glycemic response of carbohydrate foods. Various factors at both macroscopic and microscopic levels of foods can affect such digestion variables as gastric emptying rate, creation of matrix barriers to access starch during digestion, and interactions between digestive enzymes and other food components.

### 9.5.1 Protein-starch interaction

Extruded pasta products represent an excellent example of the effect of proteins in slowing starch digestion rate. Several studies have demonstrated that digestion of pasta in both healthy and diabetic subjects is characterized by low glycemic and insulinemic responses (Parillo *et al.*, 1985; Wolever *et al.*, 1986; Granfeldt and Björck, 1991). *In vitro* digestion studies on pasta (Colonna *et al.*, 1990; Fardet *et al.*, 1998, 1999) have shown that restricted swelling and the entrapment or encapsulation of starch in structured protein network-associated dense food results in decreased accessibility and, hence, lowered digestion by amylase. Furthermore, pre-incubation of pasta with pepsin (a proteolytic enzyme) enhanced starch digestibility, thereby providing support for the importance of protein components in slowing starch digestion. Even in gelatinized flour pastes in cereals such as sorghum, entrapment of starch in protein web-like structures has been seen to impede starch digestibility (Bugusu, 2003). Figure 9.4 shows such protein–starch interrelated structures in a maize flour paste where the trapped gelatinized starch is digested after free, unencumbered gelatinized starch (M. Venkatachalam and B. R. Hamaker, unpublished observations, 2006).

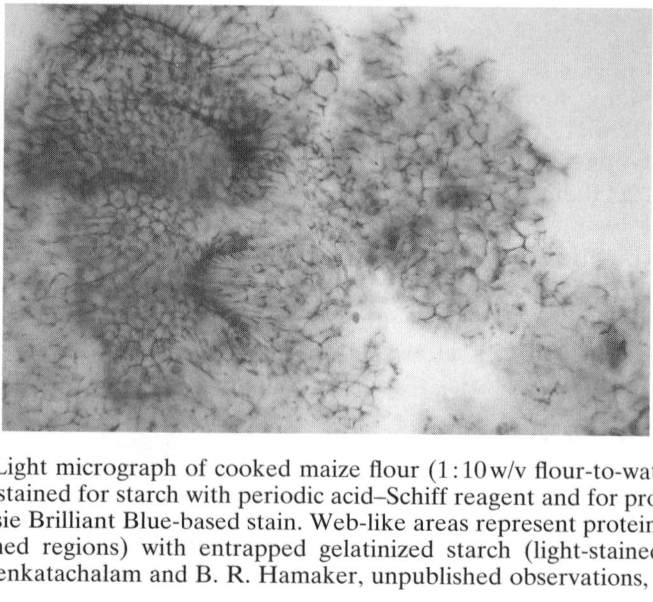

**Fig. 9.4** Light micrograph of cooked maize flour (1 : 10 w/v flour-to-water, 20 min at 100 °C) stained for starch with periodic acid–Schiff reagent and for proteins with a Coumassie Brilliant Blue-based stain. Web-like areas represent protein networks (dark-stained regions) with entrapped gelatinized starch (light-stained regions) (M. Venkatachalam and B. R. Hamaker, unpublished observations, 2005).

### 9.5.2 Lipid complexation with starch

It has been recognized that the complexation of amylose with the free fatty acids and monoglycerides in foods occurs at various stages of food preparation, storage, and even during the digestion process. Such a complex not only results in significant changes in the physicochemical and functional properties of starch – e.g. a change in the starch x-ray diffraction pattern to 'V' type, reduced solubility, increase in gelatinization temperature, retarded retrogradation during storage (Eliasson *et al.*, 1981; Biliaderis and Galloway, 1989) – but also has been shown to be less digestible in various *in vitro* and *in vivo* models (Holm *et al.*, 1983; Seneviratne and Biliaderis, 1991; Murray *et al.*, 1998). A greater resistance to digestion of amylose–lipid complexes was observed when amylose is complexed with long-chain, saturated monoglycerides compared with complexes with shorter-chain unsaturated monoglycerides (Eliasson and Krog, 1985). Murray *et al.* (1998) incorporated a mix of monostearate and monopalmitate complexed with debranched amylopectin to manufacture the V-complex in an experimental diet in dogs and compared their digestion to control and resistant starches. The authors found that the ileal and total tract digestibilities of carbohydrate for the V-complex treatment were intermediate (digestions were ranked, in terms of digestibility, as control > V-complex > RS). The same group of authors also reported that consuming a V-complex-containing diet resulted in lower carbohydrate digestibility and subsequently lower serum glucose and insulin responses than dogs fed a carbohydrate–maltodextrin-containing control diet (Patil *et al.*, 1998).

Apart from lipid–starch complexation that could modify the glycemic response, several studies have shown that co-intake of fat along with carbohydrates in a mixed meal could affect postprandial glucose response. It is believed that fat may reduce postprandial glucose by decreasing the rate of gastric emptying, at least in part related to increased stimulation of the gastrointestinal hormones [such as glucose-dependent insulin-releasing polypeptide (GIP) and glucagon-like polypeptide-1 (GLP-1)] (Morgan, 1998). Several issues, including dosage levels of fat affecting glucose response, have been described by Owen and Wolever (2003). The authors showed that fat intake along with carbohydrates in normal healthy subjects, in a dose-dependent relationship, could decrease the glycemic response; however fat consumption in a normal range (17–44% energy) does not significantly affect glycemic response. As pointed out by Owen and Wolever (2003), it is important to note that individuals with diabetes or insulin resistance should not add fat to carbohydrate meals to prevent high blood glucose surge, because studies have shown that fat addition to carbohydrate does not affect the glycemic responses in subjects with type-2 diabetes (Gannon *et al.*, 1993). Various factors – including the type and amount of fat consumed, the type of carbohydrate eaten with the fat, and the health status of subjects consuming the food – need to be taken into account when evaluating postprandial glucose and insulinemic responses to a mixed carbohydrate–lipid meal.

### 9.5.3 Dietary fiber

Several studies have shown that the use of RS in a food product not only serves as a source of fermentable fiber, but also lowers GI (Björck *et al.*, 2000). The extent and mechanism by which non-digestible carbohydrates (dietary fiber) in foods influence glycemic response is a subject of debate. There are several contradictory studies, some suggesting a role for insoluble fiber (Wolever, 1990), while several others indicate that incorporation of soluble fibers (guar gum, psyllium, β-glucans, pectin) has a significant effect on postprandial glucose response (Jenkins *et al.*, 1978; Wood *et al.*, 1990). The concept of whole-grain foods (breads, pasta, cereals) is gaining momentum and consumption of a number of grains and grain extracts has been reported to control or improve glucose tolerance and reduce insulin resistance (Hallfrisch and Behall, 2000). The structure and composition of the grain – including particle size, amount and type of fiber, viscosity effect, and amylose and amylopectin content – affect the metabolism of carbohydrates from grains. The use of the viscous fibers in lowering the glycemic response has been related to reduced gastric emptying (Jenkins, 1978; Braaten *et al.*, 1991). In the future, it may be possible to select suitable cereal genotypes for the preparation of tailor-made foods with defined glycemic and other nutritional attributes. For example, a highly viscous β-glucan-containing barley genotype (Prowashonupana) has been demonstrated to lower the glycemic response of breakfast foods (breads, porridges) significantly in healthy and diabetic volunteers (Liljeberg *et al.*, 1996; Rendell *et al.*, 2005).

### 9.5.4 Other constituents

The rate of starch digestion is seen to be influenced by several minor plant constituents (usually referred to as anti-nutrients) such as phytates, phenolic compounds (tannins), saponins, lectins, and several enzyme inhibitors. These components interfere with the catalytic activity of the glucosidase enzymes through different mechanisms, thereby limiting their action (Thompson, 1988). Fish and Thompson (1991) showed that lectin and tannic acid (from red kidney bean) individually could inhibit the starch digestive enzymes, salivary and pancreatic α-amylases; however, a combination of the two anti-nutrients abolished their inhibitory activity. The authors concluded that the effect of individual anti-nutrients may not necessarily relate to the effects observed upon consumption of the mixture of anti-nutrients as normally observed in foods. Although a majority of these minor components could potentially influence glycemic response, their practical significance has usually been limited by way of being removed or destroyed at various stages of food preparation and consumption.

Recently, there has been a renewed interest in the use of inhibitors of the human α-glucosidases to moderate carbohydrate digestion and its associated insulin response for treatment of non-insulin dependent (type-2) diabetes. Acarbose, an oligosaccharide formed by strains of the genus *Actinoplanes*, functions as an inhibitor of both α-amylase and the mucosal α-glucosidases (sucrase-isomaltase and maltase-glucoamylase) (Hiele *et al.*, 1992). It has been effective in the treatment of diabetes as it slows down digestion of disaccharides and starch (Chiasson *et al.*, 1994; Conniff *et al.*, 1994) and is used in some countries to treat diabetes. However, it has frequently been shown to have gastrointestinal side effects due to malabsorption of disaccharides. Starch blockers, purified amylase inhibitors from Great Northern beans (phaseolamin), have also shown promise in glucose homeostatis (Boivin *et al.*, 1988) and are marketed as dietary supplements (Phase 2 Starch Neutralizer™; Udani *et al.*, 2004). Unlike these blockers that need to be ingested in large quantities (4–6 g per meal) to show significant effect, trestatin (a mixture of complex oligosaccharides produced microbiologically) has been proven to be a potent inhibitor (3–6 mg per 75 g starch) of pancreatic α-amylase in several *in vitro* and *in vivo* studies (Golay *et al.*, 1991). Glycemic and insulinemic responses in healthy and diabetic volunteers were moderated after consumption of breads containing trestatin added during processing without serious gastrointestinal side effects. Although the use of enzyme inhibitors has shown promise, further studies are needed to evaluate the efficacy of these inhibitors after addition to starch-based processed foods, the dose–response relationship, and, more importantly, long-term tolerance and side effects of the use of such inhibitors.

The presence of organic acids or acid salts, such as those produced during sourdough fermentation or added during baked food preparation, has been seen to influence glycemic and insulinemic responses (Liljeberg & Björck, 1996, 1998; Liljeberg *et al.*, 1995). For example, consumption of sourdough bread (with lactic acid produced during fermentation) or breads with added calcium lactate, or sodium propionate, significantly reduced glycemic and insulinemic indexes as compared with wholemeal bread in the absence of these acids (Liljeberg *et al.*, 1995). Intake of bread with a high concentration of sodium propionate not only lowered postprandial blood glucose and insulin responses, but also significantly prolonged the duration of satiety compared with all other breads. *In vitro* digestion of these breads, however, showed a significant decrease in the rate of amylase digestion only in bread containing lactic acid. The authors concluded that the effect of acid salts such as sodium propionate on metabolic responses and satiety was due to effects other than starch hydrolysis, such as delayed gastric emptying (Liljeberg & Björck, 1996). Similar effects were observed upon addition of vinegar to a starchy meal (Liljeberg & Björck, 1998). The potential of fermentative processes or processes that incorporate organic acids to improve the nutritional features of carbohydrates need to be considered.

Recent studies in our laboratory (M. Venkatachalam, G. Zhang and B. R. Hamaker, unpublished data, 2005) show that entrapment of starch in an alginate–calcium ion biopolymer matrix effectively creates a barrier (cooked in the entrapped form) to digestion by amylases and provides a slow glucose release profile. Scanning electron microscope images of the cooked starch microspheres showed that the gelatinized starch trapped in the biopolymer matrix represents a highly dense food form that is gradually digested by the amylases from the periphery towards the center of the sphere. Various factors – including biopolymer type (alginate or blend of alginate with other polymers, such as gellan gum, chitosan, or carrageenan), biopolymer concentration, microsphere size, and calcium ion concentration – could be used to obtain biopolymer-entrapped starches with desired slow-digestion profiles. Such microspheres not only lowered glycemic response (as indicated by initial clinical studies), but may also serve as novel starch ingredients providing extended release of glucose in food products.

## 9.6 Future trends

Strategies to produce low-GI foods could include: incorporating non-digesting carbohydrates (dietary fiber, RS) into foods; starches with slow digesting properties that extend glucose release; creating proper food forms; viscosity-increasing polysaccharides that delay gastric emptying or decrease digestive enzyme access; organic acids and their salts; or anti-nutritional agents that inhibit digestion of starch and other glycemic carbohydrates. Additionally, as more research is conducted to understand the effects of low-GI foods with slow glucose release properties on health, satiety, activity levels, and mental performance, these types of slowly digestible carbohydrates may be available for consumers.

Food form will continue to be a major issue in the development of low-GI and, particularly, slow digesting foods. Highly organized, dense food forms impede starch digestion and, thereby, lower the glycemic response of starchy foods. An organized food form could simply preserve the crystalline order of starch (prevent complete gelatinization) during food processing or provide a barrier to digestive enzymes. Besides pasta (described in Section 9.5.1), whole-grain foods, wherein the cellular layers surrounding the starch granules are intact, also present an example of an organized food form with low GI. Whole-wheat-flour bread, in which some of the grain structure persists, has been reported to elicit a lower glycemic response than white bread (Liljeberg *et al.*, 1992). Similarly, legumes cooked under mild heat processing conditions (such as boiling), that had an intact cellular structure, had lower GI as compared with legumes cooked under harsher conditions (pressure cooking) or milled before cooking (Wolever *et al.*, 1987; Tovar *et al.*, 1992; Golay *et al.*, 1986). Beverages, from the point of view of providing extended energy release, represents a special challenge, because soluble glucose-containing oligosaccharides, maltodextrins, and starches tend to be rapidly digested. There is a need for a more systematic research approach to understand how glycemic carbohydrates and food form (type of matrix, concentration, cooling profile, storage conditions) influence GI and glucose release profiles, and their physiological and metabolic consequences.

## 9.7 References

ASTON L M (2006), 'Glycaemic index and metabolic disease risk', *Proc Nutr Soc*, **65**, 125–134.

AXELSEN M and SMITH U (2001), 'Treatment for diabetes', US Patent 6,316,427.

BERRY C S (1986), 'Resistant starch formation and measurement of starch that survives exhaustive digestion with amylolytic enzymes during the determination of dietary fiber', *J Cereal Sci*, **4**, 301–314.

BILIADERIS C G and GALLOWAY G (1989), 'Crystallization behavior of amylose-V complexes: structure–property relationships', *Carbohydr Res*, **189**, 31–48.

BIRD A R, BROWN I L and TOPPING D L (2000), 'Starches, resistant starches, the gut microflora and human health', *Curr Issues Intest Microbiol*, **1**, 25–37.

BJÖRCK I, LILJEBERG H and OSTMAN E (2000), 'Low glycaemic-index foods', *Br J Nutr*, **83**, S149–155.

BOIVIN M, FLOURIE B, RIZZA R A, GO V L and DIMAGNO E P (1988), 'Gastrointestinal and metabolic effects of amylase inhibition in diabetics', *Gastroenterology*, **94**, 387–394.

BRAATEN J T, WOOD P, SCOTT F W, RIEDEL K D, POSTE L and COLLINS W (1991), 'Oat gum lowers glucose and insulin after an oral glucose load', *Am J Clin Nutr*, **53**, 1425–1430.

BRAND-MILLER J C (2003), 'Glycemic load and chronic disease', *Nutr Rev*, **61**, S49–55.

BROWN I L (2004), 'Applications and uses of resistant starch', *JAOAC*, **87**, 727–732.

BUGUSU B A (2003), 'Understanding the basis of the slow starch digestion characteristic of sorghum porridges and how to manipulate starch digestion rate', Ph.D. Thesis, Purdue University, West Lafayette, Indiana, USA.

CHEN Y T, CORNBALTH M and SIDBURY J B (1984), 'Corn starch therapy in type I glycogen-storage disease', *N Engl J Med*, **310**, 171–175.

CHIASSON J L, JOSSE R G, HUNT J A, PALMASON C, RODGER N W, ROSS S A, RYAN E A, TAN M H and WOLEVER T M (1994), 'The efficacy of acarbose in the treatment of patients with non-insulin-dependent diabetes mellitus. A multicenter controlled clinical trial', *Ann Intern Med*, **121**, 928–935.

CHIU C W, HENLEY M and ALTIERI P (1994), 'Process for making amylase resistant starch from high amylose starch', National Starch and Chem. Investment Holding Corp., US Patent 5,281,276.

COLONNA P, BARRY J L, CLOAREC D, BORNET F, GOUILLOUD S and GALMICHE J P (1990), 'Enzymic susceptibility of starch from pasta', *J Cereal Sci*, **11**, 59–70.

CONNIFF R F, SHAPIRO J A and SEATON T B (1994), 'Long-term efficacy and safety of acarbose in the treatment of obese subjects with non-insulin-dependent diabetes mellitus', *Arch Intern Med*, **154**, 2442–2448.

ELIASSON A-C and KROG N (1985), 'Physical properties of amylose-monoglyceride complexes', *J Cereal Sci*, **3**, 239–248.

ELIASSON A-C, CARLSON T L-G, LARSSON K and MIEZIS Y (1981), 'Some effects of starch lipids on the thermal and rheological properties of wheat starch', *Starch/Stärke*, 1981, **33**, 130–134.

ENGLYST H N, KINGMAN S M and CUMMINGS J H (1992), 'Classification and measurement of nutritionally important starch fractions', *Eur J Clin Nutr*, **46**, S33–50.

ENGLYST H N, VEENSTRA J and HUDSON G J (1996), 'Measurement of rapidly available glucose (RAG) in plant foods: a potential in vitro predictor of the glycaemic response', *Br J Nutr*, **75**, 327–337.

EERLINGEN R C, DECEUNINCK M and DELCOUR J A (1993), 'Enzyme-resistant starch. II. Influence of amylose chain length on resistant starch formation', *Cereal Chem*, **70**, 345–350.

FANNON J E, HAUBER R J and BEMILLER J N (1992), 'Surface pores of starch granules', *Cereal Chem*, **69**, 284–288.

FARDET A, HOEBLER C B, BALDWIN P M, BOUCHET B, GALLANT D J and BARRY J L (1998), 'Involvement of the protein network in the in vitro degradation of starch from spaghetti and lasagna: a microscopic and enzymatic study', *J Cereal Sci*, **27**, 133–145.

FARDET A, ABECASSIS J, HOEBLER C, BALDWIN P M, BULEON A, BEROT S, BARRY J L and FERGUSON L R (1999), 'Influence of technological modifications of the protein network from pasta on in vitro starch degradation', *J Cereal Sci*, **30**, 133–145.

FERGUSON L R, TASMAN-JONES C, ENGLYST H and HARRIS P J (2000), 'Comparative effects of three resistant starch preparations on transit time and short-chain fatty acid production in rats', *Nutrition and Cancer*, **36**, 230–237.

FERNANDES G, VELANGI A and WOLEVER T M S (2005), 'Glycemic index of potatoes commonly consumed in North America', *Am Diet Assoc*, **105**, 557–562.

FISH B C and THOMPSON L U (1991), 'Lectin-tannin interactions and their influence on pancreatic amylase activity and starch digestibility', *J Agric Food Chem*, **39**, 727–731.

FOSTER-POWELL K, HOLT S H and BRAND-MILLER J C (2002), 'International table of glycemic index and glycemic load values', *Am J Clin Nutr*, **76**, 5–56.

GANNON M C, ERCAN N, WESTPHAL S A and NUTTALL F Q (1993), 'Effect of added fat on plasma glucose and insulin response to ingested potato in individuals with NIDDM', *Diabetes Care*, **16**, 874–880.

GÉRARD C, PLANCHOT V, COLONNA P and BERTOFT E (2000), 'Relationship between branching density and crystalline structure of A- and B-type maize mutant starches', *Carbohydr Res*, **326**, 130–144.

GOLAY A, COULSTON A, HOLLENBECK C B, KAISER L L, WURSCH P and REAVEN G M (1986), 'Comparison of metabolic effects of white beans processed into two different physical forms', *Diabetes Care*, **9**, 260–266.

GOLAY A, SCHNEIDER H, TEMLER E and FELBER J P (1991), 'Effect of trestatin, an amylase inhibitor, incorporated into bread, on glycemic responses in normal and diabetic patients', *Am J Clin Nutr*, **53**, 61–65.

GRANFELDT Y and BJÖRCK I (1991), 'Glycemic response to starch in pasta: a study of mechanisms of limited enzyme availability', *J Cereal Sci*, **14**, 47–61.

HALLFRISCH J and BEHALL K M (2000), 'Mechanisms of the effects of grains on insulin and glucose responses', *J Am Coll Nutr*, **19**, 320S–325S.

HAN J-A and BEMILLER J N (2006), 'Preparation and physical characteristics of slowly digesting modified food starches', *Carbohydr Polym*, **67**, 366–374.

HAN X Z, AO Z, JANASWAMY S, JANE J L, CHANDRASEKARAN R and HAMAKER B R (2006), 'Development of a low glycemic maize starch: preparation and characterization', *Biomacromolecules*, **7**, 1162–1168.

HIELE M, GHOOS Y, RUTGEERTS P and VANTRAPPEN G (1992), 'Effects of acarbose on starch hydrolysis. Study in healthy subjects, ileostomy patients and in vitro', *Dig Dis Sci*, **37**, 1057–1064.

HOLM J, BJÖRCK I, OSTROWSKA S, ELIASSON A C, ASP N G, LARSSON K and LUNDQUIST I (1983), 'Digestibility of amylose-lipid complexes in vitro and in vivo', *Starch/Stärke*, **35**, 294–297.

JACOBS H and DELCOUR J A (1998), 'Hydrothermal modifications of granular starch, with retention of the granular structure – a review', *J Agric Food Chem*, **46**, 2895–2905.

JENKINS D J, WOLEVER T M, LEEDS A R, GASSULL M A, HAISMAN P, DILAWARI J, GOFF D V, METZ G L and ALBERTI K G (1978), 'Dietary fibres, fibre analogues and glucose tolerance: importance of viscosity', *Br Med J*, **1**, 1392–1394.

LILJEBERG H G and BJÖRCK I M (1996), 'Delayed gastric emptying rate as a potential mechanism for lowered glycaemia after eating sourdough bread: studies in humans and rats using test products with added organic acids or an organic salt', *Am J Clin Nutr*, **64**, 886–893.

LILJEBERG H and BJÖRCK I (1998), 'Delayed gastric emptying rate may explain improved glycaemia in healthy subjects to a starchy meal with added vinegar', *Eur J Clin Nutr*, **52**, 368–371.

LILJEBERG H G, GRANFELDT Y E and BJÖRCK I M (1992), 'Metabolic response to starch in bread containing intact kernels versus milled flour', *Eur J Clin Nutr*, **46**, 561–575.

LILJEBERG H G, LONNER C H and BJÖRCK I M (1995), Sourdough fermentation or addition of organic acids or corresponding salts to bread improves nutritional properties of starch in healthy humans', *J Nutr*, **125**, 1503–1511.

LILJEBERG H G, GRANFELDT Y E and BJÖRCK I M (1996), 'Products based on a high-fiber barley genotype, but not on common barley or oats, lower post-prandial glucose and insulin responses in healthy humans', *J Nutr*, **126**, 458–466.

LUDWIG D S (2002), 'The glycemic index: physiological mechanisms relating to obesity, diabetes and cardiovascular disease', *JAMA*, **287**, 2414–2423.

MILLER J B, PANG E and BRAMALL L (1992), 'Rice: a high or low glycemic index food?', *Am J Clin Nutr*, **56**, 1034–1036.

MORGAN L M (1998), 'The role of gastrointestinal hormones in carbohydrate and lipid metabolism and homeostasis: effects of gastric inhibitory polypeptide and glucagon-like peptide-1', *Biochem Soc Trans*, **26**, 216–222.

MURRAY S, PATIL A, FAHEY G, MERCHEN N, WOLF B, LAI S-C and GAREB K (1998), 'Apparent digestibility of a debranched amylopectin-lipid complex and resistant starch incorporated into enteral formulas fed to ileal-cannulated dogs', *J Nutr*, **128**, 2032–2035.

PARILLO M, GIACCO R, RICCARDI G, PACIONI D and RIVELLESE A (1985), 'Different glycaemic responses to pasta, bread and potatoes in diabetic patients', *Diabet Med*, **2**, 374–377.

PARK J T and ROLLINGS J E (1994), 'Effects of substrate branching characteristics on kinetics of enzymatic depolymerization of mixed linear and branched polysaccharides. 1. Amylose/amylopectin alpha-amylolysis', *Biotechnol Bioeng*, **44**, 792–800.

PATIL A R, MURRAY S M, FAHEY G C, MERCHEN N R, WOLF B W, LAI C and GARLEB K A (1998), 'Apparent digestibility and glycemic responses to a debranched amylopectin-lipid complex and resistant starch incorporated into enteral formulas fed to dogs cannulated in the ileum', *FASEB J*, **12**, A210 (abstract).

QI X and TESTER R (2005), 'Compositions and uses thereof', Patent WO 2005/044284 A1.

RENDELL M, VANDERHOOF J, VENN M, SHEHAN M, ARNDT E, RAO C, GILL G, NEWMAN R and NEWMAN C (2005), 'Effect of a barley breakfast cereal on blood glucose and insulin response in normal and diabetic patients', *Plant Foods Human Nutr*, **60**, 63–67.

SEAL C J, DALY M E, THOMAS L C, BAL W, BIRKETT A M, JEFFCOAT R and MATHERS J C (2003), 'Postprandial carbohydrate metabolism in healthy subjects and those with type 2 diabetes fed starches with slow and rapid hydrolysis rates determined in vitro', *Br J Nutr*, **90**, 853–864.

SENEVIRATNE H D and BILIADERIS C G (1991), 'Action of α-amylases on amylose-lipid complex superstructures', *J Cereal Sci*, **13**, 129–143.

SHI Y-C and SEIB P A (1995), 'Fine structure of maize starches from four *wx*-containing genotypes of the W64A inbred line in relation to gelatinization and retrogradation', *Carbohydr Polym*, **26**, 141–147.

SHI Y C and TRZASKO P T (1997), 'Process for producing amylose resistant granular starch', US Patent 5,593,503, National Starch and Chem. Investment Holding Corp.

SHI Y C, CUI X, BIRKETT A M and THATCHER M G (2003), United States Patent Applications 20030219520, 20030215562.

SHIN M, SONG J and SEIB P A (2004a), 'In vitro digestibility of cross-linked starches-RS4', *Starch/Starke*, **56**, 478–483.

SHIN S I, CHOI H J, CHUNG K M, HAMAKER B R, PARK K H and MOON T W (2004b), 'Slowly digestible starch from debranched waxy sorghum starch: preparation and properties', *Cereal Chem*, **81**, 404–408.

SHIN S I, KIM H J, HA H J, LEE S H and MOON T W (2005), 'Effect of hydrothermal treatment on formation and structural characteristics of slowly digestible non-pasted granular sweet potato starch', *Starch/Stärke*, **57**, 421–430.

THOMPSON LU (1988), 'Antinutrients and blood glucose', *Food Technol*, **42**, 123–132.

THOMPSON D B (2000), 'On the non-random nature of amylopectin branching', *Carb Polym*, **43**, 223–239.

TOVAR J, GRANFELDT Y and BJÖRCK I (1992), 'Effects of processing on blood glucose and insulin responses to starch in legumes', *J Agric Food Chem*, **40**, 1846–1851.

UDANI J, HARDY M and MADSEN D (2004), 'Blocking carbohydrate absorption and weight loss: a clinical trial using Phase 2 brand proprietary fractionated white bean extract', *Altern Med Rev*, **9**, 63–69.

USDA (2005), 'Dietary Guidelines for Americans', Chapter 7, Carbohydrates, http://www.healthierus.gov/dietaryguidelines.

WEPNER B, BERGHOFER E, MIESENBERGER E, TIEFENBACHER K and NG P N K (1999), 'Citrate starch-application as resistant starch in different food systems', *Starch/Starke*, **51**, 354–361.

WOLEVER T M (1990), 'Relationship between dietary fiber content and composition in foods and the glycemic index', *Am J Clin Nutr*, **51**, 72–75.

WOLEVER T, JENKINS D J, KALMUSKY J, GIORDANO C, GIUDICI S, JENKINS A L, THOMPSON L U, WONG G S and JOSSE R G (1986), 'Glycemic response to pasta: effect of surface area, degree of cooking and protein enrichment', *Diabetes Care*, **9**, 401–404.

WOLEVER T M S, JENKINS D J A, THOMPSON L U, WONG G S and JOSSE R G (1987), 'Effect of canning on the blood glucose response to beans in patients with type 2 diabetes', *Hum Nutr Clin Nutr*, **41**, 135–140.

WOLEVER T M, JENKINS D J, JENKINS A L and JOSSE R G (1991), 'The glycemic index: methodology and clinical implications', *Am J Clin Nutr*, **54**, 846–854.

WOLF B W, LAURA L B and FAHEY G C (1999), 'Effects of chemical modification on in vitro rate and extent of food starch digestion: an attempt to discover a slowly digested starch', *J Agric Food Chem*, **47**, 4178–4183.

WOO K S and SEIB P A (2002), 'Cross-linked resistant starch. Preparation and properties', *Cereal Chem*, **79**, 819–825.

WOOD P J, BRAATEN J T, FRASER W S, RIEDEL D and POSTE L M (1990), 'Comparison of viscous properties of oat and guar gum and the effects of these and oat bran on glycemic index', *J Agric Food Chem*, **38**, 753–757.

ZHANG G, AO Z and HAMAKER BR (2006a), 'Slow digestion property of native cereal starches', *Biomacromolecules*, **7** (11), 3252–3258.

ZHANG G, VENKATACHALAM, M and HAMAKER BR (2006b), 'Structural basis for the slow digestion property of native cereal starch', *Biomacromolecules*, **7** (11), 3259–3266.

# 10

# Novel ingredients for weight loss: new developments

**J. D. Stowell, Danisco Sweeteners, UK**

## 10.1 Introduction

The quest for a magic bullet for weight loss is far from new. Throughout the last century a bewildering array of strategies emerged only to be discredited due to lack of safety or efficacy. Of the more extreme ideas, the purposeful ingestion of tapeworms must surely rank as the most bizarre. Whilst this may just be an urban legend, today's Internet abounds with articles on the subject, implicating the rich and famous and apparently still offering tapeworm eggs for sale as dietary supplements. The very thought of this is repugnant, but it does demonstrate the lengths to which some might go to achieve weight loss.

By the 1960s amphetamines had become the product of choice for appetite suppression. Ephedra is an evergreen shrub found in central Asia. It contains the alkaloids ephedrine and pseudoephedrine. It achieved remarkable popularity and, latterly, notoriety in the weight loss arena. Finally the US Food and Drug Administration (FDA) banned the sale of ephedra in dietary supplements in February, 2004 (FDA, 2004).

Increasing obesity rates combined with an ever diminishing perception of the ideal body shape, encouraged by the popular press, means that there is an ever greater disconnect between reality and expectations. This fuels the intense effort to find that magic ingredient for weight loss. Today we have the advantage of sophisticated scientific know-how combined with consumer representation and well-developed legislation. This should ensure that new ingredients reaching the market have a proven track record of safety and success, and a repeat of past failures should be avoided. However, even today there remains a disconcerting reliance on anecdote and inadequate science, particularly as evidenced by the more outrageous Internet selling techniques.

Food ingredients that facilitate weight loss fall under the spectrum of 'functional' foods as defined by the European Commission Concerted Action on Functional Food Science in Europe (FUFOSE) (Diplock *et al.*, 1999): 'A food can be regarded as 'functional' if it is satisfactorily demonstrated to affect beneficially one or more target functions in the body, beyond adequate nutritional effects in a way that is relevant to either an improved state of health and well-being and/or reduction of risk of disease'. However, the distinction between foods, supplements and medicines is becoming increasingly blurred and 'functional foods' as such do not appear as a specific category in food law either in Europe or in North America. Foods for Specified Health Use (FOSHU) in Japan do approximate to the concept of functional foods.

There are many complex aspects involved in the introduction of a new food ingredient for weight management. The area is fraught with scepticism, false hope and promises, claims and counterclaims, and highly motivated consumers fuelling industry growth. Boucher *et al.* (2001) counselled healthcare professionals to encourage their clients to resist 'the temptation to buy a "magic" pill or potion that promises effortless weight loss or weight maintenance'. Pittler and Ernst (2004), in a systematic review of dietary supplements for body weight reduction, concluded 'the evidence for most dietary supplements as aids in reducing body weight is not convincing. None of the reviewed dietary supplements can be recommended for over-the-counter use.'

It is against this background that the quest for effective strategies continues. The science is becoming increasingly sophisticated and several thorough and convincing studies have been published since the Pittler and Ernst (2004) review. Randomized, double-blind, placebo-controlled human intervention studies are important in the evaluation of individual ingredients and it is encouraging to see such studies being published (see, for example, Preuss *et al.,* 2004a, b discussed in Section 10.3.2). It is also encouraging to see major food companies such as Unilever entering the arena. The emphasis is gradually shifting from that 'magic bullet' to a more holistic approach and consumer expectations are becoming more realistic as the positive impact of a 5–10% reduction in body mass is now better understood (see Calorie Control Council websites). Most consumers know by now about the benefits of fruit, vegetables, whole grains, caloric restriction, exercise, etc., but this has had little impact on burgeoning waistlines. For example, in the USA calorie consumption increased by 450 kcal per capita per day from the mid 1960s to the 1990s (Anon., 2004). From this it is clear that some extra help is needed.

The purpose of this chapter is to provide a brief perspective on new developments in weight loss food ingredients, highlighting the different aspects that must be addressed before such ingredients could be deemed to be successful. Criteria for a successful ingredient will be listed and some of the regulatory considerations introduced. Some details of (–)-hydroxycitric acid (HCA) will be provided as an example of the approach that is being taken. Several other examples will then be outlined, together with comments on future directions. No attempt has been made to provide a comprehensive review and the reader is referred to the publications cited for further details.

## 10.2 Criteria for a successful new ingredient for weight loss

As noted above, there are many aspects to be considered when planning the introduction of a new weight loss ingredient. Some of the more obvious are listed below. Although seemingly a matter of commonsense, this simple checklist could be usefully employed to distinguish between the worthwhile and the not so worthwhile, or to identify gaps in our knowledge.

### 10.2.1 Confirmation of safety and efficacy at intended use levels

This really is the *sine qua non* of any new ingredient. It might be tempting to conclude that an ingredient is safe based on a prior history of human exposure. However, unless the historical dose and consumption patterns equate to the proposed use conditions, and unless the effects of the ingredient on specific individuals and population groups have been determined, it would be easy to miss possible adverse reactions. Nor is it acceptable to increase the dose beyond what is realistic simply in order to achieve a positive result. Evaluation of safety includes structure and exposure assessment as well as chemical characterization. Genetic toxicology, animal, metabolism and human studies all contribute to the assessment.

### 10.2.2 Data on target population groups

Again there is a temptation to declare an ingredient safe based on prior consumption by population groups unrepresentative of the target groups. Of course, such data do contribute to the totality of relevant information. However, it is important to generate data on groups representative of the target population.

### 10.2.3 Long-term effects

It is important to take into account the timeframe over which an ingredient is likely to be consumed when assessing its safety. Much information can be gained from acute toxicity studies but if the ingredient is expected to be consumed on a long-term basis then relevant data should be generated over that timeframe.

### 10.2.4 Mechanism

It is desirable but not essential to understand the mechanism(s) whereby the ingredient under evaluation mediates its effect. So long as safety and efficacy are clearly documented then there is a case that the ingredient could be marketed without unnecessary risk.

The basic mechanisms whereby weight loss ingredients mediate their effect include:

- encouraging the consumption of fewer calories;
- reducing absorption of nutrients from the digestive system, which in turn increases excretion;
- increasing the excretion of urinary metabolites;
- reducing the efficiency of conversion of nutrients into metabolizable energy. This might involve enhanced thermogenesis and/or reducing the flux through lipogenic pathways. The latter could be achieved either by competitive or allosteric enzyme inhibition or by downregulating the genes coding for the enzyme systems responsible for lipogenesis.

It is important to calculate the relative contribution each of these mechanisms might make. As an example, in the early days of the Atkins low-carbohydrate programme it was thought that urinary excretion of ketones could be responsible for the rapid weight loss seen. When calculations were undertaken it was found that urinary metabolites only accounted for a trivial proportion of the negative caloric balance. Consumption of fewer calories was actually the main reason for the successful weight loss.

### 10.2.5 Proven weight loss

For many functional foods intermediate biomarkers of efficacy need to be identified because it is impractical to measure the desired endpoint via human intervention studies. An example is the application of prebiotics and/or probiotics to reduce colon cancer risk. The incidence of colon cancer in healthy populations is low and the timeframe for its development is long. Hence, it is difficult to envisage conducting a conclusive intervention study on healthy populations. Typically the incidence of recurrence is studied in subjects who have already experienced adenomas. Complementary animal studies are also undertaken on susceptible species to which known carcinogens have been administered.

The good news for weight loss ingredients is that the endpoint is easy to measure. Weight loss is usually unequivocable. Having said this, it may be a challenge to achieve compliance in weight loss intervention studies and it may be difficult to unravel the relative contributions of individual variables.

### 10.2.6 Role in weight maintenance

Many strategies for weight loss are successful in the short term provided they encompass both caloric restriction and enhanced physical activity.

However, long-term success is notoriously elusive. Boucher *et al.* (2001) note that people participating in behavioural weight loss programmes lose an average of 8.4 kg during treatment of 20 weeks and are able to maintain, on average, two-thirds of this loss for 9–10 months after treatment. However, within 3–5 years they gradually return to their baseline weight. For a new weight loss ingredient to be truly successful it should encourage the development of habits that are sustained in the long term. Depending on the ingredient it may be practical for consumption to be ongoing or it may be more appropriately used to kick-start a change in lifestyle.

### 10.2.7 Comparison with alternative strategies

An element in the evaluation of a new weight loss ingredient or strategy should be to compare its performance with alternatives. However, in this complex area it is clear that 'one size does not fit all' so it is important that a number of products are validated, providing consumers with choice and enhancing the chances of individual success.

### 10.2.8 A word about reduced-calorie foods

Macronutrient alternatives such as intense and bulk sweeteners, bulking agents and fat replacers, and the foods into which they are formulated, can be considered as weight loss ingredients in their own right, but they are only validated as such if they actually help consumers to lose weight. The role of reduced-calorie foods in weight management has been the subject of thorough debate since intense sweeteners gathered momentum in the 1960s and particularly since the 'low-fat' trend of the 1990s failed to reverse the trend towards obesity, particularly in the USA and Europe. A recent review of the subject (Stowell, 2006) led to the following conclusion.

> Foods formulated with non-nutritive intense sweeteners and with reduced calorie bulk sweeteners and bulking agents can play an interesting role in helping consumers to improve the nutritional profile of their diets. Contrary to some reports, the main body of published data shows that these ingredients, when incorporated into foods with lower caloric density and/or reduced glycaemic impact, can actually help consumers to eat less calories. A balanced approach to weight loss and maintenance is essential for long term success.

As new ingredients aimed at weight control enter the market they will also be the subject of similar scrutiny.

## 10.3 (–)-Hydroxycitric acid

### 10.3.1 Background

*Garcinia cambogia* is an evergreen tropical shrub of the Guttiferae family native to Southeast Asia and in particular South India. It typically grows wild but is also cultivated in some areas. The fruits of *G. cambogia* are about the size of an orange but resemble a small yellowish or reddish pumpkin. The dried rinds of the fruit are used in food preparation in several Southeast Asian countries where, amongst other attributes, they are said to be effective in making meals 'more filling' (FDA, 2005a). Good use of this feature of *G. cambogia* has been made by the dietary supplement industry, particularly in the USA where supplements containing *Garcinia* extract have been promoted for appetite suppression for many years.

The active component of *Garcinia* is HCA, present at up to 30% in the fruit rind. Most of the HCA is present in the fruit as the lactone which must be converted to the acid itself in order to become active.

### 10.3.2 Conditions of use and efficacy

Many studies have been undertaken on HCA both in animals and in humans. Different preparations have been used at different levels and it has become clear that less-than-optimum strategies have been used in earlier studies making interpretation of results difficult. The clinical study involving the largest number of subjects (135) and the longest duration (12 weeks) failed to show a significantly different weight loss compared with placebo (Heymsfield *et al.*, 1998). This study involved the feeding of 1000 mg of *G. cambogia* extract containing 500 mg of HCA three times per day, 30–60 min before meals. A 1200 kcal per day diet was provided to all subjects. Subsequent criticism of this study pointed to the abnormally low calorie value of the diet as well as a lack of definition of the source of the HCA and no proof of bioavailability (Preuss *et al.*, 2004a).

The California, USA-based company, InterHealth (see Interhealth website) has undertaken detailed research on HCA in collaboration with various universities to determine the most effective product forms, dose levels and feeding strategies. They recently launched a patent pending product Super CitriMax® which is an almost completely soluble calcium and potassium salt of HCA containing 60% by weight HCA and with confirmed bioavailability (Loe *et al.*, 2001). Super CitriMax® was the subject of recent randomized, double-blind, placebo-controlled human intervention studies undertaken in India (Preuss *et al.*, 2004a, b). A pilot study (Preuss *et al.*, 2004a) involved feeding 30 obese subjects with 4667 mg Super CitriMax® per day, equivalent to 2700–2800 mg HCA in three equal doses 30–60 min before meals. The study lasted 8 weeks. An additional treatment group received the Super CitriMax® plus niacin-bound chromium (NBC) and a standardized *Gymnema sylvestre* extract (GSE). A 2000 kcal per day diet was provided to all subjects. In the HCA-fed group body weight and body mass index (BMI) decreased by 6.3%, total cholesterol, low-density lipoprotein (LDL) and triglyceride levels decreased by 6.3%, 12.3% and 8.6% respectively, whilst high-density lipoprotein (HDL) and serotonin levels increased by 10.7% and 40% respectively. Serum leptin levels decreased by 40.5% and excretion of urinary fat metabolites increased by 146–281%. The HCA/NBC/GSE group performed even better whilst the placebo group only achieved minimal positive changes.

The second study (Preuss *et al.*, 2004b) followed exactly the same protocol as Preuss *et al.* 2004a, except that it involved 60 subjects. This study achieved very similar results, with 5–6% body weight reduction in the treatment groups with only marginal or non-significant effects in the placebo group.

The bioefficacy of the calcium potassium salt of HCA has been summarized in a recent review by Downs *et al.* (2005). A convincing database is emerging for this novel ingredient. As with all new ingredients the longer-term effects need to be elucidated.

### 10.3.3 Proposed mechanism(s) of action

HCA is a competitive inhibitor of ATP-citrate lyase, an extra-mitochondrial enzyme involved in the initial steps of *de novo* lipogenesis. In this way, HCA reduces the conversion of citrate into acetyl coenzyme A, a primary step in the formation of fatty acids in the liver. Increased glycogen is produced in the liver in the presence of HCA and this may mediate satiety signals, reducing appetite (Preuss *et al.*, 2004a). In addition to this, according to Downs *et al.* (2005) HCA as the calcium potassium salt induces an increase in serotonin release and serotonin receptor reuptake inhibition (SRRI). Serotonin regulation has been proposed as a mechanism of appetite suppression.

### 10.3.4 Safety and regulatory status

The safety of HCA has been investigated in several studies, reviewed by Soni *et al.* (2004). No adverse effects have been observed either in animal toxicity tests or in human studies. Teratogenicity studies and long-term feeding studies still need to be completed.

As noted above, *G. cambogia* extract/HCA has been a component of dietary supplements in the USA for some years. In 2003 InterHealth announced that a panel of scientific experts had affirmed Super CitriMax® as GRAS (generally recognized as safe) for use in functional beverages in the USA (Interhealth website, GRAS affirmation). This is the first step towards more general food application of HCA. It seems likely that if HCA becomes a mainstream ingredient raw material supply might become an issue. This has obviously been predicted by the Ireland-based Company, Shannon Minerals Ltd, who recently submitted a premarket notification of intention to market synthetic HCA as a new dietary ingredient for dietary supplement applications. The FDA rejected this application, unconvinced of equivalence to the currently marketed HCA extracted from *G. cambogia*.

In Europe it is likely that HCA would fall under the remit of the Novel FoodsRegulation (EC) No. 258/97 although to date there is no evidence that this has been explored in any detail.

## 10.4 *Hoodia gordonii*

### 10.4.1 Background

*Hoodia gordonii* is one of several species of the genus *Hoodia* from the botanical family Asclepiadaceae. It is a cactus-like succulent plant that grows in the Kalahari desert in the southern part of Africa, mainly Botswana. The local San Bushmen have sucked on *Hoodia* as the whole fresh plant or dried whole plant for generations, principally to fight hunger and thirst during long hunting trips and at times of famine. Based on these anecdotal reports *H. gordonii* has been proposed as an anorectic agent for use by those seeking to lose or maintain weight.

### 10.4.2 Development and scientific substantiation

Whole-*Hoodia* powder contains variable amounts of fibre, organic material, antioxidants and biologically active substances including steroidal glycosides. One substance in particular is common to at least five species of *Hoodia*. This is the steroidal trisaccharide called 3-*O*-[beta-D-thevetopyranosyl-(1 → 4)-beta-D-cymaropyranosyl-(1 → 4)-beta-D-cymaropyranosyl]-12beta-*O*-tigloyloxy-14-hydroxy-14beta-pregn-5-en-20-one. It has been termed 'P57' because it was the 57th plant-derived compound investigated for commercial development by the British pharmaceutical company Phytopharm. An excellent review of the history of the development of *Hoodia* appears on the Internet (BioMolecular Sciences, Inc). P57 has been patented by Phytopharm and developed in collaboration with the CSIR (South African Council of Scientific and Industrial Research). The P57 originating from *H. gordonii*, as supplied by Phytopharm, is named P57AS3. It is this compound that is said to be responsible for the anorectic quality of the plant. Of three scientific reports on animal studies involving P57, only one has been published in a peer-reviewed journal (MacLean & Luo, 2004). The other two have only appeared in abstract form in conference presentations (Tulp *et al.*, 2001, 2002). Tulp *et al.* (2001, 2002) showed a 50% reduction in *ad libitum* food intake in rats fed *Hoodia* compared with control. The mean effective dose for appetite suppression in rats during a 4-h feeding test ranged from 1.8 to 2.7 g per kg body weight for the various *Hoodia* species. The values were similar in both lean and obese rats. Over a 2–3 week period, marked reduction in body weight was seen in the obese rats and a moderate reduction in the *Hoodia*-fed lean rats. Control rats gained weight normally during the same period. The decrease in spontaneous food intake was not due to unpalatability of the *Hoodia* diet (Phytopharm and Pfizer, unpublished observation).

MacLean and Luo (2004) recently studied the effects in rats of the steroidal glycoside P57AS3 purified from *H. gordonii*, supplied by Phytopharm and Pfizer. Intracerebroventricular injection of the purified P57AS3 resulted in an increased ATP content in the hypothalamic neurons. P57AS3 injections into the third ventricle (at doses of 0.4–40 nmol) reduced 24 hour food intake by rats by up to 60%. Subsequent experiments showed that in rats fed a low-calorie diet for 4 days, the content of ATP in the hypothalami fell by 30–50%. This effect was blocked by intracerebroventricular injections of P57AS3 (MacLean and Luo, 2004). Based on these findings, the authors hypothesize that ATP level may be a signal for the energy-sensing of satiety. More research is required to fully understand the mechanism of action of P57AS3 in weight control.

A double-blind placebo-controlled study testing P57 (reported to be from *H. Gordonii*) was carried out by Phytopharm in healthy overweight subjects. The results of this study have not yet been published and only a little information is available from the article by Habeck (2002) and from press releases on the Phytopharm website (http://www.phytopharm.co.uk). The first two stages of the study were aimed at assessing the safety, tolerability and pharmacokinetics of P57 whilst the third stage studied 19 overweight males fed either the P57 compound (at an unknown dose) or placebo twice daily for 15 days. The treatment group achieved a 30% reduction in calorie intake and a significant reduction in body fat content of 1 kg (Habeck, 2002).

### 10.4.3 Safety and regulatory status

The fact that the *Hoodia* plant has been consumed by the San Bushmen as whole fresh plant or dried whole plant for thousands of years is an element in favour of its safety. However, it is not sufficient to definitely conclude that the plant, P57 and P57AS3 from *H. gordonii* are safe for human consumption.

Since P57AS3 has been found to have similarities to the steroidal core of cardiac glycosides, long-term research is needed to determine appropriate dosage and potential contraindications, risks and side effects such as potential disturbances to heart rhythm that may be triggered by its consumption. The lack of definitive safety data has been confirmed in several communications from the US FDA. These were rejections in response to new dietary ingredient notifications as required before marketing of supplements containing *H. gordonii* (see Section 10.3.2 above). Examples are given below.

1 June 19th 2003 – A letter from the FDA to Goen Technologies Corp. that their 3/27/03 New Dietary Ingredient (NDI) notification was inadequate; attached was their 61 page notification which included a 57 page patent (US patent 6,376,657) that contained several study reports (http://

www.fda.gov/ohrms/dockets/DOCKETS/95s0316/95s-0316-rpt0186-vol133-web.pdf).

2 March 3rd 2004 – A letter from the FDA to Hoodia Products LLC that their 10/29/03 NDI notification was inadequate; attached was the 1 page NDI notification (http://www.fda.gov/ohrms/dockets/dockets/95s0316/95s-0316-rpt0218-vol156.pdf).

3 October 6th 2004 – A letter from the FDA to Awareness Corp. that their 3/23/04 NDI notification for use of dried powdered *H. gordonii* cactus pulp as a weight loss dietary supplement was inadequate; attached was their 17 page notification (http://www.fda.gov/ohrms/dockets/dockets/95s0316/95s-0316-rpt0238-01-vol173.pdf).

Similarly in Europe, the Netherlands notified the European Commission, DG Health and Consumer Protection Rapid Alert System for Food and Feed (RASFF) that attempts had been made to import slimming pills containing *H. gordonii*, unauthorized as a novel food (http:europa.eu.int/comm./food/food/rapidalert/index_en.htm).

In the USA the next step will be to submit a further premarket notification of a new dietary ingredient once adequate safety data have been published. In Europe it is becoming increasingly clear that *H. gordonii* would be considered as a novel food. This is despite earlier speculation that it might fall under the remit of medicines legislation (Feord, 2005).

### 10.4.4 Commercial activities

According to the BioMolecular Sciences, Inc. website (see references) research on the pharmacological properties of *H. gordoni*, centering on the P57 molecule, has been ongoing for the past 30 years at South Africa's CSIR. A licence agreement was signed with Phytopharm in 1997 and in 1998 Pfizer acquired an exclusive global licence for P57. It is reputed that Pfizer spent around $US 400 million on the development of P57 as a drug.

In 2003, for reasons that are not clear, Pfizer ceased work on P57 and in December 2004 an agreement with Unilever was announced (Phytopharm/Unilever, 2005). As part of the agreement Unilever agreed to initial payments to Phytopharm totalling $US 12.5 million out of a total of $US 40 million in payments plus royalties. It has been reported that Unilever could have products on the market by 2007 (e.g. *Financial Times,* 2004), probably under the Slim-Fast brand.

It is encouraging that Unilever is co-ordinating the development of *Hoodia*. As and when product(s) containing *Hoodia* reach the market consumers can be sure that a thorough approach has been taken to ensure their safety and efficacy.

This should be the end of the story so far, but unfortunately it is not. The Internet abounds with advertisements for *Hoodia*-based products for sale.

Some of these are clearly bogus even to the uninitiated but some seem to be quite genuine. Purchase of so-called *Hoodia*-based products *via* the Internet is quite straightforward but it should be borne in mind, as explained above, that these products do not yet have legal status either in Europe or the USA. This commercial activity could well undermine the long-term future of *Hoodia*. This would be most unfortunate as *Hoodia* still has the potential to become a major component in the fight against obesity.

## 10.5 Other (potential) weight loss ingredients

### 10.5.1 Green tea catechins

Green tea and its polyphenol components have been investigated as possible functional foods for a range of applications. Dulloo *et al.* (1999) investigated whether a green tea extract, by virtue of its high content of caffeine and catechin polyphenols, could increase 24-h energy expenditure and fat oxidation in humans. This was a placebo-controlled experiment and caffeine at the level in the green tea extract was also studied on its own as a second control. It was concluded that green tea has thermogenic properties and promotes fat oxidation beyond that accounted for by caffeine. Hence, green tea extract may play a role in the control of body composition *via* sympathetic activation of thermogenesis, fat oxidation or both.

In Japan, the Kao Corporation has launched a FOSHU product called 'Healthya' which is a 300 ml green tea beverage with an enhanced catechin content. The 540 mg of catechin makes the product extremely bitter. Indeed the product may curb appetite in several ways. The claim for the product is 'this product is suitable for people who are conscious of fat'.

### 10.5.2 Capsiate

Capsaicin is the pungent component of chillis. It has long been known to have a thermogenic effect (Matsumoto *et al.*, 2000), This effect is more pronounced in lean subjects than in obese subjects. As a weight loss strategy the prolonged consumption of hot chillis does not seem like a viable proposition.

Recently capsiate has been identified as a component of the nonpungent red pepper cultivar CH-19 Sweet. In a 2-week human intervention study, capsiate increased metabolic rate and promoted fat oxidation at rest, leading to the conclusion that capsiate may help to prevent obesity. Capsiate was shown to increase the levels of uncoupling protein (UCP)1 and mRNA in brown adipose tissue and UCP2 and mRNA in white adipose tissue. This suggests that the effect of capsiate may be mediated via UCP1 and UCP2 (Masuda *et al.*, 2003).

In October 2005, the Japanese food, amino acids and medical research firm Ajinomoto announced the creation of a range of foods containing capsiate. The company acquired the intellectual property rights to capsiate from fellow Japanese food and health beverage developer Morinaga & Co. and, according to the announcement, intends to conduct scientific testing to provide evidence for the future health claims it intends to make for products that it develops based on the compound (Anon., 2005).

### 10.5.3 Arabinose

L-Arabinose is a natural, poorly absorbed pentose that selectively inhibits sucrase activity. A study has shown that sucrose mediates increases in lipogenic enzymes and triacylglycerol levels in rats. This effect can be prevented by the inclusion of L-arabinose with the sucrose. The relevance for humans remains to be fully evaluated. In the meantime a commercial product is being marketed in Japan that makes use of the concept. It is presented as a vial of coffee sweetener containing L-arabinose. This product may be the forerunner to a new generation of ingredients reducing the absorption of macronutrients and hence reducing net metabolizable energy.

### 10.5.4 Calcium

Zemel (2004) has reviewed the role of calcium and dairy products in energy partitioning and weight management. He presents a convincing case that dietary calcium plays a key role in the regulation of energy metabolism. High-calcium diets attenuate adipocyte lipid accretion and weight gain during the overconsumption of an energy-dense diet, and increase lipolysis and preserve thermogenesis during caloric restriction, thereby markedly accelerating weight loss. Dairy products exert substantially greater effects than do equivalent amounts of calcium *per se*. The precise mechanisms for this effect are not yet clear. This effect has recently been confirmed in two randomized trials in obese African-American adults (Zemel *et al.*, 2005).

### 10.5.5 Red wine polyphenolics

The well publicized French paradox means that when in France one can eat and drink with abandon without fear of becoming obese. Red wine consumption has often been cited as the protective factor in this phenomenon. The good news is that there may well be a scientific basis for this happy situation. Pal *et al.* (2004) studied the impact of acute consumption of red wine polyphenolics in postmenopausal women. They found that red wine polyphenolics attenuate postprandial chylomicron and chylomicron remnant levels in plasma, possibly by delaying absorption of dietary fat.

## 10.6 Future trends

Many of us are today living in an increasingly obesogenic environment. The combination of sedentary lifestyles and ever more affordable and varied diets makes the maintenance of a caloric balance more and more of a challenge. It is difficult to deny knowledge of the value of exercise, fruit, vegetables, wholegrain and caloric restriction. However, despite this, obesity gathers momentum as the greatest epidemic ever to befall man. Whilst some prefer the word 'epidemic' to be applied only to infectious diseases, the point is well made. It is clear then that we need help, help in the form of foods that encourage us to consume less calories, help in the form of medicines that alter our metabolism in the direction of a favourable energy balance, and help by way of education on the consequences of ignoring the advice.

From this it seems that the future of novel weight loss ingredients is assured. However, it is only assured if the developers of such ingredients concentrate on sound science and do not become tempted to rush to market before proof of effect is manifest.

Satiety is mediated by a complex balance of hormonal interactions and signals (de Graaf *et al.*, 2004). We are a long way from being able to safely manipulate hormonal balance to achieve desirable body weight but investigations in this important area continue. Meanwhile the elucidation of the human genome has spawned the new science of nutrigenomics. Clearly some of us are more predisposed to obesity than others and part of the explanation is the regulation of gene expression by food components. The reader is referred to Clément (2005), Bell *et al.* (2005), Loos and Rankinen (2005) and Roche *et al.* (2005) for recent reviews on the subject.

Certainly within the next generation there is an expectation that we might manipulate gene expression through food choices in order to control body weight. Roy *et al.* (2004) studied the impact of HCA on gene expression in rats. They found several genes sensitive to HCA and in particular the genes responsible for abdominal leptin production were downregulated whilst plasma leptin was unaffected.

The pharmaceutical industry has long since recovered from the withdrawal of Fen-Phen (FDA 1997). A number of promising drugs are currently under development for the treatment of obesity. Bray and Greenway (1999) and Carpino and Hadcock (2003) have reviewed the approaches being taken.

So perhaps now the tapeworm can be allowed to rest in peace, or perhaps not? Tapeworms have been shown to impact lipid metabolism in mice in favour of lipolysis (Rath and Walkey, 1987). Maybe we can learn something useful from the physiology of and physiological response to the humble tapeworm.

The last word should go to an even older discipline. Yoga and meditation have long been proposed for the control of body weight, not because of the calories they burn but because of their impact on the psychology of food consumption. This cuts to the very heart of the issue. We do not just eat because we feel hungry but also in response to many complex psychological, social and environmental factors. A holistic approach is mandated.

## 10.7 References

ANON. (2004), 'Diet, Nutrition and the Prevention of Chronic Diseases'. Report of the joint WHO/FAO expert consultation. WHO Technical Report Series, No. 916, WHO, Geneva.

ANON. (2005), 'Ajinomoto to develop capsiate-based foods', *Nutraceuticals Int*, **10** (10), 26.

BELL C G, WALLEY A J and FROGUEL P (2005), 'The genetics of human obesity', *Nat Rev Genet*, **6**, 221–234.

BIOMOLECULAR SCIENCES, Inc, http://biomolecularsciences.com/stiflehunger.php, accessed November 2005.

BOUCHER J L, SHAFER K J and CHAFFIN J A (2001), 'Weight loss, diets, and supplements: does anything work?', *Diabetes Spectr*, **14** (3), 169–175.

CALORIE CONTROL COUNCIL websites: http://www.caloriecontrol.org and http://www.caloriescount.com, accessed November 2005.

BRAY G A and GREENWAY F L (1999), 'Current and potential drugs for treatment of obesity', *Endocr Rev*, **20** (6), 805–875.

CARPINO P A and HADCOCK J R (2003), 'Drugs to treat eating and body weight disorders', in *Burger's Medicinal Chemistry and Drug Discovery*, 6th Edition, Volume 6, Ed. Abraham D J, pp. 837–893, John Wiley, New York.

CLÉMENT K (2005), 'Genetics of human obesity', *Proc Nutr Soc*, **64**, 133–142.

DE GRAAF C, BLOM W A M, SMEETS P A M, STAFLEU A and HENDRICKS H F J (2004), 'Biomarkers of satiation and satiety', *Am J Clin Nutr*, **79**, 946–961.

DIPLOCK A T, AGGETT P J, ASHWELL M, BORNET F, FERN E and ROBERFROID M B (1999), 'Scientific concepts of functional foods in Europe: consensus document', *Br J Nutr*, **81** (Suppl. 1), 1–28.

DOWNS B W, BAGCHI M, SUBBARAJU G V, SHARA M A, PREUSS H G and BAGCHI D (2005), 'Bioefficacy of a novel calcium-potassium salt of (–)-hydroxycitric acid', *Mutat Res*, **579**, 149–162.

DULLOO A G, DURET C, ROHRER D, GIRARDIER L, MENSI N, FATHI M and CHANTRE P (1999), 'Efficacy of a green tea extract rich in catechin polyphenols and caffeine in increasing 24-h energy expenditure and fat oxidation in humans', *Am J Clin Nutr*, **70**, 1040–1045.

FDA (1995a), Untitled document, http://www.fda.gov/ohrms/dockets/dockets/95s0316/95s-0316-rpt0270-toc.htm, accessed November 2005.

FDA (1997), 'FDA announces withdrawal Fenfluramine and Dexfenfluramine', http://www.fda.gov/cder/news/phen/fenphenpr81597.htm, accessed November 2005.

FDA (2004), http://www.cfsan.fda.gov/~dms/ds-ephed.html, accessed November 2005.

FEORD J (2005), 'Food or medicine?', http://www.foodmanufacture.co.uk/news/fullstory.php/aid/1663/Food_or_medicine_.html, accessed November 2005.

*FINANCIAL TIMES* (UK, early edition, 2004), Dieting clamour fattens shares, 16 December 2004, 29.

HABECK M (2002), A succulent cure to end obesity, *Drug Discov. Today*, **7** (5), 280–281.

HEYMSFIELD S B, ALLISON D B, VASSELLI J R, PIETROBELLI A, GREENFIELD D and NUNEZ C (1998), '*Garcinia cambogia* (hydroxycitric acid) as a potential antiobesity agent. A randomized controlled trial', *JAMA*, **280** (18), 1596–1600.

INTERHEALTH website: http://www.interhealthusa.com/products/supercitrimax.aspx, accessed November 2005.

INTERHEALTH website, GRAS affirmation: http://www.interhealthusa.com/news/citrimax_Gras1.aspx, accessed November 2005.

LOE Y C, BERGERON N and SCHWARZ J-M (2001), 'Gas chromatography/mass spectrometry method to quantify blood hydroxycitrate concentration', *Anal Biochem*, **292**, 148–154.

LOOS R J F and RANKINEN T (2005), 'Gene–diet interactions on body weight changes', *J Am Diet Assoc*, **105** (5), (Suppl. 1), S29–S34.

MACLEAN D B and LUO L G (2004), 'Increased ATP content/production in the hypothalamus may be a signal for energy-sensing of satiety: studies on the anorectic mechanism of a plant steroidal glycoside', *Brain Res*, **1020**, 1–11.

MASUDA Y, HARAMIZU S, OKI K, OHNUKI K, WATANABE T, YAZAWA S, KAWADA T, HASHIZUME S and FUSHIKI T (2003), 'Upregulation of uncoupling proteins by oral administration of capsiate, a nonpungent capsaicin analog' *J Appl Physiol*, **95**, 2408–2415.

MATSUMOTO T, MIYAWAKI C, UE H, YUASA T, MAYATSUJI A and MORITANI T (2000), 'Effects of capsaicin-containing yellow curry sauce on sympathetic nervous system activity and diet-induced thermogenesis in lean and obese young women', *J Nutr Sci Vitaminol*, **46** (6), 309–315.

PAL S, NAISSIDES M and MAMO J (2004), 'Polyphenolics and fat absorption', *Int J Obes*, **28**, 324–326.

Phytopharm/Unilever (2005), http://miranda.hemscott.com/servlet/HsPublic?context=ir.access&ir_option=RNS_NEWS&item=24507083576851&ir_client_id=3054, accessed November 2005.

PITTLER M H and ERNST E (2004), 'Dietary supplements for body-weight reduction: a systematic review', *Am J Clin Nutr*, **79**, 529–536.

PREUSS H G, BAGCHI D, BAGCHI M, SANYASI RAO C V, SATYANARAYANA S and DEY D K (2004a), 'Efficacy of a novel, natural extract of (–)-hydroxycitric acid (HCA-SX) and a combination of HCA-SX, niacin-bound chromium and *Gymnema sylvestre* extract in weight management in human volunteers: a pilot study', *Nutr Res*, **24**, 45–58.

PREUSS H G, BAGCHI D, BAGCHI M, RAO C V S, DEY D K and SATYANARAYANA S (2004b), 'Effects of a natural extract of (–)-hydroxycitric acid (HCA-SX) and a combination of HCA-SX plus niacin-bound chromium and *Gymnema sylvestre* extract on weight loss', *Diabetes Obes Metab*, **6**, 171–180.

RATH E A and WALKEY M (1987), Fatty acid and cholesterol synthesis in mice infected with the tapeworm *Hymenolepis microstoma*, *Parasitology*, **95** (1), 79–92.

ROCHE H M, PHILLIPS C and GIBNEY M (2005), 'The metabolic syndrome: the crossroads of diet and genetics', *Proc Nutr Soc*, **64**, 371–377.

ROY S, RINK C, KHANNA S, PHILLIPS C, BAGCHI D, BAGCHI M and SEN C K (2004), 'Body weight and abdominal fat gene expression profile in response to a novel hydroxycitric acid-based dietary supplement', *Gene Expr*, **11**, 251–262.

SONI M G, BURDOCK G A, PREUSS H G, STOHS S J, OHIA S E and BAGCHI D (2004), 'Safety assessment of (–)-hydroxycitric acid and Super CitriMax, a novel calcium/potassium salt', *Food Chem Toxicol*, **42**, 1513–1529.

STOWELL J D (2006), 'Calorie control and weight management', in *Sweeteners and Sugar Alternatives in Food Technology*, Ed. Mitchell H L, Blackwell, Oxford, pp. 432.

TULP O L, HARBI N A and DERMARDEROSIAN A (2002), 'Effect of Hoodia plant on weight loss in congenic obese LA/Nutl//-cp rats. *FASEB J*, **16** (4), A648.

TULP O L, HARBI N A, MIHALOV J and DERMARDEROSIAN A (2001), 'Effect of Hoodia plant on food intake and body weight in lean and obese LA/Ntul//-cp rats', *FASEB J*, **15** (4), A404.

ZEMEL M B (2004), 'Role of calcium and dairy products in energy partitioning and weight management', *Am J Clin Nutr*, **79** (Suppl.), 907S–912S.

ZEMEL M B, RICHARDS J, MILSTEAD A and CAMPBELL P (2005), 'Effects of calcium and dairy on body composition and weight loss in African-American adults', *Obes Res*, **13** (7), 1218–1225.

# Part III

# Dairy ingredients and lipids for weight control

# 11

# Dietary and supplemental calcium and its role in weight loss: weighing the evidence

**G. Gerstner, Jungbunzlauer Ladenburg GmbH, Germany and M. de Vrese, Federal Research Center for Nutrition and Food, Germany**

## 11.1 Introduction: role of dietary and supplementary calcium in weight control

The recommended daily intake of calcium (1000 mg/day for most adults, 1200 mg/day for pregnant women) has been set to meet the requirements of bone-health and the prevention of osteoporosis. Beyond this, calcium plays an essential role in numerous other vital functions: regulation of cell membrane fluidity and permeability, nerve conduction, muscle contraction and blood clotting. Calcium has anti-hypertensive properties and the consumption of calcium in sufficient amounts may reduce the risk of colon cancer. Various studies over the last few years have shown that increased calcium intake can significantly fight overweight and obesity.

In the following sections the question will be addressed as to whether a role for calcium in weight control is substantiated by facts gained from epidemiological studies and the results of *in vitro*, animal and human intervention studies, showing either a positive role for calcium in lipid metabolism and weight control, or no effect at all. In order to understand these effects, the role of calcium in the regulation of energy metabolism is to be examined. This comprises effects on cellular energy metabolism (the Zemel hypothesis) and the reduction of energy intake by the formation of poorly absorbable calcium soaps and a potential calcium effect on appetite.

Section 11.4 compares dietary calcium from milk products with calcium supplements and calcium-fortified food, and deals with quantitative aspects. Section 11.5 gives an overview of the calcium salts used for functional food products. Some conclusions, a short outlook on future trends and recommendations for further references are given at the end of the chapter.

## 11.2 Determining the role of calcium in weight control

Recently, an anti-obesity effect of dietary calcium has been postulated (for reviews see Teegarden (2003), Zemel (2002) and Zemel and Miller (2004a)). Although first observations in rats and men showing an inverse relation between calcium intake, adipocyte intracellular calcium and obesity had already been published at the end of the 1980s (Draznin *et al.*, 1988), this idea has never been more popular in the scientific community since the publication of the papers of Zemel and colleagues (Xue *et al.*, 1998, 2001, Zemel *et al.* 1995, 2000). These publications were based to a major extent on investigations on obese and insulin-resistant mutant mice ('agouti mouse') and led to an intensive re-examination and extended interpretation of data from several epidemiological studies.

### 11.2.1 Epidemiological and intervention studies showing a role for calcium in weight management

Data from the US NHANES III (Third National Health and Nutrition Examination Survey), the CSFII study (Continuing Survey of Food Intake by Individuals), the CARDIA study, the Quebec Family Study and the HERITAGE (Health, Risk Factors, Exercise, Training and Genetics) Family Study showed accordingly a significant inverse relationship between calcium consumption and body weight, body mass index (BMI; BMI = body weight/body length, $kg/m^2$), body fat distribution and the prevalence of obesity respectively (Table 11.1).

Zemel and co-workers (2000), who re-examined data from 380 women (of about 7000) from the NHANES III study, found less body fat and a lower risk for obesity in people with the highest calcium intake after controlling for energy intake and physical activity, and the risk of being in the highest BMI quartile was reduced by 85% at the highest quartile of calcium intake. The anti-obesity effect of calcium has been demonstrated in black and in white people of both sexes, although in the HERITAGE Family Study the strongest effects occurred in white women and black men (Loos *et al.*, 2004): the former exhibited a significant inverse relationship between calcium and BMI, percentage body fat and total abdominal fat, the latter between calcium intake and leanness.

An inverse relationship between BMI and dietary calcium or consumption of milk and dairy products was also found in adult women when the data from the CSFII study (Albertson *et al.*, 2003), as well as data in a sample of the cross-sectional Portuguese Health Interview Survey 1998–1999 (Marques-Vidal *et al.*, 2005), were re-examined. Two other long-term observational studies examined the effect of milk consumption on body composition and also on several physiological parameters. In the Quebec Family Study, abdominal circumference was negatively associated with dairy products consumption (Drapeau *et al.*, 2004, Jacqmain *et al.*, 2003), whereas in the prospective CARDIA study, an inverse relation-

**Table 11.1** Human studies showing significant anti-obesity effects of increased calcium intake

| Subjects | Period | Verum group | Results | References |
|---|---|---|---|---|
| A. Re-examination of earlier epidemiological studies | | | | |
| | | | *Inverse association between:* | |
| NHANES III | c-s | | calcium intake and risk of being in the highest BMI quartile | Zemel *et al.*, 2000 |
| HERITAGE Family Study | c-s | | calcium intake and BMI, % body fat and (black men) obesity | Loos *et al.*, 2004 |
| CSFII study | c-s | | intake of dairy calcium and BMI | Albertson *et al.*, 2003 |
| Portuguese Health Interview Survey | c-s | | dairy intake and BMI | Marques-Vidal. *et al.*, 2006 |
| Quebec Family Study | c-s | | dairy consumption and abdominal circumference | Jacqmain *et al.*, 2003 |
| CARDIA study | 10 years | | dairy intake and obesity | Pereia *et al.*, 2002 |
| B. Re-examination of prior observation and intervention studies with skeletal endpoints | | | | |
| | | | *Significant inverse relationship between:* | |
| 150 + 198 women 19–26 years (2 cohorts) | c-s | | calcium intake and BMI | Davies *et al.*, 2000 |
| 70 + 216 midlife women (2 cohorts) | 8 years/ 21 years | | calcium intake and midlife weight gain | |
| | | | *In the verum compared with the placebo group:* | |
| 216 women >65 years | 4 years | +1.2 g/day Ca; same energy intake | significantly more weight loss over 4 years | Davies *et al.*, 2000 |
| Young healthy women, 19–26 years | 3 years | +1.5 g/day Ca | less fat/more lean body mass | Barger-Lux *et al.*, 2001 |

**Table 11.1** *Continued*

| Subjects | Period | Verum group | Results | References |
|---|---|---|---|---|
| C. Observation/intervention studies relating nutrient (or especially calcium) intake to body composition | | | | |
| | | | *Significant inverse relationship between:* | |
| 54 normal weight women, 18–30 years | 2 years | | energy-adjusted Ca intake and change in weight/fat | Lin *et al.*, 2000 |
| Midlife Caucasian women | c-s | | calcium intake in midlife and BMI/body fat* | Lovejoy *et al.*, 2001 |
| Midlife African American women | c-s | | no calcium effect | |
| Puerto Rican children | c-c | | dairy product (~ calcium) intake and obesity | Tanasecu *et al.*, 2000 |
| 53 white preschool children, initially 2 years old | until 8 years | | calcium intake and body fat accumulation* | Carruth and Skinner, 2001<br>Skinner *et al.*, 2003 |
| African-American women | c-s | | calcium intake and BMI | Buchowski *et al.*, 2002 |
| 80 obese, 10–14 years; Ca below recommendations | c-s | | calcium intake and overweight/obesity | Lelovics, 2004 |
| 35 non-obese adults (mean 31 years) | — | | Ca intake is positively associated with fat oxidation** | Melanson *et al.*, 2003 |
| | | | *In the verum compared with the placebo group:* | |
| African-American hypertensive males + NIDD | 1 year | +2 servings yoghurt/day | 4.5 kg less body fat ($p < 0.01$)* | Zemel *et al.*, 1990 |
| 32 obese adults | 24 weeks | Standard diet (450 mg/day Ca, 500 kcal/day deficit) + 800 mg/day Ca supplement | Significantly more weight loss (–8.4% vs. –6.4%) | Zemel and Miller, 2004 |

* % or kg body fat were assessed by dual energy x-ray absorptiometry (DEXA); ** measured by whole-room indirect calorimetry.
c-s = cross-sectional, c-c = case control, NIDD = non-insulin dependent diabetic

ship was found between milk and dairy products intake and several parameters associated with insulin resistance, including obesity (Pereia *et al.*, 2002).

Although positive results were independent of whether calcium intake itself was estimated in the respective study or whether milk was taken as a measure of calcium intake, the approach for assessing calcium intake may be criticised, as calcium was not the prime test parameter in the studies mentioned. This criticism is, however, weakened by the fact that evidence also came from studies relating nutrient intake to body composition and from the re-analysis of clinical observational studies and controlled intervention trials, with the primary focus on the calcium effect on bone mass or blood pressure respectively (Table 11.1). By reverting to the same pool of studies with skeletal endpoints, Davies and colleagues (2000) and Heaney (2003) re-examined data from 780 women of young, middle and older age (four observational studies and one randomised controlled trial) or from 348 young women (19–26 years) from two cohorts respectively. Overall the authors found a significant negative association between calcium intake and body weight. The weight increase per year of women of middle age was also negatively associated with calcium consumption (Heaney, 2003). Young women at the lower (25%) quartile of calcium intake had a 15% prevalence to overweight, whereas a high calcium intake according to the recommended dietary intake (RDA) was associated only with a 4% prevalence (Heaney, 2003), and the odds ratio (OR) for being overweight was 2.25 when calcium intake was below the median (Davies *et al.*, 2000). Davies *et al.* also calculated from the results of the intervention studies, that the daily consumption of a 1500 mg calcium supplement would reduce body weight significantly as compared with a placebo group and that 3% of the weight change can be explained by the level of calcium intake, whereby an increase of calcium intake by 1 g accounts for a weight reduction of 8 kg. The re-examination of further clinical studies (six observational studies and three clinical trials, with skeletal or circulation endpoints) by the same group confirmed the above-mentioned results in terms of quality and quantity (Heaney *et al.*, 2002).

Despite these, overall, quite consistent results, it must be stated explicitly that re-examination of previous studies and, in particular, of observational studies provides, for several reasons, not the strongest evidence for an anti-obesity effect of calcium.

The original goal of these studies was not to investigate the effects of calcium on weight loss, therefore the study design and, in particular, the choice of the independent variables and primary study parameters are often not optimised for the problem of interest. Another problem is that some of the studies are included and re-used in various combinations for several re-examinations and meta-analyses of the calcium effect, which leads only to an apparently increased statistical power. Finally, if associations are derived from observational studies, no evidence of causality can be ascertained, even if the data allow for control of possible confounding factors such as energy intake or physical activity. A high or low intake of dairy products (and thus of calcium) could, for example, be simply the consequence of a lifestyle that favours a lower or higher body weight.

Therefore it is particularly important that, in recent years, some studies have been published that test explicitly the effect of calcium on body weight, body fat and the efficacy of weight-reduction diets. An epidemiological, population-based, cross-sectional observation study in 357 male and 470 female Tehranian adults aged 18–74 years showed an inverse association between milk, cheese and yoghurt consumption (assessed with the use of a 168-item semi-quantitative food-frequency questionnaire) and parameters of the metabolic syndrome – including waist circumference and obesity (Azadbakht *et al.*, 2005). Subjects in the highest compared with the lowest quartile of dairy intake had lower odds of having enlarged waist circumference (OR = 0.63 vs. 1; $p < 0.001$) and a lower prevalence of obesity (17 vs. 23%; $p < 0.04$). The ratios became weaker after adjustment for calcium intake, indicating that the effect of dairy consumption on waist girth and obesity is only partly mediated by dietary calcium.

Numerous smaller observational studies of recent years, with between 35 and 80 participating subjects and observation periods of between 2 months and 8 years, relating nutrient or especially calcium intake to body composition, consistently revealed that a high calcium intake from the regular diet in childhood and adulthood as well as supplemental calcium is associated with a lower body weight (or BMI), less body fat due to a shift from fat to lean body mass and less age-dependent weight gain in midlife (Table 11.1). Moreover, calcium increased the efficacy of energy-reduced weight-reduction diets.

There are only a small number of (prospective) intervention trials in humans using calcium supplementation and body weight gain as independent and dependent study variables. In an earlier, placebo-controlled intervention trial in diabetic African-American males, the intake of ~300 mg/day calcium as yoghurt (two servings per day) throughout 1 year also increased body fat loss significantly by 4.5 kg (Zemel and Zemel, 1990). Zemel and co-workers (2004) also reported significantly greater weight loss (–10.9%) in subjects on a standard energy-deficient diet plus dairy products compared with subjects on the same standard diet alone or plus calcium supplements from other sources (–8.6% or –6.4% respectively; $p < 0.01$, $n = 32$, 24 weeks). Consumption of calcium and milk products enhanced particularly truncal fat loss, as shown in a randomised controlled study on 34 obese adults (Zemel *et al.*, 2005). Addition of three servings per day of calcium-fortified low-fat yoghurt to an energy-reduced (–500 cal/day) low-calcium diet over 12 weeks increased weight loss by 22%, body fat loss by 61% and central fat loss by 81%.

### 11.2.2 Epidemiological and intervention studies showing no calcium effect

However, not all cell culture and animal experiments confirmed the mechanism of the calcium effect proposed by Zemel and co-workers, and not all epidemiological studies and intervention trials observed positive effects of calcium supplements and/or milk products on body weight. Feeding normal or energy-dense diets differing in calcium content (0.2–1.8%) to normal and obese rats and mice (Paradis and Cabanac, 2005, Zhang and Tordoff, 2004) had no significant effect on energy intake, body weight or body fat and did not show the inverse relationship between 1,25-dihydroxy-vitamin $D_3$ or parathyroid hormone (PTH) and body weight that is propounded by Zemel and co-workers (Shi *et al.*, 2001). In addition, the core of Zemel's hypothesis, that a diet-induced decrease of intracellular calcium concentration in the adipocytes would enhance lipolysis and decrease fat deposition in adipocytes could not be confirmed in any of these studies. For example, when intracellular calcium in white adipose tissue was increased artificially by adrenergic stimulation, this was even associated with enhanced lipolysis (Boschmann *et al.*, 2002). This coincides with findings made by Barr and co-workers (2004). Repeating the analysis of Zemel *et al.* (2000), but using the data from 6878 instead of 380 women, as in the NHANES III study, they did not observe a significant association between a low calcium or milk product intake and the risk of being in the highest quartile for body fat. A lack of relationship between calcium intake and BMI was also found in an observational study on 65 adult and 78 infant Pima Indians (Venti *et al.*, 2005). In this case the authors explain the negative study results with the fact that Pima Indians are genetically prone to becoming obese, and that this could conceal a weak calcium effect. The Fourth Tromso study, a Norwegian population study on 9252 men and 9662 women, even showed a positive association between calcium intake and BMI in men and an unexpected negative association between vitamin D intake and BMI in both sexes (Kamycheva *et al.*, 2003). In addition, in a longitudinal observation study in 1200 adolescents weight gain over 3 years was even directly proportional to the number of dairy product servings per day (Berkey *et al.*, 2005).

In two recently published randomised controlled intervention trials on obese adults, high-calcium, energy-restricted diets (2400 or 1400 mg/day calcium, mainly from dairy products) caused the same (Bowen *et al.*, 2005) or a non-significantly higher (+20%; Thompson *et al.*, 2005) loss of body weight and body fat, compared with the same energy-restricted diets containing 500 or 800 mg/day calcium respectively.

Furthermore, administration of 1 g/day 'extra calcium' did not promote postpartum loss of body weight and fat in lactating and non-lactating mothers (Wosje and Kalkwarf, 2004). The same calcium dose increased weight and fat loss in 100 pre- and postmenopausal women following an energy-restricted diet over 25 weeks; however, this increase was not significant (Shapses *et al.*, 2004).

### 11.2.3 How to weigh up the differing study outcomes

All in all there is, at this point in time, some confusion about the extent and importance of the postulated role of supplemental calcium or dairy products in weight management. One comment (Clifton, 2005) concludes from the recently published studies that did not find a calcium effect, that this may be 'the beginning of the end for the dietary calcium and obesity hypothesis'. This is certainly not correct, as the author does not explain or consider otherwise the findings of the numerous studies with a positive outcome.

On the other hand it is still completely unclear how the different outcomes of the 'positive' and 'negative' studies come about. Erroneous estimates of calcium intake are certainly not the explanation, because in both fractions there are small and observational studies in which regular consumption of dairy products and other calcium sources was estimated according to food-frequency questionnaires, as well as controlled intervention trials with defined and controlled administration of supplemental calcium. Also, with respect to other factors – such as, ethnicity, age, the pre- or post-menopausal stage of women, weight or sex of the subjects, the energy provided (i.e. normocaloric or calorie-restricted diets) and the calcium content of the basal diet or the amount of supplemental calcium – the positive and negative studies do not differ completely. Other parameters such as the nutritional, calcium or vitamin D status of the study subjects, the bioavailability of calcium from different sources as well as the influence of other diet components (except for milk and dairy components) were usually not taken into consideration.

It seems rather likely that the influence of calcium on body weight and body fat is in any case rather small, and that therefore already small differences between studies concerning design, study population or other factors not included in the compilation of the results, could decide on whether an effect is apparent or even statistically significant. Beyond that, those studies that were originally designed to address other topics, and which were then re-analysed, need to be interpreted particularly cautiously. In addition, cross-sectional/observational studies are not usually suited to uncovering causal relationships, but show only associations.

In order to examine the role of dietary calcium in weight management, more well-designed longer-term intervention studies with a sufficient number of participants, defined endpoints and well-characterised target groups are required, as well as knowledge of the underlying mechanisms. It will be, after all, not so much a question of whether calcium has an anti-obesity effect or not (in reality there is mostly an 'under certain conditions yes, otherwise no'), but rather in which target group can calcium play a role in weight management, and to what extent, and how this impact is modified by other factors.

## 11.3 Mechanisms: calcium and the regulation of energy metabolism

How does calcium work? Although the physiological or cell-biology basis for the changes in body weight and body fat has not been fully elucidated, a hypothesis has been developed by Zemel and co-workers (2000), based largely on experiments in the obese agouti mutant mouse (Jones *et al.*, 1996, Shi *et al.*, 2001, Xue *et al.*, 1998, 2001, Zemel *et al.*, 1995). The agouti protein is involved in the development of the wild-type coat colour of agoutis (South-American guinea pig-like rodents), mice and other mammals. Furthermore, it plays a role in the regulation of food intake. Over-expression of this protein due to a vital mutation in the encoding gene locus in mice not only leads to a yellowish coat colour, but also to body fat accumulation, insulin resistance and hyperinsulinaemia with aging. Feeding highly palatable diets to these animals causes overeating and leads to obesity, an effect that can be prevented by increasing the calcium content of the diets, e.g. from 0.4 to 1.2% (Zemel *et al.*, 2000).

According to Zemel's hypothesis, consumption of relatively large amounts of dietary calcium increases circulating [$Ca^{2+}$] and decreases counter-regulatory serum concentrations of the calcitropic hormones PTH and, as a consequence, vitamin D (calcitriol, 1,25-dihydroxy-vitamin $D_3$). Calcitriol increases intracellular [$Ca^{2+}$] in cultured human adipocytes when added to the cell-culture medium. This means for the above-mentioned metabolic steps, that the decreased serum calcitriol in turn down-regulates $Ca^{2+}$ influx into adipocytes and thereby reduces intracellular [$Ca^{2+}$] (Fujita and Palmieri, 2000, Palmieri *et al.*, 1998, Shi *et al.*, 2001, Zemel *et al.*, 2000). Intracellular calcium is involved in the regulation of several key enzymes of fat and energy metabolism, including fatty acid synthase. Decreased adipocyte intracellular [$Ca^{2+}$] thereby stimulates lipolysis, fatty acid oxidation (Melanson *et al.*, 2003) and in some studies the expression of uncoupling protein 2 and thereby thermogenesis. According to these mechanisms, increased body core temperature was observed in mice fed a high-calcium diet (Zemel *et al.*, 2000). At the same time lipogenic gene expression and fatty acid synthase activity are inhibited, but a contribution of *de novo* lipogenesis in the development of obesity in humans remains doubtful (Hellerstein, 1999). All these effects result in decreased adipocyte lipid accumulation (Shi *et al.*, 2001), weight and body fat reduction and an overall shift of dietary energy from adipose tissue to lean body mass.

Other studies, however, did not support these proposed mechanisms. Feeding normal or energy-dense diets differing in calcium content (0.2–1.8%) to normal and obese rats and mice had no significant effect on energy intake, body weight and body fat, and did not show the inverse relationship between 1,25-dihydroxy-vitamin $D_3$ or PTH and body weight (Paradis and Cabanac, 2005, Zhang and Tordoff, 2004). Papakonstantinou and co-workers (2003) observed less weight gain and less body fat in rats on a high- (2.4%) compared with a low- (0.4%) calcium diet. They, however, did not find the increase in body core temperature as predicted by Zemel, and the observed effects on fat and weight were explained simply by increased faecal excretion of fat.

This brings up again an idea proposed a longer time ago, according to which the divalent cation calcium prevents the intestinal absorption of part of the dietary fat and increases faecal lipid loss and sterol excretion forming insoluble fatty acid soaps and bile salts (Denke *et al.*, 1993, Drenick, 1961, Vaskonen *et al.*, 2001, 2002, Vaskonen 2003, Welberg *et al.*, 1994). By the same mechanism calcium may enhance a cholesterol-lowering effect of other food components, e.g. plant sterols (Vaskonen *et al.*, 2001). The extent of this effect increased with an increasing proportion of long-chain saturated fatty acids in the diet, whereby, with Western eating habits, the energy excretion with fat is probably around 1 and 3% of the daily energy supply, i.e. around 30 and 90 kcal/day. In a study by Shahkhalalili and co-workers (2001) calcium fortification of chocolate doubled calcium ingestion from 950 to 1855 mg/day and increased faecal fat excretion by ~36 kcal/day (4.04 g/day). This effect seems small, but in the long run it can contribute a significant share to fat and weight loss. From the above data a body-fat reduction by 1–4 kg/year is calculated, although other studies find weaker effects (Table 11.2).

**Table 11.2** Effect of a 300 mg (one serving) increment in regular calcium intake on body weight and body fat (according to Heaney *et al.* (2002))

| Group | Period | ΔBody weight* | ΔBody fat* | Reference |
|---|---|---|---|---|
| Children | 2–96 month | | –1.0 kg | Carruth and Skinner, 2001 |
| Young women | 8 years | –2.5 kg | | Davies *et al.*, 2000 |
| Middle-aged women | 1 year | –0.11 kg/year | | Davies *et al.*, 2000 |
| Elderly women | 1 year | –0.16 kg/year | | Davies *et al.*, 2000 |
| Adult women | n.a. | –3 kg | | Zemel *et al.*, 2000 |
| African-American men | 1 year | | –4.9 kg | Zemel *et al.*, 1990 |

* Differences between groups or highest versus lowest quartiles in cross-sectional studies, or differences per year in longitudinal and intervention studies.

A third possible mechanism, which may slightly contribute to weight reduction as well, has been the subject of a recent publication (Ping-Delfos *et al.*, 2004). In a randomised, blind, controlled cross-over study with a sequential-meal design, 11 overweight or obese subjects (mean BMI 31 kg/m$^2$) consumed isocaloric high (543 mg calcium and 349 IU vitamin D) and low (248 mg calcium and 12 IU vitamin D) dairy calcium breakfasts followed by a very low calcium (48 mg calcium and 25 IU vitamin D) standard lunch. High calcium intake did not affect hunger and satiety immediately after the meal, but did significantly reduce spontaneous food intake over the subsequent 24 h.

## 11.4 Dietary versus supplementary calcium and weight control

Many of the above-cited papers, which compare dairy calcium with calcium supplements or calcium-fortified non-dairy food, show a somewhat greater effect of the former. This suggests that other milk components may modulate the weight-loss effect of calcium or have an effect of their own. These dairy components are possibly whey proteins and peptides, which may work synergistically with calcium to alter lipid metabolism and/or to affect post-prandial satiety.

On the other hand, these studies also show that calcium has an anti-obesity effect of its own that is independent from other components of the diet. However, based on the results of the available positive studies and without exact knowledge of the mechanism, it is not possible to answer the question as to what extent this calcium effect is independent from the level of the 'normal' dietary calcium intake. According to our current understanding it could make sense to increase calcium intake above that of the recommended intake by using calcium-fortified food and/or calcium supplements in order to optimise intake for an anti-obesity effect.

In addition, the contribution of the different mechanisms (i.e. the Zemel mechanism versus the formation of calcium soaps) to the overall calcium effect is not clear, although answering this question may be of a certain relevance for the development of calcium supplements and calcium-fortified food. The use of highly water-soluble complex calcium salts and the addition of caseinophosphopeptides improves calcium bioavailability, increases calcium absorption and thus promotes lipolysis, fatty acid oxidation and increased loss of lipids from adipocytes according to Zemel's hypothesis, while the formation of calcium soaps and thus the intestinal fat excretion would be reduced.

Independent of the answer to these questions, some quantitative information can be given to the extent of the anti-obesity effects of calcium. A quantitative re-analysis of the data from Davies and Heaney (Davies *et al.*, 2000), using simple bivariate and multiple regression models, revealed that calcium intake accounted for ~3% of the variation in BMI in young women and that each 100 mg increment in daily calcium intake would decrease average BMI by 0.3 kg/m$^2$ (according to a regression coefficient of 0.003). The apparent weakness of this association may be partly due to the fact, that the respective studies had not been designed to investigate the effect of calcium on body weight, but had skeletal end-points. Indeed, other studies showed somewhat greater effects in adults (Table 11.2).

The actual importance of these effects becomes evident regarding population means (i.e. for weight, BMI or body fat). In young women, an increase in calcium intake by 600 mg/day from 500 to 1100 mg/day causes a drop in mean BMI of 1.8 kg/m$^2$ (–8%), but decreases the predicted prevalence of overweight (BMI > 26 kg/m$^2$) substantially by 78% from 16.6 to 3.6% and the prevalence of obesity (BMI > 30 kg/m$^2$) by 84% from 0.99 to 0.16% of that age group (Heaney *et al.*, 2002). Midlife weight gain decreased by 97% from 0.4 kg/year to 0.01 kg/year comparing women with 25% of the recommended calcium intake with those who had the recommended calcium intake (Heaney, 2003); 3.5–4.5% less body fat in pre-school boys and girls (body fat ~18–21%), correlates to one additional serving of calcium per day (300 mg), means a drop in body fat of –20% (Carruth and Skinner, 2001).

## 11.5 Using calcium in functional food products

Generally, functional foods are neither dietetic products nor food supplements, but processed foods with distinctive added-value features such as health and well-being. In order to be able to differentiate themselves from the established products, food companies use specific health claims, among which the link between calcium and bone health is one of the most widely used and accepted claims worldwide. According to Leatherhead Food International (2005), the functional foods market in the five major European markets, the United States, Japan and Australia had a combined turnover of US$ 9.9 billion in 2003. Leatherhead uses a strict definition, measuring only products that make genuine functional health claims. By country, this can be broken down as follows: Japan, 45.3%; United States, 26.9%; France, 7.2%; UK, 7.1%; Spain, 5.5%; Germany, 4.9%; Italy, 1.9%; Australia, 1.2%. Total sales are expected to increase by 16% per annum over the next 5 years to reach US$ 21 billion by 2008, with Japan accounting for the lion's share. The global market can also be segmented by health benefit. Allowing for sector overlap, a breakdown analysis reveals that gut health products dominate, with sales of about US$ 5.7 billion (38%), ahead of immune function with US$ 4.7 billion (32%), heart health with US$ 2.55 billion (17%) and bone health with US$ 1.95 billion (13%).

### 11.5.1 General aspects: calcium sources used, applications, market segmentation

Table 11.3 gives an overview of the calcium salts significantly used for functional food products in Europe and the United States, their calcium contents, main application areas and typical fortified product examples (baby food, clinical nutrition and dietetic food applications are not considered in this table).

Nowadays, practically every type of foodstuff does have a fortified line already. Looking at the ingredients list, it is evident that there is not 'the' calcium source but rather a range of different products used commercially:

- inorganic salts such as calcium carbonate, calcium chloride and calcium phosphates;
- organic salts such as calcium lactate, calcium lactate gluconate and (tri-)calcium citrate;
- natural calcium salts such as milk calcium (mainly consisting of calcium phosphate);

With regard to total volumes used in the industry, the inorganic salts calcium phosphate and especially calcium carbonate are clearly dominating due to their high calcium content combined with a low price level. However, in addition to economic considerations, technological aspects such as solubility, stability, ease of processing and taste on the one hand, as well as nutritional aspects such as palatability and bioavailability on the other hand, are vital when choosing the appropriate calcium salt.

### 11.5.2 Technological aspects

*Solubility and dispersibility*

As summarised in Table 11.3, insoluble forms of calcium (calcium carbonate, calcium phosphate, milk calcium) are preferred in non-liquid applications such as cereals and energy bars and can even be used at high concentration levels. However, when liquid formulations are to be fortified, solubility, stability and taste of ingredients are much more important. As displayed in Table 11.3, there are organic calcium salts with good solubility like calcium lactate and those with excellent solubility like calcium lactate gluconate, but their drawback is a comparably low calcium content (13%). Calcium chloride (27% calcium) displays good solubility, but its use is limited to applications with low fortification levels due to its bitter and salty taste. On the other hand, other inorganic salts with a high calcium content, for example calcium carbonate and calcium phosphate, are poorly soluble and for that reason can only be used in specific liquid applications. Tricalcium citrate offers a good combination, having a high calcium level (21%) and moderate solubility (0.9 g/l).

**Table 11.3** Calcium (Ca) salts significantly used for fortification in functional food products in Europe and the United States and current product examples from retail

| Ca salt | Ca content (%) | Solubility (g/l water, RT) | Main applications | Product example | Ca content of product (mg/100 g) |
|---|---|---|---|---|---|
| Ca carbonate | 40 | Insoluble | Cereals, dairy and soy products, energy bars | Whole grain flakes with vitamins, fibres and minerals | 182 |
| Ca chloride 2aq | 27 | 970 | Sports drinks | Non-carbonated sports drink beverage | 24 |
| Ca gluconate | 9 | 35 | Beverages | Juice drink with Ca | 42 |
| Ca lactate 5aq | 13 | 66 | Beverages | Fruit juice lemonade plus Ca | 24 |
| Ca lactate gluconate | 13 | 400 | Beverages, dairy products | Carbonated soft drink with vitamin C and Ca | 62 |
| Ca phosphate | 17–36 | Insoluble | Cereals, dairy and soy products, juices, energy bars | Soy milk with Ca | 120 |
| Milk Ca | 9–28 | Insoluble | Dairy products, energy bars | Milk drink with vitamin D and Ca | 120 |
| Tricalcium citrate 4 aq | 21 | 0.9 | Beverages, dairy and soy products | Kids dairy dessert with Ca | 130 |

RT, room temperature; aq, $H_2O$.

Solubility is strongly influenced by the pH of the system since the solubility of calcium salts typically increases with decreasing pH (Clydesdale, 1988). According to final calcium-fortified liquid products available in European and US supermarkets (Gerstner 2002a, 2004), slightly soluble to insoluble calcium salts (calcium carbonate, calcium phosphate, milk calcium, tricalcium citrate) can be used in the following liquid product categories.

1 Clear beverages at low dosage levels and, preferably, pH below 4.5 (typically ≤50 mg total calcium/100 ml).
2 Cloudy beverages at pH values below 4.5, such as orange juice (typically ≤146 mg total calcium/100 ml).
3 Milk and dairy drinks (typically 130–180 mg total calcium/100 ml).
4 Soy drinks (typically 75–140 mg total calcium/100 ml).

In contrast to the beverages of category 1, where calcium salts are dissolved, calcium salts used for the beverages of categories 2–4 are predominantly dispersed. In order to further increase solubility, dissolving or ease of dispersion, particularly fine (micronised) powders have been developed. In the case of tricalcium citrate, particle sizes are <70 μm at a low and <20 μm at a high fortification level. Why are dispersed systems preferred in categories 2–4? One of the main reasons is the lower price for tricalcium citrate, calcium carbonate and calcium phosphate compared with more soluble (organic) calcium forms. In any case, the feasibility of calcium addition has to be considered as cloudy beverages, milk and soy products represent a complex food matrix from the technological point of view.

*Taste*

Generally, high levels of calcium, particularly insoluble forms like carbonates and phosphates, tend to produce a chalky mouthfeel, form sediments and may promote astringency or bitter taste in the final product (Flynn and Cashman, 1999). Calcium lactate may impart some bitter notes at high concentrations, comparable with characteristics found for calcium chloride (Tordoff, 1996). Calcium carbonate may come across as soapy or lemony. Calcium phosphate has a bland flavour, but imparts a gritty mouthfeel. Negative effects of calcium on taste can be masked with chelating agents (e.g. tripotassium citrate) and the use of stabilisers (e.g. carrageenan), as well as with the addition of flavourings. Tricalcium citrate and calcium lactate gluconate are considered to be among the most neutral tasting salts in most applications and can be applied at high dosage levels.

With regard to calcium lactate gluconate, Technical University Munich-Weihenstephan has performed detailed studies on taste properties (Gerstner, 2002b). Triangle taste panels with trained students and scientists have detected and evaluated differences between fortified and non-fortified samples at different calcium lactate gluconate concentrations. In apple juice for example, fortification with calcium lactate gluconate could not be detected at up to 150 mg added calcium/100 ml. For cloudy juices (category

2), tricalcium citrate and its derivative calcium citrate malate are the preferred choices due to their good compatibility with fruit-based juices and their low effect on taste.

*Ease of processing and stability*
It is known that using highly soluble calcium salts at high concentrations may lead to adverse effects in dairy and soy applications, especially during the heating step (Flynn and Cashman, 1999, Reddy *et al.*, 1999). The addition of mineral salts and especially of calcium has a strong impact on the functionality of these products. With higher-solubility salts more free calcium ions are in solution and available for reaction than with lower-solubility salts and so complications in the form of gelation and calcium sediments can develop during processing, heat treatment or shelf life. This is the case if phosphates and proteins naturally contained in milk and soy beverages react with available calcium. Thus, although it might be easier to add highly soluble calcium salts rather than insoluble calcium salts to milk and soy products, higher amounts of calcium might be difficult to achieve without control of pH and addition of stabilisers and chelating agents (Flynn and Cashman, 1999, Reddy *et al.*, 1999). In contrast to the other calcium salts, tricalcium citrate is an interesting physical anomaly as it is less soluble at higher temperatures. Due to this inverse solubility, tricalcium citrate is less reactive during the heating process, thus minimising precipitates, fouling and cleaning intervals (Gerstner, 2004).

Among the soluble calcium forms, calcium lactate gluconate has the highest solubility of all commonly used organic calcium salts, which is the main functional advantage of this product (Table 11.3). Its solubility is synergistically enhanced to approximately 400 g/l water and well beyond that of the relatively highly soluble single components calcium lactate (66 g/l) and calcium gluconate (35 g/l). The reason for this phenomenon of extremely high solubility is believed to be the ability of mixtures of lactate and gluconate ions to form metastable complexes with calcium ions in solution, which provides additional stability benefits in food and beverage applications. At the Technical University Munich-Weihenstephan, calcium lactate gluconate was tested for important processing parameters such as the dissolution characteristics of highly concentrated solutions (K.-H. Engel, personal communication, 2002). Concentrations of up to 50% could be reached within minutes without negative consequences on colour or odour, and with only a slight influence on pH. In storage stability tests, solutions with concentrations of 5, 10 and 30% calcium lactate gluconate remained stable at room temperature for at least 1 week. These characteristics significantly reduce the time needed for adding calcium during processing. High dissolubility and stability can also be deciding factors as to when calcium lactate gluconate is used in concentrates or instant preparations.

It is also possible to combine insoluble with more soluble salts to control costs while having acceptable solubility/dispersibility in the final product. In this respect, calcium-fortified products contain combinations such as calcium phosphate–calcium lactate, calcium carbonate–tricalcium citrate as well as tricalcium citrate–calcium lactate gluconate (Gerstner 2002a, 2004).

### 11.5.3 Nutritional aspects

*Calcium bioavailability of tricalcium citrate compared with calcium carbonate and calcium phosphate*

Any nutrient's effectiveness depends on its bioavailability, which means how well the human body absorbs and utilises it. On average, only about 10–30% of calcium is absorbed from a mixed diet by healthy adults (National Research Council, 1989). Several different factors influence this level, among others, the type of calcium salt used for fortification purposes.

A review on calcium citrate and bone health has been published recently (Edelstein, 2004). Various scientific studies have shown that organic calcium salts outperform inorganic calcium sources such as calcium carbonate and calcium phosphate with regard to their relative bioavailability. Accordingly, the US National Institutes of Health recommended calcium citrate for supplementation, especially for older individuals where absorbability can be a limiting factor due to reduced gastric acid production (National Institutes of Health, 1994).

Researchers at the University of Texas conducted a meta-analysis of calcium bioavailability, which evaluated 15 studies on the bioavailability of two of the most common forms of calcium supplements, tricalcium citrate and calcium carbonate (Sakhaee *et al.*, 1999). All but one study showed significantly greater absorption of calcium from tricalcium citrate than from calcium carbonate, ranging from +5 to +97%. Based on the statistical evaluation of all 15 studies, the authors confirmed this superior bioavailability of tricalcium citrate and calculated it to be, on average, +22 to +27% compared with calcium carbonate, regardless of whether the supplement was taken on empty stomach or co-administered with meals.

Absorption of calcium from soy milk fortified with tricalcium phosphate reached only 75% of the efficiency of absorption of calcium from cows' milk (Heaney *et al.*, 2000). Similarly, calcium phosphate has also been described in scientific studies to display lower bioavailability than tricalcium citrate or its derivative calcium citrate malate. In commercially marketed calcium-fortified orange juices, bioavailability was 48% greater for calcium citrate malate than for a tricalcium phosphate–calcium lactate blend (Heaney *et al.*, 2005). In long-term clinical studies with elderly women, tricalcium citrate displayed a significant, almost three times higher absorption than calcium phosphate (Riggs *et al.*, 1998).

*Effect of calcium lactate gluconate on bone density*

Besides tricalcium citrate, calcium lactate gluconate is among the most intensively researched organic calcium salts with regard to bioavailability.

Its superior effect on fractional absorption rate of calcium, calcium bioavailability biomarkers (urinary and serum ionised calcium and PTH) and bone mineral density (BMD) have been reviewed previously (Gerstner, 2003).

The main purpose of the recommended high calcium intake is osteoporosis prevention. Therefore, an increase in BMD or bone stability is a better criterion for the efficacy of a calcium salt than its absorbability. Calcium lactate gluconate, when administered to 19 non-menopausal women with osteoporosis during or after a hormone therapy, significantly reduced bone fracture rate (Almustafa *et al.*, 1992). Moreover, in a study in 50 Chinese women, aged 62–92 years, calcium lactate gluconate increased BMD of the hip more than exercise (Lau *et al.*, 1992). Additional evidence of beneficial effects on bone health of calcium lactate gluconate (via Calcium Sandoz®) was supplied by a meta-analysis of Schaafsma *et al.* (2001). The authors compared 16 clinical studies in elderly and late postmenopausal women (mean age 58–79 years), who were supplemented for 12–48 months with 500–1250 mg/day calcium as calcium lactate gluconate, calcium carbonate, calcium citrate and other salts. Without exception, intake of Calcium Sandoz® calcium lactate gluconate increased BMD of the lumbar spine between +0.2 to +1.8%, whereas other supplements, even very well absorbable salts such as calcium citrate malate, partly decreased BMD. Thus, supplementation with calcium lactate gluconate is likely to improve bone health more effectively than calcium citrate malate or calcium carbonate.

### 11.5.4 Calcium-rich functional food products with anti-obesity claims

Although the majority of calcium-fortified functional food products have the purpose of providing calcium in sufficient amounts to contribute to the prevention of osteoporosis, there are some products on the market bearing an anti-obesity claim. Three prominent examples from large dairy companies that have been found in supermarkets in 2005 are shown in Table 11.4.

However, these products contain relatively little calcium (≤300 mg/serving, the Dannon product is without supplemental calcium). Therefore for two of the products three to four servings per day are recommended in order to provide a daily dose of 600–900 mg calcium. Such an amount was sufficient in clinical studies to have significant effects on weight and fat metabolism. For the third product no recommendation of several servings per day is given. Hence, although it contains double the amount of calcium compared with a conventional yoghurt, the postulated anti-obesity effect is based on its low energy content (32 cal/serving), supplemental dietary fibre and green tea extract, as well as the recommendation of physical activity.

Besides the calcium originating from the dairy basis, the Yoplait yoghurt had been fortified with tricalcium phosphate, whereas for the Nestlé dairy

**Table 11.4** Examples of products rich in calcium and with anti-obesity claims (purchased in 2005)

| Product | Weight loss claim | Nutrition facts | |
|---|---|---|---|
| Light 'n Fit® non-fat yogurt Blackberry, Dannon, USA | Slim down with yogurt. Lose more weight as part of a reduced calorie diet. Dairy products, like Light 'n Fit® yogurt, have been shown in studies to help you lose more weight and burn more fat than just cutting calories alone.* *3–4 servings daily (providing at least 600 mg of calcium per day) as part of a high-calcium, reduced-calorie diet | Labelled per serving (170 g): | |
| | | Calories | 90 |
| | | Fat | 0 g |
| | | Sodium | 95 mg |
| | | Potassium | 270 mg |
| | | Carbohydrates | 16 g |
| | | Protein | 6 g |
| | | Calcium | 15% DV (150 mg) |
| | | Phosphorus | 15% |
| | | Vitamin A | 6% DV |
| | | Vitamin D | 20% DV |
| | | Riboflavin | 15% DV |
| | | Vitamin B12 | 10% DV |
| Thick & Creamy Vanilla, Yoplait, USA | Burn more fat Recent research shows that dairy foods, like Yoplait, may help you burn more fat and lose more weight than cutting calories alone.* *3 servings of dairy daily in a reduced-calorie diet. Check out www.YoplaitUSA.com for more ways to develop a healthy and effective weight loss plan. | Labelled per serving (170 g): | |
| | | Calories | 190 |
| | | Fat | 3.5 g |
| | | Cholesterol | 15 mg |
| | | Sodium | 100 mg |
| | | Potassium | 310 mg |
| | | Carbohydrates | 32 g |
| | | Protein | 7 g |
| | | Calcium | 30% DV (300 mg) |
| | | Phosphorus | 15% |
| | | Vitamin A | 15% DV |
| | | Vitamin D | 20% DV |
| Sveltesse Line-Activ® milk drink strawberry, Nestlé, Switzerland | Helps to keep your waistline! A delicious milk drink, which – in combination with a balanced diet and regular physical exercise – helps to keep your waistline. Sveltesse Line-Activ® supports the fat metabolism and thus contributes to a healthy and light diet. Each bottle contains dietary fibres, green tea and double as much calcium as a regular yoghurt drink. | Labelled per serving (88 g): | |
| | | Calories | 32 |
| | | Fat | 0.1 g |
| | | Sodium | 0.03 g |
| | | Carbohydrates | 4.8 g |
| | | Protein | 1.8 g |
| | | Calcium | 26% EU-RDA (211 mg) |
| | | Fibre | 2.6 g |

DV, US daily value, which is 1000 mg for calcium; EU-RDA, recommended daily allowance in the European Union according to Council Directive 90/496/EEC (1990), which is 800 mg for calcium.

drink milk minerals had been used to increase calcium levels. The question of which calcium salt has the best anti-obesity properties in functional foods and drinks cannot be answered, as long as the contribution of the Zemel mechanism and the formation of calcium soaps to the overall calcium effect remains unclear. The former effect requires the use of highly water-soluble complex calcium salts to increase serum calcium concentration, the latter a high calcium concentration in the intestine.

## 11.6 Conclusions and future trends

Since the first studies with the model of the agouti mouse and the re-analysis of older epidemiological studies brought forward the hypothesis of an anti-obesity effect of calcium, numerous further animal experiments, epidemiological studies and intervention trials on humans have been published. Nevertheless, an anti-obesity effect of calcium can no longer be taken as given, as in the last few years a similar number of investigations have been published that did not find such an effect of calcium, at least not a statistically significant one. In the opinion of the authors of this chapter, the main reason for this is that the anti-obesity effect of calcium is rather moderate (meaning that overweight and obesity are not due to calcium deficiency) and that it depends furthermore on numerous factors, endogenous and environmental, which are not, by any means, all known. Therefore, studies of apparently similar design might have opposite results. Verification of the calcium effect is required in large clinical studies on healthy subjects and on those with disorders in their lipid metabolism as well as elucidation of the underlying mechanisms.

Besides Zemel's hypothesis, that decreased intracellular calcium levels brought about by increased dietary calcium would promote lipolysis, fatty acid oxidation and the reduction of intracellular fat depots in adipose tissue, two other mechanisms have been suggested as explanations of an anti-obesity effect: increased faecal lipid loss due to the formation of calcium soaps in the intestine as well as a decreased or later food intake after a previous calcium-rich meal. The contribution, however, of the different mechanisms to the overall calcium effect is unclear, although it is of critical importance to decide whether calcium intake should be increased by consuming highly water-soluble complex calcium salts and the addition of caseinophosphopeptides. Due to their high bioavailability, these complex calcium compounds, like calcium lactate gluconate, indeed support the Zemel mechanism, but it needs to be elucidated whether they also play a role in the formation of calcium soaps and thus intestinal fat excretion.

Therefore, in the opinion of these authors, among others, it is at present not justified to recommend an increased consumption of calcium-rich food or calcium supplements as a crucial part of a public-health strategy for weight management purposes. On the other hand, it seems quite justified to develop low-calorie foods for the purpose of maintaining weight reduction, and to fortify them with functional food components with weight reducing properties, where calcium can also provide a relevant contribution to health. Alongside this, the desirability of a plentiful calcium supply from milk products, other (fortified) foods and calcium supplements remains without question, particularly for osteoporosis prevention, but also for its potential cancer-preventive effects and its favourable effect on blood pressure.

## 11.7 Sources of further information and advice

Studies of the role of calcium in weight loss or the prevention of overweight and obesity are a rather recent, still developing field of research. It is absolutely necessary to be prepared to question once again findings that in the past were thought to have been verified. Therefore, researchers who are interested in this field and who want to extend their knowledge, need to resort to reviewing articles published in scientific journals and the original literature cited in these articles, as well as any other original contributions, which can, for example, be obtained from scientific data banks such as Medline (http://www.ncbi.nlm.nih.gov/entrez/query.fcgi). Monographs on this topic in books are hardly available. Furthermore, the National Dairy Council in the United States has a website (http://www.nationaldairycouncil.org/healthyweight/science.asp) that provides references exclusively for studies showing a positive impact of calcium and dairy products in weight management. The site contains short descriptions of the respective studies, links to the original abstracts and another link to an issue of the *Dairy Council Digest* with the title: 'Dairy foods' role in achieving a healthy weight. Some food producers also have websites where specific information on calcium and weight management are addressed, most notably General Mills, USA (http://www.yoplait.com/health_archive_boost.aspx and http://www.sogoodgirls.com). With regard to information on supplemental calcium and obesity and on how to use calcium salts in functional food products, food ingredients manufacturer Jungbunzlauer, Switzerland offers a dedicated download area in the Special Salts product group (http://www.jungbunzlauer.com/services/downloads.html).

On the other hand the scientific literature on the topic of overweight, obesity and lipid metabolism is so extensive, and there are so many monographs, that it is virtually impossible to select a short list of representative books or review articles. Therefore only one book published in 2004 by Woodhead Publishing Limited is to be mentioned, with the title '*Food, Diet and Obesity*'. It gives a comprehensive overview of the topic and contains a chapter on 'Calcium and obesity' (Barr, 2004).

## 11.8 References

ALBERTSON A M, GOOD C K, HOLSCHUH N M and ELDRIDGE E L (2003), 'The relationship between dietary calcium intake and body mass index in adult women: data from the Continuing Survey of Food Intake by Individuals 1994–96', *FASEB J.*, **17**, A289.

ALMUSTAFA M, DOYLE F H, GUTTERIDGE D H, HAND D J, DAVIS T M, SPINKS T J, FREEMANTLE C and JOPLIN G F (1992), 'Effects of treatments by calcium and sex hormones on vertebral fracturing in osteoporosis', *Q. J. Med.*, **83**, 283–294.

AZADBAKHT L, MIRMIRAN P, ESMAILLZADEH A and AZIZI F (2005), 'Dairy consumption is inversely associated with the prevalence of the metabolic syndrome in Tehranian adults', *Am. J. Clin. Nutr.*, **82**, 523–530.

BARGER-LUX M J, DAVIES K M, HEANEY R P, CHIN B K and RAFFERTY K (2001), 'Calcium supplementation may attenuate accumulation of fat in young women', *J. Bone Miner. Res.*, **16**, S219.

BARR S I (2004), 'Calcium and obesity', in Mela D. (Ed.), '*Food, Diet and Obesity*', Cambridge, Woodhead, pp. 431–447.

BARR S I, FULGONI V L and PEREIRA M A (2004), 'Relationship of calcium or dairy product intakes on percent bod fat, BMI, and anthropometric measures in NHANES-III', *FASEB J.*, **18** (5 Part II), A873.

BERKEY C S, ROCKETT H R, WILLETT W C and COLDITZ G A (2005), 'Milk, dairy fat, dietary calcium, and weight gain: a longitudinal study of adolescents', *Arch. Pediatr. Adolesc. Med.*, **159**, 543–550.

BOSCHMANN M, KRUPP G, LUFT F C, KLAUS S and JORDAN J (2002), 'In vivo response to alpha(1)-adenoreceptor stimulation in human white adipose tissue', *Obes. Res.*, **10**, 555–558.

BOWEN J, NOAKES M and CLIFTON P M (2005), 'Effect of calcium and dairy foods in high protein, energy-restricted diets on weight loss and metabolic parameters in overweight adults', *Int. J. Obes. Relat. Metab. Disord.*, **29**, 957–965.

BUCHOWSKI M S, SEMENYA J and JOHNSON A O (2002), 'Dietary calcium intake in lactose maldigesting intolerant and tolerant African-American women', *J. Am. Coll. Nutr.*, **21**, 47–54.

CARRUTH B R and SKINNER J D (2001), 'The role of dietary calcium and other nutrients in moderating body fat in preschool children', *Int. J. Obes. Relat. Metab. Disord.*, **25**, 559–566.

CLIFTON P (2005), 'The beginning of the end for the dietary calcium and obesity hypothesis', *Obes. Res.*, **13**, 1301.

CLYDESDALE F M (1988), 'Minerals interactions in foods', in Smith K T (Ed.), '*Handbook of Trace Minerals in Foods: Their Relationship to Health and Nutrition*', New York, Marcel Dekker, pp. 57–94.

DAVIES K M, HEANEY R P, RECKER R R, LAPPE J M, BARGER-LUX M J, RAFFERTY K and HINDERS S (2000), 'Calcium intake and body weight', *J. Clin. Endocrinol. Metab.*, **85**, 4635–4638.

DENKE M A, FOX M M and SCHULTE M C (1993), 'Short-term dietary calcium fortification increases fecal saturated fat content and reduces serum lipids in men', *J. Nutr.*, **123**, 1047–1053.

DRAPEAU V, DESPRES J P, BOUCHARD C, ALLARD L, FOURNIER G, LEBLANC C and TREMBLAY A (2004), Modifications in food group consumption are related to long-term body weight changes', *Am. J. Clin. Nutr.*, **80**, 29–37.

DRAZNIN B, SUSSMAN K E, ECKEL R H, KAO M, YOST T and SHERMAN N A (1988), 'Possible role of cytosolic free calcium concentrations in mediating insulin resistance of obesity and hyperinsulinemia', *J. Clin. Invest.*, **82**, 1848–1852.

DRENICK E J (1961), 'The influence of ingestion of calcium and other soap-forming substances on fecal fat', *Gastroenterology*, **41**, 242–244.

EDELSTEIN S (2004), 'Calcium citrate and bone health', in Remacle, C. and Reusens B. (Eds), '*Functional Foods, Ageing and Degenerative Disease*', Cambridge, Woodhead, pp. 174–183.

FLYNN A and CASHMAN K (1999), 'Calcium', in Hurrel, R. (Ed.), '*The Mineral Fortification of Foods*', Surrey, Leatherhead Food International Ltd, pp. 18–53.

FUJITA T and PALMIERI G M A (2000), 'Calcium paradox disease: calcium deficiency prompting secondary hyperparathyroidism and cellular calcium overload', *J. Bone Miner. Metab.*, **18**, 109–125.

GERSTNER G (2002a), 'The challenge of calcium fortification of beverages', *Innov. Food Technol.*, **14**, 26–28.

GERSTNER G (2002b), 'Calcium lactate gluconate – the innovative solution for extra calcium', *Innov. Food Technol.*, **16**, 20–21.

GERSTNER G (2003), 'How can we get more calcium?', *Int. Food Ingredients*, **3**, 24–26.

GERSTNER G (2004), 'Feasibility of calcium fortification in dairy and soy drinks', *Wellness Foods Europe*, **3**, 24–29.

HEANEY R P (2003), 'Normalizing calcium intake: projected population effects for body weight', *J. Nutr.*, **133**, S268–270.

HEANEY R P, DAVIES K M and BARGER-LUX M J (2002), 'Calcium and weight: clinical studies', *J. Am. Coll. Nutr.*, **21**, S152–155.

HEANEY R P, DOWELL M S, RAFFERTY K and BIERMAN J (2000), 'Bioavailability of the calcium in fortified soy imitation milk, with some observations on method', *Am. J. Clin. Nutr.*, **71**, 1166–1169.

HEANEY R P, RAFFERTY K, DOWELL M S and BIERMAN J (2005), 'Calcium fortification systems differ in bioavailability', *J. Am. Diet. Assoc.*, **105** (5), 807–809.

HELLERSTEIN M K (1999), 'De novo lipogenesis in humans: metabolic and regulatory aspects', *Eur. J. Clin. Nutr.*, 53, S53–65.

JACQMAIN M, DOUCET E, DESPRES J-P and BOUCHARD C (2003), 'Calcium intake, body composition, and lipoprotein-lipid concentrations in adults', *Am. J. Clin. Nutr.*, **77**, 1448–1452.

JONES B H, KIM J H, ZEMEL M B, WOYCHIK R P, MICHAUD E J, WILKISON W O and MOUSTAID N (1996), 'Upregulation of adipocyte metabolism by *agouti* protein: possible paracrine actions in yellow mouse obesity', *Am. J. Physiol.*, **20**, E192–196.

KAMYCHEVA E, JOAKIMSEN R M and JORDE R (2003), 'Intakes of calcium and vitamin D predict body mass index in the population of Northern Norway', *J. Nutr.*, **133**, 102–106.

LAU E M, WOO J, LEUNG P C, SWAMINATHAN R and LEUNG D (1992), 'The effects of calcium supplementation and exercise on bone density in elderly Chinese women', *Osteoporos. Int.*, **2**, 168–173.

LEATHERHEAD FOOD INTERNATIONAL (2005), '*Key Players in the International Functional Foods Industry*', Surrey, Leatherhead Food International Ltd.

LELOVICS Z (2004), 'Relation between calcium and magnesium intake and obesity', *Asia Pac. J. Clin. Nutr.*, **13**, S144.

LIN Y C, LYLE R M, MCCABE L D, MCCABE G P, WEAVER C M and TEEGARDEN D (2000), 'Dairy calcium is related to changes in body composition during a two-year exercise intervention in young women', *J. Am. Coll. Nutr.*, **19**, 754–760.

LOOS R J, RANKINEN T, LEON A S, SKINNER J S, WILMORE J H, RAO D C and BOUCHARD C (2004), 'Calcium intake is associated with adiposity in Black and White men and White women of the HERITAGE Family Study', *J. Nutr.*, **134**, 1772–1778.

LOVEJOY J C, CHAMPAGNE C M, SMITH S R, DE JONGE L and XIE H (2001), 'Ethnic differences in dietary intakes, physical activity, and energy expenditure in middle-aged, premenopausal women: the Healthy Transitions study', *Am. J. Clin. Nutr.*, **74**, 90–95.

MARQUES-VIDAL P, GONCALVES A and DIAS C M (2006), 'Milk intake is inversely related to obesity in men and in young women: data from the Portuguese Health Interview Survey 1998–1999', *Int. J. Obes.*, **30**, 88–93.

MELANSON E L, SHARP T A, SCHNEIDER J, DONAHOO W T, GRUNWALD G K and HILL J O (2003), 'Relation between calcium intake and fat oxidation in adult humans', *Int. J. Obes.*, **27**, 196–203.

NATIONAL INSTITUTES OF HEALTH (1994), 'Optimal calcium intake', *NIH Consens Statement Online*, June 6–8, **12** (4), 1–31 (http://www.ncbi.nlm.nih.gov/books/bv.fcgi?rid=hstat4.chapter.13595).

NATIONAL RESEARCH COUNCIL (1989), 'Calcium', in '*Recommended Dietary Allowances*' 10th edition, Report of the Subcommittee on the Tenth Edition of the RDA, Food and Nutrition Board and the Commission on Life Sciences, Nutrition Research Council. Washington DC, National Academy Press, pp. 174–184.

PALMIERI G M A, NUTTING D F, BHATTACHARYA S K, BERTORINI T E and WILLIAMS J C (1998), 'Parathyroid ablation in dystrophic hamsters', *J. Clin. Invest.*, **68**, 646–654.

PAPAKONSTANTINOU E, FLATT W P, HUTH P J and HARRIS R B S (2003), High dietary calcium reduces body fat content, digestibility of fat and serum vitamin D in rats', *Obes. Res.*, **11**, 387–394.

PARADIS S and CABANAC M (2005), 'Calcium deficiency cannot induce obesity in rats', *Physiol. Behav.*, **85**, 259–264.

PEREIA M A, JACOBS D R JR, VAN HORN L, SLATTERY M L, KARTASHOV A I and LUDWIG D S (2002), 'Dairy consumption, obesity, and the insulin resistance syndrome in young adults: the CARDIA Study', *JAMA*, **287**, 2081–2089.

PING-DELFOS W C, SOARES M J and CUMMINGS N K (2004), 'Acute suppression of spontaneous food intake following dairy calcium and vitamin D', *Asia Pac. J. Clin. Nutr.*, **13**, S82.

REDDY S, SHER A, VAN VADEHRA D and WREDAL E R (1999), 'Calcium complex and a process of making a food fortified with calcium', US Patent 5, 928, 691.

RIGGS B L, O'FALLON W M, MUHS J, O'CONNOR M K, KUMAR R and MELTON L J (1998), 'Long term effects of calcium supplementation on serum parathyroid hormone level, bone turnover and bone loss in elderly women', *J. Bone Miner. Res.*, **13**, 168–174.

SAKHAEE K, BHUKET T, ADAMS-HUET B and RAO D S (1999), 'Meta-analysis of calcium bioavailability: A comparison of calcium citrate with calcium carbonate', *Am. J. Ther.*, **6**, 313–321.

SCHAAFSMA A, DE VRIES P J F and SARIS W H M (2001), 'Delay of natural bone loss by higher intakes of specific minerals and vitamins', *Crit. Rev. Food. Sci. Nutr.*, **41**, 225–249.

SHAHKHALALILI Y, MURSET C, MEIRIM I, DURUZ E, GUINCHARD S, CAVADINI C and ACHESON K (2001), 'Calcium supplementation of chocolate: effect on cocoa butter digestibility and blood lipids in humans', *Am. J. Clin. Nutr.*, **73**, 246–252.

SHAPSES S A, HESHKA S and HEYMSFIELD S B (2004), 'Effect of calcium supplementation on weight and fat loss in women', *J. Clin. Endocrinol. Metab.*, **89**, 632–637.

SHI H, DIRIENZO D and ZEMEL M B (2001), 'Effects of dietary calcium on adipocyte lipid metabolism and body weight regulation in energy-restricted aP2-agouti transgenic mice', *FASEB J.*, **15**, 291–293.

SKINNER J D, BOUNDS W, CARRUTH B R and ZIEGLER P (2003), 'Longitudinal calcium intake is negatively related to children's body fat indexes', *J. Am. Diet Assoc.*, **103**, 1626–1631.

TANASECU M, FERRIS A M, HIMMELGREEN D A, RODRIGUEZ P and PEREZ-ESCAMILLA R (2000), 'Biobehavioral factors are associated with obesity in Puerto Rican children', *J. Nutr.*, **130**, 1734–1742.

TEEGARDEN D (2003), 'Calcium intake and reduction in weight or fat mass', *J. Nutr.*, **133**, S249–251.

THOMPSON W G, ROSTAD HOLDMAN N, JANZOW D J, SLEZAK J M, MORRIS K L and ZEMEL M B (2005), 'Effect of energy-reduced diets high in dairy products and fiber on weight loss in obese adults', *Obes. Res.*, **13**, 1344–1353.

TORDOFF M G (1996), 'Some basic psychophysics of calcium salt solutions', *Chem. Senses*, **21**, 417–424.

VASKONEN T (2003), 'Dietary minerals and modification of cardiovascular risk factors', *J. Nutr. Biochem.*, **14**, 492–506.

VASKONEN T, MERVAALA E, SEPPANEN-LAAKSO T and KARPPANEN H (2001), 'Diet enrichment with calcium and magnesium enhances the cholesterol-lowering effect of plant sterols in obese Zucker rats', *Nutr. Metab. Cardiovasc. Dis.*, **11**, 158–167.

VASKONEN T, MERVAALA E, SUMUVUORI V, SEPPANEN-LAAKSO T and KARPPANEN H (2002), 'Effects of calcium and plant sterols on serum lipids in obese Zucker rats on a low-fat diet', *Br. J. Nutr.*, **87**, 239–245.

VENTI C A, TATARANNI A and SALBE A D (2005), 'Lack of relationship between calcium intake and body size in an obesity-prone population', *J. Am. Diet Assoc.*, **105**, 1401–1407.

WELBERG J W, MONKELBAAN J G, DE VRIES E G, MUSKIET F A, CATS A, OREMUS E T, BOERSMA-VAN EK, VAN RIJSBERGEN H, VAN DER MEER R, MULDER N H and KLEIBEUKER J H (1994), 'Effects of supplemental dietary calcium on quantitative and qualitative fecal fat excretion in man', *Ann. Nutr. Metab.*, **38**, 185–191.

WOSJE K S and KALKWARF H J (2004), 'Lactation, weaning, and calcium supplementation: effects on body composition in postpartum women', *Am. J. Clin. Nutr.*, **80**, 423–429.

XUE B, GREENBERG A G, KRAEMER F B and ZEMEL M B (2001), 'Mechanism of intracellular calcium inhibition of lipolysis in human adipocytes', *FASEB J.*, **15**, 2527–2529.

XUE B, MOUSTAID-MOUSSA N, WILKISON W O and ZEMEL M B (1998), 'The *agouti* gene product inhibits lipolysis in human adipocytes via a $Ca^{2+}$ dependent mechanism', *FASEB J.*, **12**, 1391–1396.

ZEMEL M B (2002), 'Regulation of adiposity and obesity risk by dietary calcium: mechanisms and implications', *J. Am. Coll. Nutr.*, **21**, S146–151.

ZEMEL M B, KIM J H, WOYCHIK R P, MICHAUD E J, KADWELL S H, PATEL I R and WILKISON W O (1995), 'Agouti regulation of intracellular calcium: Role in the insulin resistance of viable yellow mice', *Proc. Natl. Acad. Sci. USA*, **92**, 4733–4737.

ZEMEL M B and MILLER S L (2004), 'Dietary calcium and dairy modulation of adiposity and obesity risk', *Nutr. Rev.*, **62**, 125–131.

ZEMEL M B, RICHARDS J, MATHIS S, MILSTEAD A, GEBHARDT L and SILVA E (2005), 'Dairy augmentation of total and central fat loss in obese subjects', *Int. J. Obes.* (*Lond.*), **29**, 391–397.

ZEMEL M B, SHI H, GREER B, DIRIENZO D and ZEMEL P C (2000), 'Regulation of adiposity by dietary calcium', *FASEB J.*, **14**, 1132–1138.

ZEMEL M B, THOMPSON W, MILSTEAD A, MORRIS K and CAMPBELL P (2004), 'Calcium and dairy acceleration of weight and fat loss during energy restriction in obese adults', *Obes. Res.*, **12**, 582–590.

ZEMEL M B, ZEMEL P C, BRYG R J and SOWERS J R (1990), 'Dietary calcium induces regression of left ventricular hypertrophy in hypertensive non-insulin-dependent diabetic blacks', *Am. J. Hypertens.*, **3**, 468–473.

ZHANG Q and TORDOFF M G (2004), 'No effect of dietary calcium on body weight of lean and obese mice and rats', *Am. J. Physiol. Regul. Integr. Comp. Physiol.*, **286**, R669–R677.

# 12

# Conjugated fatty acids, body composition and weight control

**J. L. Sebedio, UMR, 1019, INRA-Université d'Auvergne, France**

## 12.1 Introduction

Conjugated linoleic acid or CLA is a collective name that has been used to describe positional and geometrical isomers of linoleic acid (18:2n-6) having two conjugated double bonds; some of these are shown in Fig. 12.1. Over the past two decades and especially since the discovery of Ha *et al.* (1987), who reported that an extract from grilled ground beef later identified as CLA had biological effects, numerous studies have been carried out first on animals and lately in humans demonstrating the possible implications of CLA isomers on health. A large number of studies both in animals and humans have been carried out on mixtures of CLA isomers synthesised by chemical means, others have investigated pure isolated isomers and only very few have studied the natural CLA mixtures. A recently published book gives a summary of the studies carried out up to 2003 (Sebedio *et al.*, 2003). These studies have shown that CLA could have an effect on the immune system (Cook *et al.*, 2003), on atherosclerosis (Kritchevsky, 2003), on mammary cancer (Banni *et al.*, 2003), and on body composition (Keim, 2003). This chapter will only deal with the possible effect on CLA isomers on body composition and the data obtained from both animals and humans will be discussed to evaluate the potential utilisation of CLA in body fat reduction and weight control. We will first look at the sources of CLA, then at the actual consumption of CLA by humans, and we will describe the data obtained in both animals and humans. We will then discuss the possibility of incorporating CLA in functional foods.

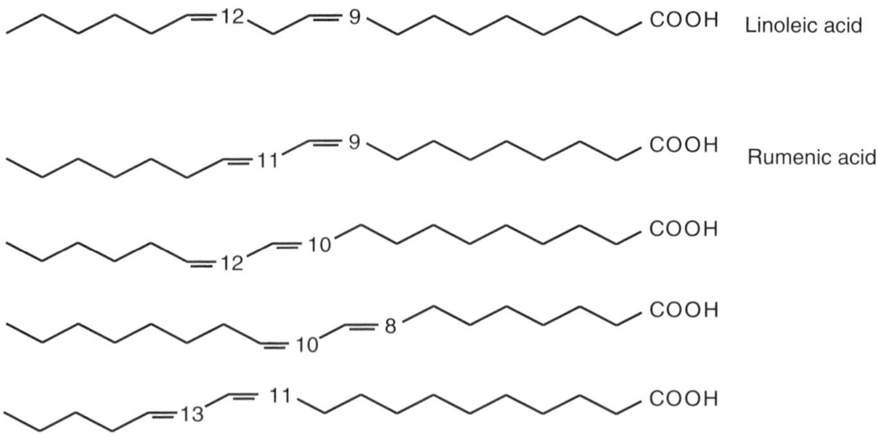


**Fig. 12.1** Structures of some CLA isomers.

## 12.2 Sources of conjugated linoleic acid and estimated daily intake

### 12.2.1 Natural sources

In food, CLA is found in products from ruminants such as milk and meat, and products made from them such as cheese and cultured dairy products (Parodi, 2003). CLA has been shown to be produced in the rumen as a result of biohydrogenation from linoleic acid, a polyunsaturated fatty acid that is found in the pasture. Rumenic acid or 9c,11t-18:2 is the major CLA isomer produced. Biohydrogenation also produces 11t-18:1 fatty acid or vaccenic acid. CLA has also been shown to be produced in the mammary gland by Δ9 desaturation of vaccenic acid which passed via the circulatory system to the mammary gland and adipose tissue (Corl *et al.*, 2001). The second most important CLA isomer, the 7t,9c-18:1, has been shown to be only produced in the mammary gland (Corl *et al.*, 2002). Linolenic acid, a fatty acid present in the pasture, does not directly produce rumenic acid but contributes to its level by giving vaccenic acid which can then be converted to the 9c,11t isomer.

As previously discussed the major CLA isomer in dairy and meat products is rumenic acid or 9c,11t-18:2. This isomer represents more than 70% of the total CLA isomers (Table 12.1). It is accompanied by a mixture of other *cis,cis*, *cis,trans*, and *trans,trans* isomers. Some earlier studies reported CLA content of dairy products but it is only since the development of sample preparation and sophisticated chromatographic methods (Christie, 2003) that the problems of co-eluting peaks and artefact formation could be avoided. Direct gas-liquid chromatographic analysis does not allow separation of the different isomers. However, these can be resolved satisfactorily by using silver nitrate high-performance liquid chromatography (Sehat

**Table 12.1** CLA content and content of 9c,11t (% of total isomers) in samples of butter, cheese and beef fat (adapted from Parodi, 2003)

| CLA | Butter ($n = 1$) | Cheese ($n = 16$) | Beef ($n = 20$) |
|---|---|---|---|
| 9c,11t (%) | 76.5 | 83.5 | 72.0 |
| Σtt | 9.4 | 6.3 | 12.3 |
| Σcc | 4.8 | 0.7 | — |
| Total (mg/g fat) | 5.0 | 9.3 | 2.7 |

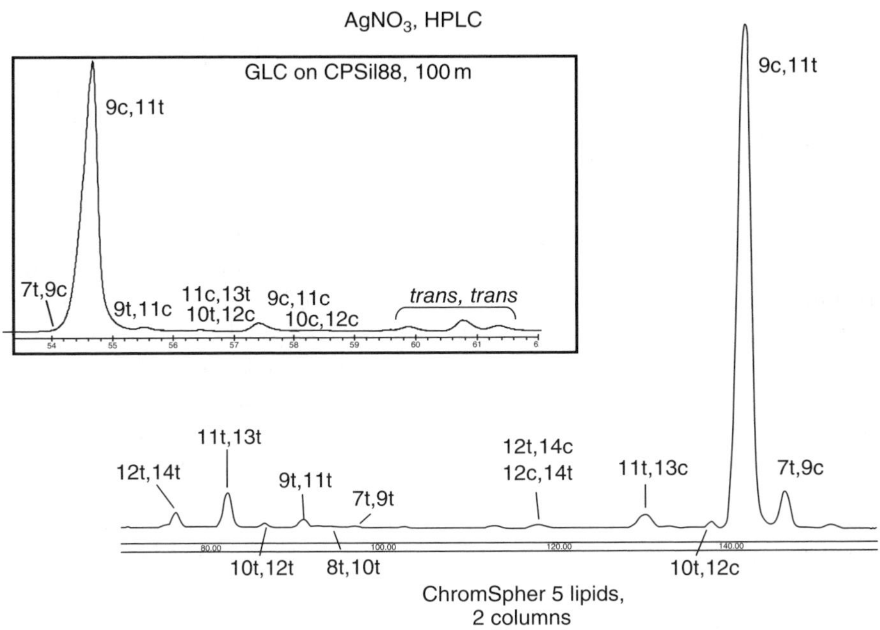


**Fig. 12.2** Silver nitrate high-performance liquid chromatographic analysis ($AgNO_3$-HPLC) on two ChromSpher 5 lipids columns and gas liquid chromatographic analysis (GLC) on a 100-m CPSil88 column of fatty acid methyl esters of milk lipid (P. Juaneda and J. L. Sebedio, unpublished data, 2002).

*et al*., 1998), as reported in Fig. 12.2. As shown in Table 12.1 the CLA content in food products is low and it will be important to take this into account when discussing the data obtained from the human studies. Very similar CLA contents were reported for different countries, the quantities ranging from 1.0 to 28.7 mg/g of fat (Table 12.2). Of importance is the fact that the level of CLA in these products can be modulated by different factors such as the breed of the animal and the lactation number, and especially by the diet (Parodi, 2003). However, cows fed the same diet can exhibit large differences in milk CLA content (Parodi, 2003). The effect of the diet is

**Table 12.2** CLA content (minimum and maximum, in mg/g fat), cows' milk from different countries (adapted from Parodi, 2003)

| Country | Number | Minimum (mg/g fat) | Maximum (mg/g fat) | Sample type |
|---|---|---|---|---|
| Australia | 17 | 10.3 | 18.5 | Cows (summer, fall) |
| Austria | 13 | 5.2 | 14.4 | Butter |
| France | 198 | 2.1 | 15.6 | Butter |
| Germany | 909 | 1.0 | 10.5 | Butter (barn-fed cows) |
| | 593 | 4.9 | 18.9 | Butter (pasture-fed cows) |
| Italy | 12 | 6.3 | 16.7 | Butter |
| Ireland | 23 | 5.6 | 18.2 | Butter |
| Netherlands | 63 | 3.6 | 13.3 | Butter |
| Switzerland | 11 | 7.1 | 10.8 | Milk(June–Sept lowland grazing) |
| | 21 | 19.2 | 28.7 | Milk(June–Sept highland grazing) |
| United Kingdom | 21 | 6.0 | 14.4 | Butter |

illustrated in Table 12.2 for Germany and Switzerland. For the study carried out in Germany, preparing a butter from milk from pasture-fed cows resulted in almost triple the mean CLA content compared with butter prepared using milk from barn-fed cows. Similar results were reported for the study carried out in Switzerland when comparing milk from highland and lowland grazing cows. Milk from goats and sheep also contains similar quantities of CLA but their contribution to the daily intake would only be of importance for a number of countries from the Mediterranean region.

Feeding strategies to enrich CLA content of milk have also been studied. Basically, two methods have been used to modify the CLA content of milk fat. The first one is to use techniques that increase the level of substrates for CLA and vaccenic acid synthesis in the rumen and the second is to modify the rumen microbial activity. Plant oils – primarily from cereals and oilseeds – fish oils, and pasture feeding were used to elevate milk fat CLA concentration. For more details, readers are referred to the comprehensive review of Stanton *et al.* (2003). As an example, Corl *et al.* (2003) have obtained a butter containing about 16% vaccenic acid (11t-18:1) and around 4% of 9c,11t-18:2 compared with 1.3% of 11t-18:1 and 0.5% 9c,11t-18:2 in the control butter by feeding cows with a corn-based total mix ration (control butter) while the cows producing the high-*trans* milk were fed with the same ration supplemented with 2 g/100 g sunflower oil and 1 g/100 g fish oil.

Daily intakes of CLA isomers have been estimated in different countries, as reported in Table 12.3, using different techniques such as utilisation of national dietary survey data, food frequency questionnaires, dietary assessment, and 7-day dietary records. The daily intake is quite low and interestingly two studies that have compared men and women found a lower CLA intake for women; this may result from a lower intake of meat and dairy

**Table 12.3** Estimated daily intake of CLA in different countries (adapted from Parodi, 2003)

| Country | CLA intake (mg) |
|---|---|
| Australia | 500–1500 |
| Germany | Men, 430 |
| | Women, 350 |
| | Women, 246 |
| Sweden | (323)* |
| | (160) |
| USA | Men, 3–486 (176) |
| | Women, 1–399 (104) |
| | Men, 0–454 (212) |
| | Women, 0–520 (150) |

* Values in parentheses represent means.

products in the latter. Daily intakes range from 0 to about 400–500 mg in most of the countries studied, except in Australia where larger intakes (up to 1.5 g/day) have been observed (Table 12.3).

### 12.2.2 Industrial sources

CLA supplements have mainly been sold as soft-gel capsules since 1995 in the United States and, more recently, in different European countries and Japan. Recently, Saebo (2003) reported the composition of 17 commercial CLA capsules sampled in January-March 2002 in different countries. Conjugated acid mixtures are usually obtained by alkali isomerisation of linoleic acid followed by a purification process in order to remove contaminants – such as polymers, sterols, and sometimes heavy metals – that could arise from the isomerisation process if mineral acids are used in a stainless steel reactor. Sunflower and safflower oils are the two types of starting material used for the isomerisation process. Products may be classified as four- or two-isomer mixtures. The two-isomer product is a mixture of the 9c,11t-18:2 and the 10t,12c-18:2 in about equal quantities while the four-isomer product is a mixture of 9c,11t-, 10t,12c-, 8t,10c- and 11c,13t-18:2 isomers. Furthermore, most of the products contain between 60 and 80% CLA as free fatty acids (Table 12.4). Further work is being carried out in order to produce triacylglycerols (Saebo, 2003).

## 12.3 Effect of conjugated linoleic acid on body composition

A large part of the studies so far developed has been carried out using animal models and only a few intervention studies on humans have been reported. Earlier studies on animals and on humans were done using a

**Table 12.4** Content of CLA (% of total fatty acids) and 10t,12c–18:2 isomer (% of CLA) in supplements sampled in 2002 (adapted from Saebo, 2003)

| Product | Country | CLA (%) | 10t,12c (%) |
|---|---|---|---|
| 1 | Norway | 80.1 | 47.8 |
| 2 | Norway | 78.6 | 47.1 |
| 3 | Norway | 69.1 | 46.7 |
| 4 | Norway | 78.3 | 48.7 |
| 5 | Norway | 76.4 | 46.6 |
| 6 | USA | 71.4 | 46.3 |
| 7 | USA | 74.8 | 43.1 |
| 8 | USA | 77.9 | 48.5 |
| 9 | USA | 70.8 | 44.4 |
| 10 | USA | 79.6 | 45.3 |
| 11 | USA | 72.0 | 44.4 |
| 12 | USA | 74.3 | 43.6 |
| 13 | USA | 61.5 | 28.5 |
| 14 | USA | 76.3 | 48.4 |
| 15 | USA | 1.2 | 47.8 |
| 16 | South Africa | 51.7 | 16.5* |
| 17 | Norway | 57.7 | 29.9* |

* Contains 16.1 and 16.5% of 11c,13t respectively.

50:50 mixture of 9c,11t- and 10t,12c-18:2 isomers (Fig. 12.3). Later studies using single isomers enabled the determination of which isomer was the active one and which one(s) may have some adverse effects. A recent intervention study on humans published in 2005, for the first time compared a butter naturally low in CLA (0.4g CLA/100g butter) with a butter enriched in CLA (4.2g CLA/100g butter) (Desroches *et al.*, 2005).

### 12.3.1 Animal studies

Many studies on different animal species such as mice, rats, and pigs (e.g. Ostrowska *et al.*, 1999; Park *et al.*, 1999b; Gavino *et al.*, 2000; Bouthegourd *et al.*, 2002; Evans *et al.*, 2002; Wang and Jones, 2004), have shown that CLA may affect body composition, mainly by a reduction of body fat and sometimes by enhancement of fat-free mass (Fig. 12.4). It was also shown by feeding and withdrawing CLA in mice that the process is reversible, but the body fat accumulation in mice previously fed the CLA was smaller than that of the control and did not appear to return to control levels even after 8 weeks (Park *et al.*, 1999a) when tissue CLA had returned to control levels. The effect of CLA on body composition was dependent on the species and mice seem to be the most reactive (Pariza *et al.*, 2001). It was then demonstrated using fractions enriched with one or other isomer that body composition changes were associated with the 10t,12c-18:2 isomer (Park *et al.*,

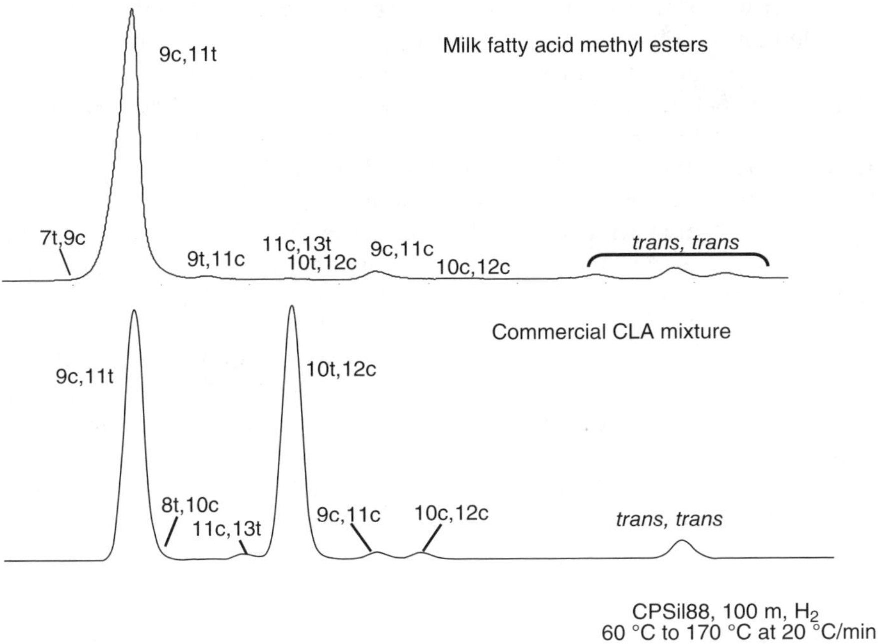


**Fig. 12.3** Gas liquid chromatographic analyses of CLA isomers in milk (top) and of a commercial CLA mixture (bottom) (P. Juaneda and J. L. Sebedio, unpublished data, 2002).

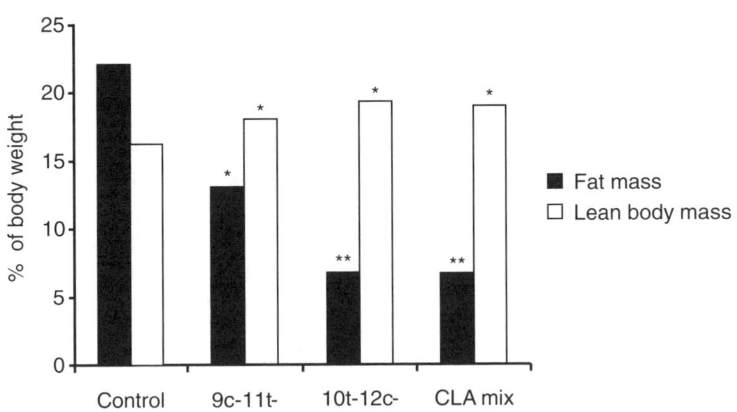


**Fig. 12.4** Effect of feeding pure CLA and a CLA mixture on body composition of female mice; **significantly different from control and from 9c,11t (adapted from Park *et al.*, 1999b).

1999b). It was also found that CLA reduced fat deposition in male AKR/J mice fed either a low-fat diet or a high-fat diet (West *et al.*, 1998). Studies carried out on animals, and also on cell cultures, have shown that the 10t,12c isomer may act at different levels (Pariza *et al.*, 2001). CLA was reported to alter energy balance by increasing energy expenditure (West *et al.*, 1998). In fully differentiated 3T3-L1 adipocytes, CLA supplementation was shown to reduce the lipoprotein lipase (LPL) activity, one of the key enzymes in lipid metabolism (Park *et al.*, 1997). Treatment of 3T3-L1 adipocytes with the 10t,12c isomer also resulted in a dose-dependent decrease in the expression of the stearoyl coenzyme A (CoA) desaturase, an important enzyme in lipogenesis (Choi *et al.*, 2000). The 10t,12c isomer also affects pre-adipocyte differentiation (Kang *et al.*, 2003), inhibits proliferation, reduces triglyceride accumulation and induces apoptosis in 3T3-L1 pre-adipocytes (Evans *et al.*, 2000).There are also *in vivo* data to support the suggestion that CLA supplementation reduces adipose tissues by apoptosis in mice (Tsuboyama-Kasaoka *et al.*, 2000). Another study on rats also suggested that CLA reduced adipose tissue cell size rather than cell number (Azain *et al.*, 2000).

### 12.3.2 Human studies

The data obtained from the human studies so far carried out do not give a clear picture compared with studies using the different animal models and it is therefore difficult to determine if any of the CLA isomers or a mixture of them have an effect on body composition in humans. As shown in Table 12.5, most of the studies differed in subject gender, initial body weight (obese and non-obese subjects), duration, the nature of the isomers, the length of the treatment, and also the methods utilised to evaluate the effect of the treatment. Most studies used isomers in gelatine capsules while one study (Malpuech-Brugère *et al.*, 2004) used synthetic triacylglycerols in a functional food and another (Desroches *et al.*, 2005) used a butter enriched in CLA in comparison with a butter low in CLA.

As an example, in obese men and women (Fig. 12.5) (Blankson *et al.*, 2000), a decrease in fat mass was observed even at the lowest dosage (1.7 g/day of mixed CLA), while an increase in lean body mass was only detected at the highest CLA dosage. However it is somewhat surprising that an intermediate amount (5.1 g/day) did not have any effect on body composition. Interestingly, in the study of Malpuech-Brugère *et al.* (2004) feeding the isolated isomers at 1.5 and 3.0 g/day for 18 weeks did not result in any changes in body composition in overweight men. In fact it is impossible to compare these two intervention studies considering the differences in the protocols. By looking at the results reported in Table 12.5, one may suggest that in non-obese subjects (body mass index, BMI <25), CLA has little or no effect on body composition, except in the study of Thom *et al.* (2001) where exercise was associated with the treatment. On the contrary, feeding

**Table 12.5** Effect of feeding CLA on body composition in humans

| Gender | BMI (kg/m$^2$) | CLA (g/day) | Duration (weeks) | Effects | References |
|---|---|---|---|---|---|
| M/F | >30 | 2.8 | 24 | Exercise effect | Atkinson, 1999 |
| F | <25 | 3.9 | 9 | No | Zambell *et al.*, 2000 |
| M/F | >25 and <35 | 1.7–6.8 | 12 | ↓Fat mass | Blankson *et al.*, 2000 |
| M/F | 30 | 3.4 | 12 | No | Berven *et al.*, 2000 |
| M/F | <25 | 4.2 | 12 | ↓3.8% fat mass | Smedman and Vessby, 2001 |
| M/F | <25 | 1.8 | 12 | ↓4% fat mass | Thom *et al.*, 2001 |
| M/F | <30 | 0.7–1.4 | 4 + 4 | ↓Fat mass | Mougios *et al.*, 2001 |
| M/F | >30 | 4.2 | 4 | ↓Abdominal diameter | Riserus *et al.*, 2001 |
| | 25 | 6 + training | 4 | No | Kreider *et al.*, 2002 |
| F | <30 | 2.1 | 6 | No | Petridou *et al.*, 2003 |
| M/F | 28 | Weight loss then 1.8–3.6 | 3<br>13 | No effect of CLA on body weight regain | Kamphuis *et al.*, 2003 |
| M | <30 | 1.5–3<br>9c11t/10t,12c | 18 | No | Malpuech-Brugère *et al.*, 2004 |
| M | >30 | 3<br>9c,11t | 12 | No | Riserus *et al.*, 2004a |
| M | >30 | 0.6–2.4<br>9c,11t/10t,12c | 13 | No | Tricon *et al.*, 2004 |
| M/F | <30 | 3.6 | 52 | ↓5% fat mass | Gaullier *et al.*, 2004 |
| MF | 30 | 3.4 | (52) + 52 extension study | No effect after first 52 weeks on CLA | Gaullier *et al.*, 2005 |
| M | 31 | Butter enriched in CLA vs butter low in CLA | 4 (cross-over) | No | Desroches *et al.*, 2005 |

BMI, body mass index.

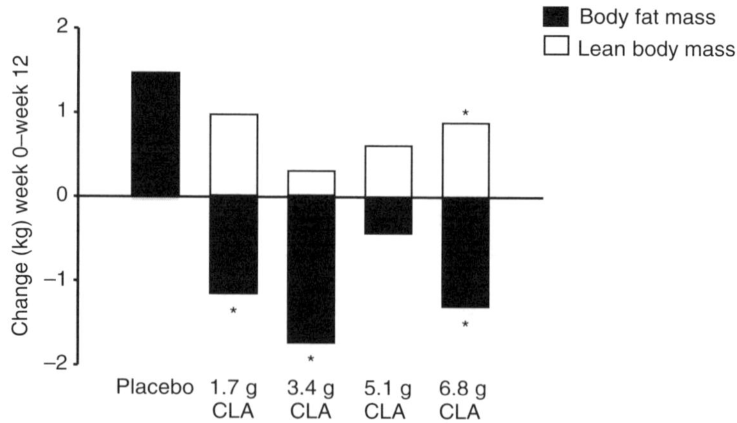


**Fig. 12.5** Effect of feeding CLA on body composition of humans; *different from placebo (adapted from Blankson *et al.* (2000)).

obese men with CLA most often resulted in a loss of fat mass but the effects were small if we consider the amount of isomers fed to the subjects (up to 6–7 g/day).

Only the studies of Gaullier *et al.* (2004, 2005) examined the long-term effects of feeding 3.4 g/day of a mixture of CLAs for two consecutive periods of 52 weeks. During the first period of 52 weeks CLA fed as free fatty acid or as triacylglycerol (CLA-TG) reduced the fat mass as well as body weight and BMI in both CLA groups, but only the CLA-TG group was different from the placebo for body weight and BMI. The same participants were included in an extension trial for another 52 weeks in order to evaluate the safety of using a CLA supplement for a long period. Feeding 3.4 g of CLA per day to volunteers who had already had the treatment for 52 weeks did not lead to further decrease in either fat mass or body weight. However, body weight and fat mass decreased in the subjects administered the placebo during the initial period.

## 12.4 Safety issues

### 12.4.1 In animals

The first adverse effects of feeding CLA, and especially the 10t,12c-18:2 isomers, were reported for animals and described for mice by Tsuboyama-Kasaoka *et al.* (2000). In C57BL/6J mice, supplementation with a 1% equimolar mixture of the 9c,11t and 10t,12c isomers reduced fat mass but the liver was massively enlarged. Histological analysis revealed a macrovesicular steatosis. Further studies (Clement *et al.*, 2002) showed that mice fed with 10t,12c-enriched CLA developed lipoatrophy, hyperinsulinaemia and fatty liver while the 9c,11t isomer had little or no effect (Clement *et al.*, 2002; Degrace *et al.*, 2003). While adipose tissue mass was shown to decrease after feeding CLA for 6 days, plasma levels of leptin and adiponectin decreased after 2 days of feeding, and hyperinsulinaemia developed on day 6 (Poirier *et al.*, 2005). CLA was shown to alter the capacity of pancreatic islets to secrete insulin and the increase in insulin secretion was correlated to an increase in beta cell mass and number, leading to liver steatosis (Poirier *et al.*, 2005). Degrace *et al.* (2003) demonstrated using C57BL/6J mice that the steatosis was not due to an alteration of the liver lipoprotein production. A three-fold decrease in plasma triacylglycerol and induction of mRNA expression of low-density lipoprotein receptors suggest an increase in the lipoprotein clearance at the level of liver. Further work also indicated that the steatosis was not due to impaired fatty acid oxidation as in fact in the liver, fatty acid oxidation capacities were increased when mice were fed the 10t,12c isomer, which increased both liver carnitine palmitoyl-transferase I and acyl-CoA oxidase gene expression for example (Degrace *et al.*, 2004).

### 12.4.2 In humans

Earlier human studies carried out by Berven *et al.* (2000) on overweight and obese subjects, using gel capsules, only reported small adverse events as a result of feeding CLA isomers for 12 weeks. In this study, blood lipids, haematological parameters, blood electrolytes, and liver safety parameters did not change significantly within the groups during the study. However, three subjects in each treatment reported adverse events such as diarrhoea or gastritis heartburn. No adverse events were also reported in the study of Malpuech-Brugère *et al.* (2004) when feeding pure isomers of CLA in a food matrix. In the study of Gaullier *et al.* (2005), who fed CLA isomers as free fatty acids (CLA-FFA) or triacylglycerols (CLA-TG) to healthy overweight subjects for 1 year, followed by a dose of 3.4 g CLA/day as TG for 1 year, similar adverse events such as gastrointestinal pains were reported. However, serum high-density lipoprotein (HDL) cholesterol decreased in the group previously fed CLA-TG. Serum lipoprotein a, Lp(a) also tended to increase in both CLA groups after 24 months. In addition to Lp(a) an increase in the leukocyte and thrombocyte counts was also observed; the authors indicated that these changes were within the normal ranges but may indicate the presence of an inflammatory or immunological response to CLA supplementation. Serum insulin level increased in the CLA-TG group while no modifications were found in the CLA-FFA group.

In a study on subjects with type 2 diabetes, Moloney *et al.* (2004) showed that a supplementation of 3.0 g/day of CLA for 8 weeks resulted in an increase in fasting glucose concentration and reduction of insulin sensitivity. CLA also reduced fibrinogen concentrations but had no effect on C-reactive protein and interleukin-6. In another study (Belury *et al.*, 2003), also with subjects having type 2 diabetes, the quantity of 10t,12c isomer in plasma was inversely correlated with changes in body weight and in serum leptin. Unfortunately no information was available on body composition and insulin sensitivity. Concerns were raised by the findings of the group of Smedman, who carried out studies on a high-risk group of abdominally obese men. None of the studies carried out by this group showed any effects of CLA on body weight or BMI even if CLA resulted in a slight decrease in body fat, particularly of abdominal fat in obese men. On the contrary, CLA isomer induced lipid peroxidation, as reported in Fig. 12.6. Administration of a CLA mixture to obese men at 4.2 g/day for 1 month resulted in an increase of both 8-isoprostaglandin $F_{2\alpha}$ ($PGF_{2\alpha}$) and of 15-oxo dihydro-$PGF_{2\alpha}$ as indicators of non-enzymic and enzymatic arachidonic acid oxidation, respectively, (Basu *et al.*, 2000) as compared with the control group. However, these peroxidation parameters went back to their original values 2 weeks after cessation of the treatment (Fig. 12.6). In another feeding trial on 60 men with metabolic syndrome, the same team observed the same effect on lipid peroxidation parameters when pure 10t, 12c-18:2 was administered (Fig. 12.7) indicating that the effect observed during the first study could be due to the 10t,12c isomer (Riserus *et al.*, 2002b). Furthermore, feeding this pure isomer also resulted in an increase of C-reactive protein by 110% compared with placebo. The increase in 8-iso-PGF2α was also independently related to insulin resistance and oxidative stress seems closely related to insulin resistance. The 10t,12c-18:2 isomer was also found to induce hyperproinsulinaemia which as reported by the

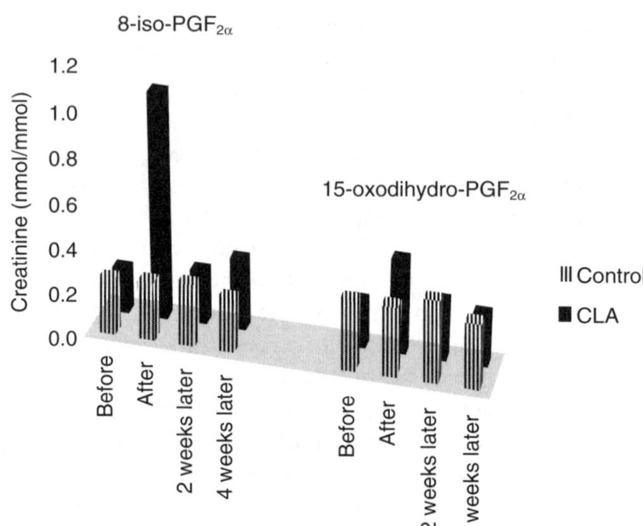


**Fig. 12.6** Effect of feeding and of withdrawing CLA to humans on the excretion of 8-isoprostaglandin $F_{2\alpha}$ ($PGF_{2\alpha}$) and of 15-oxodihydro-$PGF_{2\alpha}$ in urine.

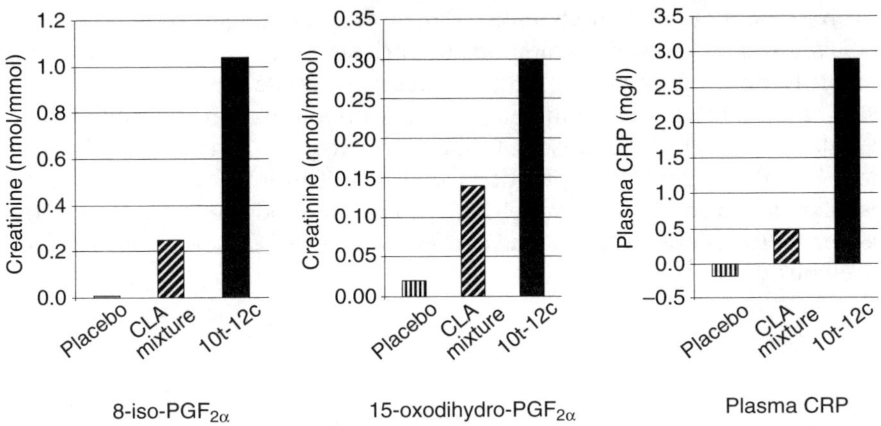


**Fig. 12.7** Effect of feeding pure 10t,12c and a CLA mixture on plasma C-reactive protein (CRP) and on the excretion of 8-iso-$PGF_{2\alpha}$ and of 15-oxodihydro-$PGF_{2\alpha}$ in urine.

authors may predict diabetes and cardiovascular disease (Riserus *et al.*, 2004b). Interestingly, a similar effect of an enriched 9c,11t fraction (increased insulin resistance, lipid peroxidation compared with placebo) was observed without affecting serum lipids or glucose concentration (Riserus *et al.*, 2004b) while 10t,12c was shown to increase glycaemia and decrease HDL cholesterol (Riserus *et al.*, 2002a). The authors, however, think that further work with a larger group is needed before any conclusions about the effect of the 9c,11t isomer in obese men can be drawn. In contrast, a study carried out on healthy subjects (Noone *et al.*, 2002) indicated that a mixture of CLA improved plasma triacyglycerol concentrations with no adverse effects on insulin and glucose metabolism.

## 12.5 Conclusions: conjugated linoleic acid and functional foods

If we consider what has been published on the effects of CLA in animals and humans, the consumption of food containing CLA does not seem to provide enough active component to exert any beneficial activity. As demonstrated for mammary cancer and for atherosclerosis (Sebedio *et al.*, 2003) the active component is the 9c,11t-18:2, and increasing the daily consumption of CLA up to 3 g/day would hardly be possible either by increasing the amount of products containing CLA or/and by enriching products from ruminant origin for example. As previously underlined, a lot of consideration has been given to the second solution and strategies have been proposed not only to enrich milk and meat from ruminants but also pig and chicken tissues. However, methods of enrichment practised for ruminants are different from those used in the latter case. While the fatty acid precursors of CLA are fed to ruminants, ClA mixtures containing both the 9c,11t- and the 10t,12c-18:2 isomers are usually given to pigs and chickens (Watkins and Li, 2003). This latter practice would result in introducing the 10t,12c isomer in the food chain, which may not be a good idea considering the adverse effects observed in some cases with the 10t,12c isomer, as discussed previously.

## 12.6 References

ATKINSON R L (1999), 'Conjugated linoleic acid for altering body composition', in YURAWECZ M P, MOSSOBA M M, KRAMER J K B, PARIZA M W, NELSON G J (Eds), *Advances in Conjugated Linoleic Acid Research*, volume 1. Champaign, AOCS Press, pp. 348–353.

AZAIN M J, HAUSMAN D B, SISK M B, FLATT W P and JEWELL D E (2000), 'Dietary conjugated linoleic acid reduces rat adipose tissue cell size rather than cell number', *J. Nutr.*, **130**, 1548–1554.

BANNI S, HEYS S D and WAHLE K W J (2003), 'Conjugated linoleic acids as anticancer nutrients: studies in vivo and cellular mechanisms', in Sebedio J L, Christie W W, Adlof R (Eds), *Advances in Conjugated Linoleic Acid Research*, volume 2. Champaign, AOCS Press, pp. 267–282.

BASU S, RISERUS U, TURPEINEN A and VESSBY B (2000), 'Conjugated linoleic acid induces lipid peroxidation in men with abdominal obesity', *Clin. Sci.*, **99**, 511–516.

BELURY M A, MAHON A and BANNI S (2003), 'The conjugated linoleic acid (CLA) isomer, t10c12-CLA, is inversely associated with changes in body weight and serum leptin in subjects with type 2 diabetes mellitus', *J. Nutr.*, **133**, 257S–260S.

BERVEN G, BYE A, HALS O, BLANKSON H, FAGERTUN H and THOM E (2000), 'Safety of conjugated linoleic acid (CLA) in overweight or obese volunteers', *Eur. J. Lipid Sci. Technol.*, **102**, 455–462.

BLANKSON H, STAKKESTAD J A, FAGERTUN H, THOM E, WADSTEIN J and GUDMUNDSEN O (2000), 'Conjugated linoleic acid reduces body fat mass in overweight and obese humans', *J. Nutr.*, **130**, 2943–2948.

BOUTHEGOURD J C, EVEN P C, GRIPOIS D, TIFFON B, BLOUQUIT M F, ROSEAU S, LUTTON C, TOME D and MARTIN J C (2002), 'A CLA mixture prevents body triglyceride accumulation without affecting energy expenditure in Syrian hamsters', *J. Nutr.*, **132**, 2682–2689.

CHOI Y, KIM Y C, HAN Y B, PARK Y, PARIZA M W and NTAMBI J M (2000), 'The trans-10,cis-12 isomer of conjugated linoleic acid downregulates stearoyl-CoA desaturase 1 gene expression in 3T3-L1 adipocytes', *J. Nutr.*, **130**, 1920–1924.

CHRISTIE W W (2003), 'Analysis of conjugated linoleic acid: an overview', in SEBEDIO J L, CHRISTIE W W, ADLOF R (Eds), *Advances in Conjugated Linoleic Acid Research*, volume 2, Champaign, AOCS Press, pp. 1–12.

CLEMENT L, POIRIER H, NIOT I, BOCHER V, GUERRE-MILLO M, KRIEF S, STAELS B and BESNARD P (2002), 'Dietary trans-10,cis-12 conjugated linoleic acid induces hyperinsulinemia and fatty liver in the mouse', *J. Lipid Res.*, **43**, 1400–1409.

COOK M E, BUTZ D, LI G, PARIZA M, WHIGHAM L and YANG M (2003), 'Conjugated linoleic acid enhances immune responses but protects against the collateral damage of immune events' in SEBEDIO J L, CHRISTIE W W, ADLOF R (Eds), *Advances in Conjugated Linoleic Acid Research*, volume 2. Champaign, AOCS Press, pp. 283–291.

CORL B A, BAUMGARD L H, DWYER D A, GRIINARI J M, PHILLIPS B S and BAUMAN D E (2001), 'The role of delta 9-desaturase in the production of cis9,trans11 CLA', *J. Nutr. Biochem.*, **12**, 622–630.

CORL B A, BAUMGARD L H, GRIINARI J M, DELMONTE P, MOREHOUSE K M, YURAWECZ M P and BAUMAN D E (2002), 'Trans7-cis9 CLA is synthesized endogenously by delta 9-desaturase in dairy cows', *Lipids*, **37**, 681–688.

CORL B A, BARBANO D M, BAUMAN D E and IP C (2003), 'Cis-9, trans-11 CLA derived endogenously from trans-11 18 : 1 reduces cancer risk in rats', *J. Nutr.*, **133**, 2893–2900.

DEGRACE P, DEMIZIEUX L, GRESTI J, CHARDIGNY J M, SEBEDIO J L and CLOUET P (2003), 'Association of liver steatosis with lipid oversecretion and hypotriglyceridemia in C57BL/6j mice fed trans-10, cis-12 linoleic acid', *FEBS Lett.*, **546**, 335–339.

DEGRACE P, DEMIZIEUX L, GRESTI J, CHARDIGNY J M, SEBEDIO J L and CLOUET P (2004), 'Hepatic steatosis is not due to impaired fatty acid oxidation capacities in C57BL/6j mice fed the conjugated trans-10, cis-12-isomer of linoleic acid', *J. Nutr.*, **134**, 861–867.

DESROCHES S, CHOUINARD P Y, GALIBOIS I, CORNEAU L, DELISLE J, LAMARCHE B, COUTURE P and BERGERON N (2005), 'Lack of effect of dietary conjugated linoleic acids naturally incorporated into butter on the lipid profile and body composition of overweight and obese men', *Am. J. Clin. Nutr.*, **82**, 309–319.

EVANS M, GEIGERMAN C, COOK J, CURTIS L, KUEBLER B and MCINTOSH M (2000), 'Conjugated linoleic acid suppresses triglyceride accumulation and induces apoptosis in 3T3-L1 preadipocytes', *Lipids*, **35**, 899–910.

EVANS M, BROWN J and MCINTOSH M (2002), 'Isomer-specific effects of conjugated linoleic acid (CLA) on adiposity and lipid metabolism', *J. Nutr. Biochem.*, **13**, 508.

GAULLIER J M, HALSE J, HOYE K, KRISTIANSEN K, FAGERTUN H, VIK H and GUDMUNDSEN O (2004), 'Conjugated linoleic acid supplementation for 1 y reduces body fat mass in healthy overweight humans', *Am. J. Clin. Nutr.*,**79**, 1118–1125.

GAULLIER J M, HALSE J, HOYE K, KRISTIANSEN K, FAGERTUN H, VIK H and GUDMUNDSEN O (2005), 'Supplementation with conjugated linoleic acid for 24 months is well tolerated by and reduces body fat mass in healthy overweight humans', *J. Nutr.*, **135** (4), 778–784.

GAVINO V C, GAVINO G, LEBLANC M J and TUCHWEBER B (2000), 'An isomeric mixture of conjugated linoleic acids but not pure cis-9,trans-11-octadecadienoic acid affects body weight gain and plasma lipids in hamsters', *J. Nutr.*, **130**, 27–29.

HA Y L, GRIMM L K and PARIZA M W (1987), 'Anticarcinogens from fried ground beef: heat altered derivatives of linoleic acid', *Carcinogenesis*, **8**, 1881–1887.

KAMPHUIS M M, LEJEUNE M P, SARIS W H and WESTERTERP-PLANTENGA M S (2003), 'The effect of conjugated linoleic acid supplementation after weight loss on body weight regain, body composition, and resting metabolic rate in overweight subjects', *Int. J. Obes. Relat. Metab. Disord.*, **27**, 840–847.

KANG K, LIU W, ALBRIGHT K J, PARK Y and PARIZA M W (2003), 'Trans-10,cis-12 CLA inhibits differentiation of 3T3-L1 adipocytes and decreases PPAR gamma expression', *Biochem. Biophys. Res. Commun.*, **303**, 795–799.

KEIM N L (2003), 'Conjugated linoleic acid and body composition' in SEBEDIO J L, CHRISTIE W W, ADLOF R (Eds), *Advances in Conjugated Linoleic Acid Research*, volume 3, Champaign, AOCS Press, pp. 316–324.

KREIDER R B, FERREIRA M P, GREENWOOD M, WILSON M and ALMADA A L (2002), 'Effects of conjugated linoleic acid supplementation during resistance-training on body composition. Bone density, strength, and selected hematological markers', *J. Strength Cond. Res.*, **3**, 325–334.

KRITCHEVSKY D (2003), 'Conjugated linoleic acid in experimental atherosclerosis', in SEBEDIO J L, CHRISTIE W W, ADLOF R (Eds), *Advances in Conjugated Linoleic Acid Research*, volume 3, Champaign, AOCS Press, pp. 292–301.

MALPUECH-BRUGÈRE C, VERBOEKET-VAN D E VENNE W P, MENSINK R P, ARNAL M A, MORIO B, BRANDOLINI M, SAEBO A, LASSEL T S, CHARDIGNY J M, SEBEDIO J L and BEAUFRERE B (2004), 'Effects of two conjugated linoleic acid isomers on body fat mass in overweight humans', *Obes. Res.*, **12**, 591–598.

MOLONEY F, YEOW T P, MULLEN A, NOLAN J J and ROCHE H M (2004), 'Conjugated linoleic acid supplementation, insulin sensitivity, and lipoprotein metabolism in patients with type 2 diabetes mellitus', *Am. J. Clin. Nutr.*, **80**, 887–895.

MOUGIOS V, MATSAKAS A, PETRIDOU A, RING, S, SAGREDOS A, MELISSOPOULOU A, TSIGILIS N and NIKOLAIDIS M (2001), 'Effect of supplementation with conjugated linoleic acid on human serum lipids and body fat', *J. Nutr. Biochem.*, **12**, 585–594.

NOONE E, ROCHE H M, NUGENT A P and GIBNEY M J (2002), 'The effects of dietary supplementation using isomeric blends of conjugated linoleic acid on lipid metabolism in healthy human subjects', *Br. J. Nutr.*, **88**, 243–251.

OSTROWSKA E, MURALITHARAN M, CROSS R F, BAUMAN D E and DUNSHEA F R (1999), 'Dietary conjugated linoleic acids increase lean tissue and decrease fat deposition in growing pigs', *J. Nutr.*, **129**, 2037–2042.

PARIZA M W, PARK Y and COOK M E (2001), 'The biologically active isomers of conjugated linoleic acid', *Prog. Lipid Res.*, **40**, 283–298.

PARK Y, ALBRIGHT K J, LIU W, STORKSON J M, COOK M E and PARIZA M W (1997), 'Effect of conjugated linoleic acid on body composition in mice', *Lipids*, **32**, 853–858.

PARK Y, ALBRIGHT K J, STORKSON J M, LIU W, COOK M E and PARIZA M W (1999a), 'Changes in body composition in mice during feeding and withdrawal of conjugated linoleic acid', *Lipids*, **34**, 243–248.

PARK Y, STORKSON J M, ALBRIGHT K J, LIU W and PARIZA M W (1999b), 'Evidence that the trans-10,cis-12 isomer of conjugated linoleic acid induces body composition changes in mice', *Lipids*, **34**, 235–241.

PARODI P W (2003), 'Conjugated linoleic acid in food', in SEBEDIO J L, CHRISTIE W W, ADLOF R (Eds), *Advances in Conjugated Linoleic Acid Research*, volume 2, Champaign, AOCS Press, pp. 101–122.

PETRIDOU A, MOUGIOS V and SAGREDOS A (2003), 'Supplementation with CLA: isomer incorporation into serum lipids and effect on body fat of women', *Lipids*, **38**, 805–811.

POIRIER H, ROUAULT C, CLEMENT L, NIOT I, MONNOT M C, GUERRE-MILLO M and BESNARD P (2005), 'Hyperinsulinaemia triggered by dietary conjugated linoleic acid is associated with a decrease in leptin and adiponectin plasma levels and pancreatic beta cell hyperplasia in the mouse', *Diabetologia*, **48**, 1059–1065.

RISERUS U, BERGLUND L and VESSBY B (2001), 'Conjugated linoleic acid (CLA) reduced abdominal adipose tissue in obese middle-aged men with signs of the metabolic syndrome: a randomised controlled trial', *Int. J. Obes. Relat. Metab. Disord.*, **25**, 1129–1135.

RISERUS U, ARNER P, BRISMAR K and VESSBY B (2002a), 'Treatment with dietary trans10cis12 conjugated linoleic acid causes isomer specific insulin resistance in obese men with the metabolic syndrome', *Diabetes Care*, **25**, 1516–1521.

RISERUS U, BASU S, JOVINGE S, FREDRIKSON G, ARNLOV J and VESBY B (2002b), 'Supplementation with conjugated linoleic acid causes isomer-dependent oxidative stress and elevated C-protein', *Circulation*, **106**, 1925–1929.

RISERUS U, VESSBY B, ARNLOV J and BASU S (2004a), 'Effects of cis-9,trans-11 conjugated linoleic acid supplementation on insulin sensitivity, lipid peroxidation, and proinflammatory markers in obese men', *Am. J. Clin. Nutr.*, **80**, 279–283.

RISERUS U, BESSBY B, ARNER P and ZETHELIUS B (2004b), 'Supplementation with trans10cis12-conjugated linoleic acid induces hyperproinsulinaemia in obese men: close association with impaired insulin sensitivity', *Diabetologia*, **47**, 1016–1019.

SAEBO A (2003), 'Commercial synthesis of conjugated linoleate', in Sebedio JL, Christie WW, Adlof R (Eds), *Advances in Conjugated Linoleic Acid Research*, volume 2, Champaign, AOCS Press, pp. 71–81.

SEBEDIO J L, CHRISTIE W W and ADLOF R (2003), '*Advances in Conjugated Linoleic Acid Research*, volume 2, Champaign, AOCS Press.

SEHAT N, KRAMER J K, MOSSOBA M M, YURAWECZ M P, ROACH J A, EULITZ K, MOREHOUSE K M and KU Y (1998), 'Identification of CLA isomers in cheese by gas chromatography, silver ion high performance liquid chromatography and mass spectra reconstructed ion profiles', *Lipids*, **33**, 963–971.

SMEDMAN A and VESSBY B (2001), 'Conjugated linoleic acid supplementation in humans – metabolic effects', *Lipids*, **36**, 773–781.

STANTON C, MURPHY J, MCGRATH E and DEVERY R (2003), 'Animal feeding strategies for conjugated linoleic acid enrichment of milk', in SEBEDIO J L, CHRISTIE W W, ADLOF R (Eds) '*Advances in Conjugated Linoleic Acid Research*, volume 2, Champaign, AOCS Press, pp. 123–145.

THOM E, WADSTEIN J and GUDMUNDSEN O (2001), 'Conjugated linoleic acid reduces body fat in healthy exercising humans', *J. Int. Med. Res.*, **29**, 392–396.

TRICON S, BURDGE G C, KEW S, BANERJEE T, RUSSELL J J, JONES E L, GRIMBLE R F, WILLIAMS C M, YAQOOB P and CALDER P C (2004), 'Opposing effects of cis-9,trans-11 and trans-10,cis-12 conjugated linoleic acid on blood lipids in healthy humans', *Am. J. Clin. Nutr.*, **80**, 614–620.

TSUBOYAMA-KASAOKA N, TAKAHASHI M, TANEMURA K, KIM H J, TANGE T, OKUYAMA H, KASAI M, IKEMOTO S and EZAKI O (2000), 'Conjugated linoleic acid supplementation reduces adipose tissue by apoptosis and develops lipodystrophy in mice', *Diabetes*, **49**, 1534–1542.

WANG Y W and JONES P J (2004), 'Conjugated linoleic acid and obesity control: efficacy and mechanisms', *Int. J. Obes. Relat. Metab. Disord.*, **28**, 941–955.

WATKINS B A and LI Y (2003), 'CLA in functional food: enrichment of animal products', in SEBEDIO J L, CHRISTIE W W, ADLOF R (Eds), *Advances in Conjugated Linoleic Acid Research*, volume 2, Champaign, AOCS Press, pp. 174–188.

WEST D B, DELANY J P, CAMET P M, BLOHM F, TRUETT A A and SCIMECA J (1998), 'Effects of conjugated linoleic acid on body fat and energy metabolism in the mouse', *Am.J. Physiol.*, **275**, R667–R672.

ZAMBELL K L, KEIM N L, VAN LOAN M D, GALE B, BENITO P, KELLEY D S and NELSON G J (2000), 'Conjugated linoleic acid supplementation in humans: effects on body composition and energy expenditure,' *Lipids*, **35**, 777–782.

# 13

# Omega-3 fatty acids and other polyunsaturated fatty acids and weight control

**M. Sörhede Winzell and B. Ahrén, Lund University, Sweden**

## 13.1 Introduction

Over the past decades, clinical investigations have evaluated the effects of polyunsaturated fatty acids (PUFAs), with particular interest in the omega-3 (or n-3) PUFAs, and their potential role in preventing metabolic diseases (Simopoulos, 1999, Manco *et al.*, 2004, Riccardi *et al.*, 2004, Nettleton and Katz, 2005). Over the past century, there has been a shift in the type of fat being consumed and today diets contain large amounts of saturated fat, high levels of omega-6 (or n-6) PUFAs and trans-fatty acids. The ratio between omega-6 and omega-3 PUFAs has increased tremendously due to decreased fish consumption in combination with increased intake of omega-6 PUFAs, owing mainly to the use of vegetable oils in cooking.

High intake of dietary fats, in particular saturated fats, may lead to the development of obesity, insulin resistance and type 2 diabetes (Arner *et al.*, 1991; Taniguchi *et al.*, 1992; Shulman, 2000; Zraika *et al.*, 2002). This seems to be closely connected to the accumulation of triglycerides in non-adipocytes – including hepatocytes, myocytes and pancreatic β-cells – a phenomenon that has been called lipotoxicity (Zhou *et al.*, 2000; Unger, 2003). Lipotoxicity is associated with increased endogenous glucose production from the liver, impaired insulin-stimulated glucose uptake in skeletal muscle and blunted glucose-stimulated insulin secretion from pancreatic β-cells (Unger and Orci, 2000, Unger and Zhou, 2001). The PUFAs may, however, exert different effects on metabolism, for example: (1) regulating fuel partitioning within the cell by stimulating β-oxidation and inhibiting lipogenesis; (2) altering membrane stability and fluidity and thereby affecting insulin signalling; (3) regulating gene transcription mainly via fatty acid regulated transcription factors such as the peroxisomal proliferator-activated receptors (PPARs) and the sterol regulatory element binding protein-1 (SREBP-1) (Clarke and Jump, 1994; Krey *et al.*, 1997; Nakatani *et al.*, 2003; Sampath and Ntambi, 2004). PUFAs may therefore have the capacity to prevent or counteract the detrimental effects of high-fat diets on body weight and whole-body metabolism.

It is important to determine optimal doses of PUFAs for prevention and treatment of metabolic diseases including overweight and obesity. This chapter will focus on the effect of various PUFAs, in particular the omega-3 PUFAs, on the control of body weight and whether dietary supplementation with these fatty acids may improve insulin resistance and type 2 diabetes.

## 13.2 Determining the role of omega-3 fatty acids and other polyunsaturated fatty acids in weight control

The positive effects of omega-3 PUFAs were observed early on among Greenland Inuits, who, despite high fat intake, displayed low mortality from coronary heart disease (Dyerberg *et al.*, 1975). Other epidemiological studies have reported lower prevalence of obesity, type 2 diabetes and cardiovascular diseases in populations consuming large amounts of omega-3 PUFAs from fatty fish (Mouratoff *et al.*, 1969; Kromann and Green, 1980). Subsequent studies have demonstrated that dietary supplementation of omega-3 PUFAs exerts positive effects in several metabolic diseases including coronary heart disease, hypertension, arteriosclerosis, diabetes and inflammatory diseases (Terry *et al.*, 2003; Din *et al.*, 2004; Calder, 2004; Ruxton *et al.*, 2004).

### 13.2.1 Definition, structure and metabolism

The PUFAs are fatty acids containing two or more double bonds. These fatty acids are essential since they cannot be produced in the human body and must therefore be provided in the diet. There are two main types of PUFA, the omega-3 and the omega-6 fatty acids. In the omega-3 PUFAs, the first double bond is located between the third and the fourth carbons, counting from the methyl end of the carbon chain; in the omega-6 PUFA the double bond is located between the sixth and the seventh carbons (Fig. 13.1).

Animals cannot, in general, produce omega-3 or omega-6 fatty acids since they lack the enzymes needed for insertion of the double bonds, whereas in plants these fatty acids are produced via Δ12- and Δ15-desaturase activity. The simplest members of the omega-6 and omega-3 fatty

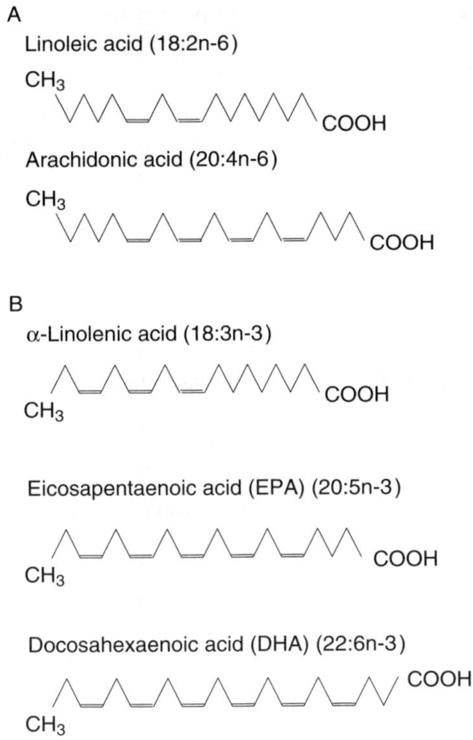


**Fig. 13.1** Schematic structures of common (A) omega-6 and (B) omega-3 PUFAs.

acids are linoleic acid (18:2n-6) and α-linolenic acid (18:3n-3), respectively (Fig. 13.1). Although mammalian cells do not synthesise linoleic acid and α-linolenic acid, these fatty acids are metabolised by desaturation and elongation reactions (Fig. 13.2). Linoleic acid is converted into γ-linolenic acid (18:3n-6), which in turn can be elongated to produce arachidonic acid (20:4n-6) (Fig. 13.2). The same group of enzymes have the ability to metabolise α-linolenic acid and convert it into eicosapentaenoic acid (EPA; 20:5n-3). There is thus a competition between the omega-6 and the omega-3 fatty acids in the enzymatic reactions and also for their metabolisation. The Δ6-desaturase reaction is the rate-limiting step, and this enzyme has α-linolenic acid as its preferred substrate. In the next reaction step, EPA can be further converted through elongation to docosahexaenoic acid (DHA; 22:6n-3) (Fig. 13.2). These long-chain, more unsaturated forms of linoleic acid and α-linolenic acid are in turn substrates for the production of important biological molecules, which will be discussed later in this chapter.

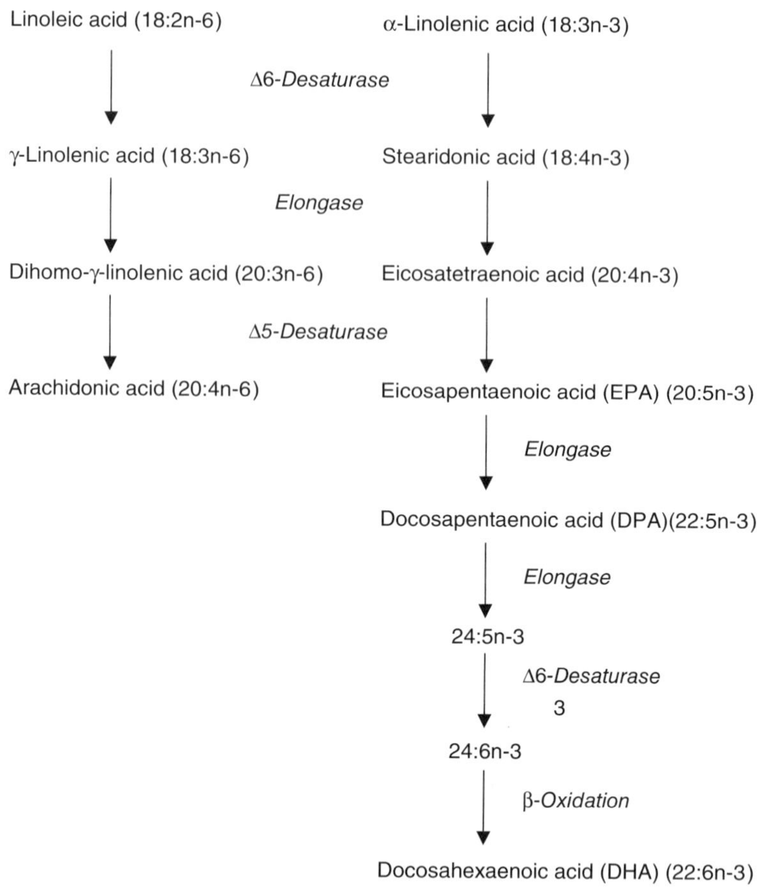


**Fig. 13.2** Metabolic pathways for conversion of linoleic acid and α-linolenic acid into longer derivatives in mammalian cells.

### 13.2.2 Dietary sources

The different forms of the PUFAs are found in different food sources (Table 13.1). Plant seed oils like corn oil, sunflower oil and safflower oil are rich in omega-6 PUFAs, constituting up to 75% of the fatty acid content. Most plant oils are richer in omega-6 PUFAs than in omega-3 PUFAs (Table 13.2). Sunflower and safflower oil exist in two different forms, one rich in monounsaturated fat and one rich in PUFAs. Linoleic sunflower oil is available as liquid oil and it is also used in margarine. Because of the high levels of PUFAs in these oils, they are susceptible to oxidation during commercial usage, especially frying, and so they are hydrogenated to a more stable form. Thus, important dietary sources of omega-6 PUFAs are the vegetable oils and margarines. Green plant tissues are rich in α-linolenic acid (18:3n-3), constituting more than 50% of the fatty acids. This is, however,

**Table 13.1** Food sources of different omega-3 and omega-6 PUFAs

| Type of PUFA | Structure | Source |
|---|---|---|
| Omega-3 | α-Linolenic acid | Walnuts, flaxseed oil, canola oil |
| | EPA | Fatty fish, fish oil |
| | DHA | Fatty fish, fish oil |
| Omega-6 | Linoleic acid | Corn, safflower, soybean and sunflower oil |
| | γ-Linolenic acid | Seed oils of borage, blackcurrant and evening primrose |
| | Arachidonic acid | Meat, eggs |

**Table 13.2** PUFA content in vegetable oils

| Vegetable oil | PUFA content (% by weight) | 18:2 Linoleic acid (n-6) | 18:3 γ-Linoleic acid (n-6) α-Linolenic acid (n-3) |
|---|---|---|---|
| Canola oil | 29.6 | 20.3 | 9.3 |
| Corn oil | 54.7 | 53.5 | 1.2 |
| Flaxseed oil | 66 | 12.7 | 53.3 |
| Safflower oil | 74.6 | 74.6 | 0 |
| Soybean oil | 57.9 | 51.1 | 6.8 |
| Sunflower oil | 65.7 | 65.7 | 0 |

not a significant source of omega-3 PUFAs since the total fat content is very low (Table 13.3). α-Linolenic acid is abundant in plant oils derived from flaxseed, soybean and rapeseed (Table 13.2). The longer forms of omega-3 PUFAs are more readily found in fatty fish like salmon, herring and mackerel, but also are also found in lean fish liver – which contains large amounts of EPA and DHA (Table 13.3). Nuts contain considerable amounts of omega-3 PUFAs and walnuts, in particular, are rich in α-linolenic acid (Feldman, 2002).

The composition of dietary fatty acids has changed over the last 100 years (Simopoulos, 1995). The total intake of fat and the amount of saturated fats have increased as well as the omega-6 PUFAs, while the intake of omega-3 PUFAs has decreased. Studies in Palaeolithic nutrition suggest that the hunter–gatherer populations consumed equal amounts of omega-6 and omega-3 PUFAs (Eaton *et al.*, 1998). Today the ratio between these fatty acids is 10–20:1 in the Western diet (Simopoulos, 1999). The reason for the decreased intake of omega-3 PUFAs is mainly a reduced intake of fish. In fact, modern agriculture results in decreased omega-3 PUFA content in many foods – including vegetables, meats, eggs and even in cultured fish – due to the industrial production of animal feed with high contents of omega-6-rich grains (Crawford, 1968, Simopoulos, 1999). The increased amount of omega-6 compared with omega-3 PUFAs in standard diets may have

**Table 13.3** Food sources of omega-3 fatty acids

| Source | Omega-3 fatty acid (% by weight) |
|---|---|
| Seafood | |
| Mackerel | 1.8–5.3 |
| Herring | 1.2–3.1 |
| Salmon, tuna, trout | 0.5–1.6 |
| Halibut | 0.4–0.9 |
| Shrimp, cod | 0.2–0.5 |
| Plaice, flounder, haddock | 0.2 |
| Nuts and seeds | |
| Almonds | 0.4 |
| Flaxseed | 22.8 |
| Peanuts | 0.003 |
| Walnuts, black | 3.3 |
| Walnuts, English | 6.8 |
| Vegetables | |
| Broccoli (raw) | 0.1 |
| Kale (raw) | 0.2 |
| Lettuce | 0.1 |
| Radish seeds | 0.7 |
| Seaweed, Spirulina (dried) | 0.8 |
| Soybeans, green (raw) | 3.2 |
| Soybeans, mature seeds sprouted | 2.1 |
| Spinach (raw) | 0.1 |

profound effects on human health since studies have indicated that omega-6 PUFAs may shift the physiological status into a prothrombotic, proaggregatory status with increased vasoconstriction and decreased bleeding time (Calder, 2005). The omega-3 PUFAs on the other hand seem anti-inflammatory, antithrombotic and hypolipidaemic, and may thus have beneficial effects in the prevention and/or treatment of several metabolic diseases (Calder, 2005).

The dietary PUFA intake is rather similar throughout Western societies. In Sweden and Finland the PUFAs represent around 5% of the total energy consumption (Becker, 1999, Valsta, 1999) and in the United States the intake averages 7%. The omega-3 PUFAs represent ~0.7% of the energy intake, mainly deriving from intake of vegetable oils. The ratio of omega-6 and omega-3 fatty acids is thus approximately 10:1 (Kris-Etherton *et al.*, 2000). The dietary sources of PUFAs are mainly vegetable oils and linoleic acid is the major form, constituting 84–89%, while around 10% are represented by α-linolenic acid. The intake of highly unsaturated PUFAs, like the EPA and DHA found in fatty fish, is low, being 0.1–0.65 g/day in the United States. In the United Kingdom the pattern is similar with increasing consumption of linoleic acid (omega-6) and an estimated omega-3 intake of 0.1–0.5 g/day (Sanders, 2000). However, in Malaysian adults the eating pattern is different. The total fat intake range is 22–26%, while in Western countries it is 35–40%, and the PUFAs constitute only around 4% of the fats. The PUFAs consumed are mainly omega-6 linoleic acid and the omega-6:omega-3 ratio is approximately 10, similar to that in Europe and the United States (Tkw, 1997).

### 13.2.3 Food intake and body weight control

High-fat food intake is considered to be one of the major causes of the development of obesity and obesity-associated insulin resistance (Astrup, 2001; Riccardi *et al.*, 2004). Laboratory animal studies and epidemiological studies in humans have demonstrated that consumption of high-fat dense diets, a typically Western diet, results in insulin resistance and obesity (Storlien *et al.*, 2000; Astrup, 2001; Winzell and Ahren, 2004). There are however, studies indicating that different types of fat have different effects on whole-body energy metabolism and glucose homeostasis, and inclusion of dietary oils containing PUFAs have been proposed to exert positive effects both in patients and in animal models of type 2 diabetes (Malasanos and Stacpoole, 1991; Storlien *et al.*, 1991). There are studies demonstrating that PUFAs, in particular the omega-3 PUFAs (EPA and DHA), are less effective in promoting obesity compared with saturated fats (Shillabeer and Lau, 1994; Azain, 2004). The mechanisms behind these observations probably involve modulation of fuel partitioning since PUFAs down-regulate lipogenesis and stimulate fat oxidation, because these fatty acids regulate the expression of several genes involved in lipid metabolism (Clarke, 2004; Sampath and Ntambi, 2004). Reduction in body fat content has been observed in rodents fed a diet containing fish oil (Ruzickova *et al.*, 2004; Ikemoto *et al.*, 1996), demonstrating that omega-3 PUFAs decreased the visceral fat by inhibiting both hypertrophy and hyperplasia of the fat cells.

In contrast, the effect of omega-3 PUFA on human body weight control is rather limited. However, in a recent study, overweight men and women were assigned to a daily fish meal, a weight-loss programme or the two in combination for 16 weeks and the effects on body weight and the plasma glucose and lipid profile were investigated (Mori *et al.*, 1999). The fish meal did not in itself reduce the body weight of these obese subjects, but the dietary fish component significantly improved the outcome of the weight-loss programme in that body weight was reduced in combination with improved glucose and insulin levels as well as the serum lipid profile. In another study, 17 subjects (healthy, obese and type 2 diabetic) entered a 5-week diet programme with diets rich in either saturated fats or PUFAs (Summers *et al.*, 2002). Both energy and fat intake appeared to be reduced in the subjects on the PUFA-rich diets, although body weight was not altered. The abdominal subcutaneous fat area was reduced in the group consuming the PUFA-rich diet, and this coincided with improved insulin sensitivity. The results indicate that PUFAs are effective in altering body fat content, which may have beneficial effects on energy metabolism.

### 13.2.4 Clinical studies on the effect of polyunsaturated fatty acids on glucose control and dyslipidaemia

The effect of omega-3 fatty acids on glycaemic control in humans is controversial. Several studies and reviews have indicated that omega-3 PUFAs have adverse effects in that these fatty acids induce elevated basal plasma glucose, and this was particularly pronounced in patients with type 2 diabetes consuming large amounts of fish oil (>10 g fish oil/day) (Borkman *et al.*, 1989; Friday *et al.*, 1989; Vessby, 1989). However, in other studies with lower doses of omega-3 PUFAs, ranging from 1–2 g/day, glucose homeostasis was maintained within normal ranges (Westerveld *et al.*, 1993; Luo *et al.*, 1998; Sirtori *et al.*, 1998). Luo *et al.* (1998) demonstrated that a moderate intake of omega-3 PUFAs (1.8 g/day) in type 2 diabetic men resulted in a significant reduction in plasma triglyceride levels. There were, however, no effects on fasting glycaemia or $HbA_{1c}$. During the 2-month study, body weight and energy intake remained stable. In addition, in other studies, which included patients with hypertension and dyslipidaemia, no adverse effects on plasma glucose levels were observed (Grundt *et al.*, 1995; Toft *et al.*, 1995). In both human and animal studies, dietary omega-3 PUFA supplementation was found to result in reduced circulating triglyceride levels, which may be one explanation for the improved insulin sensitivity observed after fish-oil feeding (Mori *et al.*, 1999; Sirtori *et al.*, 1998). The triglyceride-lowering effect is the most consistent and reproducible finding in both animal and human studies with omega-3 PUFAs and fish oil. Two meta-analyses of trials with omega-3 PUFAs or fish oil in patients with type 1 and type 2 diabetics, as well as in healthy controls, demonstrated that dietary fish oils have no statistically significant effect on glycaemic control but the supplementation efficiently reduced plasma triglyceride levels (Friedberg *et al.*, 1998; Montori *et al.*, 2000). There is thus strong evidence suggesting no adverse effects of fish oil or omega-3 PUFAs on glycaemia, and beneficial effects on plasma lipids, when consumed in moderate doses (1–3 g/day).

Animal studies have demonstrated that various dietary fat subtypes can modulate insulin action indicating that PUFAs have positive effects on insulin sensitivity (Storlien *et al.*, 1991, 2000). One study, where rats were fed isocaloric high-fat diets with different types of fatty acids, demonstrated that diets rich in saturated fat resulted in insulin resistance while rats fed a high level of PUFAs with a low omega-6 : omega-3 ratio had normal insulin action (Storlien *et al.*, 1991). It is thus possible that saturated fatty acids affect the cellular membranes in a negative way resulting in impaired insulin action and that this can be prevented by the addition of unsaturated fatty acids to the diet (Ma *et al.*, 2004). PUFAs may thus, at least in animal models, affect glycaemic control by improving insulin sensitivity.

## 13.3 Effects of omega-3 fatty acids and other polyunsaturated fatty acids on energy metabolism and other factors connected to weight control

The mechanism behind the benefits of omega-3 PUFAs on energy metabolism is at present not completely understood. There are, however, many possibilities since these fatty acids have many different roles in a cell. For example, apart from being an energy source, fatty acids build up the cellular membranes, regulate gene expression and function as signalling molecules and as precursors for complex biologically active molecules such as, for example, eicosanoids (Simopoulos, 1999, Ruxton *et al.*, 2004). Since omega-3 PUFAs exert positive effects in many different diseases there have been implications for a common pathway for the effects. One mechanism that has been presented is the ability of omega-3 PUFAs to affect the biochemical composition of biological membranes (Ma *et al.*, 2004). Indeed, the cellular fatty acids composition is a mirror of the ingested types of fatty acids. Incorporation of PUFAs into lipid membranes results in altered interaction between the lipids and the membrane proteins (Ma *et al.*, 2004). There are, however, other possibilities that need to be considered – including the digestion and absorption of the fatty acids.

### 13.3.1 Digestion and absorption of fatty acids

The length and the degree of saturation of fatty acids influence the biophysical properties of the lipids. This has, for example, effects on the digestion and absorption of the fatty acids from the intestine (Small, 1991). Different sources of fat are composed of different types of triglycerides. Triglycerides are digested in the intestinal lumen by lipases to produce fatty acids and monoacylglycerol and the absorption of fatty acids from the intestinal lumen is generally an efficient process. After absorption, the fatty acids are taken up by the enterocytes where the triglycerides are reconstructed, packed in chylomicrons and very-low-density lipoproteins (VLDLs) and secreted into the lymph. From the lymph, the triglycerides are transported to various capillary beds where they bind to the capillary surface. Here, they are hydrolysed by lipoprotein lipase and the surrounding adipocytes or muscle cells take up the free fatty acids. However, the triglycerides containing long-chain PUFAs like arachidonic acid or EPA are poor substrates for lipoprotein lipase. Instead, they appear to be good substrates for hepatic lipase, and thus acylglycerols containing long-chain PUFAs are returned and metabolised by the liver. To be able to study the uptake and the destiny of the PUFAs, rats were fed purified triglycerides containing oleic acid and long-chain PUFAs (Fahey *et al.*, 1985). The results showed that the uptake of the PUFAs was significantly slower than the uptake of saturated or monounsaturated fatty acids. This demonstrates that the PUFAs are absorbed and metabolised at a lower rate, which may influence both appetite and satiety, two factors that are of great importance in weight control.

### 13.3.2 Effect on ectopic lipid accumulation

Studies in cell culture systems have demonstrated that fatty acids have effects on adipocyte proliferation and differentiation (Azain, 2004). Feeding rats a high-fat diet rich in PUFAs demonstrated no difference in pre-adipocyte replication compared with rats fed a normal diet, while a diet rich in saturated fats accelerated the replication (Shillabeer and Lau, 1994). Furthermore, the size of the adipose tissue was reduced in PUFA-fed rats compared with rats fed saturated fat and this was due to less efficient storage of triglycerides (Shillabeer and Lau, 1994). Thus, the diet containing saturated fat induced expansion of the adipose tissue more efficiently than the diet containing PUFAs; possible mechanisms for these effects are that PUFAs do not induce pre-adipocyte replication to the same extent and are less efficiently incorporated in triglycerides.

Feeding a diet rich in saturated fats results in accumulation of triglycerides, not only in adipose tissue but also in non-adipocytes and this phenomenon, called lipotoxicity, has been found to correlate to the onset of insulin resistance (Unger, 1995; Boden and Shulman, 2002). There are, however, studies indicating that diets enriched with PUFAs improve insulin sensitivity in both rodents and humans (Storlien *et al.*, 1991; 2000, Summers *et al.*, 2002). One possible mechanism of action is that PUFAs prevent the accumulation of lipids in non-adipocytes. In rodents, fish oil prevented lipid accumulation in adipose tissue more efficiently compared with other dietary oils, and it was suggested that omega-3 PUFAs increase fatty acid oxidation and inhibit triglyceride synthesis through affecting expression of specific genes involved in these metabolic pathways (Jump *et al.*, 1994).

### 13.3.3 Regulation of gene expression by polyunsaturated fatty acid

Fatty acids are converted to fatty acyl coenzyme A (CoA) rapidly after entering a cell. The fatty acid derivatives are then shunted into different cellular pathways such as oxidation for production of energy, membrane synthesis, elongation and/or desaturation, or production of signalling molecules. PUFAs have an important function in regulating gene expression. Several transcription factors such as PPARs, SREBPs, hepatocyte nuclear factor-4$\alpha$ (HNF-4$\alpha$) and liver X receptors (LXRa) have PUFAs as ligands (Krey *et al.*, 1997; Worgall *et al.*, 1998). The fatty acids bind to PPARs resulting in altered expression of genes involved in fatty acid degradation and oxidation, which in turn leads to reduced intracellular accumulation of triglycerides. Transcription of genes encoding lipogenic enzymes such as fatty acid synthase (FAS), acetyl-CoA carboxylase (ACC), and stearoyl-CoA desaturase (SCD) is down-regulated, while transcription of enzymes involved in fatty acid oxidation such as acyl-CoA oxidase (ACO), medium-chain acyl-CoA dehydrogenase (MCAD), carnitine palmitoyl transferase 1 (CPT-1), acyl-CoA synthase (ACS) and uncoupling protein 2 (UCP-2) is up-regulated (Krey *et al.*, 1997; Nakatani *et al.*, 2003; Levy *et al.*, 2004; Ide, 2005). This leads to pleiotrophic and complex actions of PUFAs involving a large variety of intracellular regulatory pathways. SREBP-1 is another transcription factor that regulates fatty acid metabolism in the liver in that its activation results in increased transcription of genes involved in lipogenesis (Horton *et al.*, 2002). Recent data have shown that rats fed a diet enriched with fish oil had reduced effect and expression of SREBPs in the liver (Xu *et al.*, 2001; Nakatani *et al.*, 2003). The overall effect of PUFAs on gene expression results in accelerated oxidation of fat and reduced lipogenesis.

### 13.3.4 The mechanism of polyunsaturated fatty acid in insulin resistance and type 2 diabetes

The molecular effects of PUFAs are such that these fatty acids may have an impact on the regulation of insulin sensitivity (Lombardo and Chicco, 2006). There are indeed indications that omega-3 PUFAs may have positive effects on glucose tolerance by reducing insulin resistance, as demonstrated in rodent models of obesity (Storlien *et al.*, 2000). Rats fed a high-fat diet supplemented with a low ratio of omega-6:omega-3 PUFA maintained normal insulin action, while rats fed a diet containing high levels of saturated and monounsaturated fats showed insulin resistance in several tissues (Storlien *et al.*, 1991). Feeding fish oil to mice, providing 5–10% of the daily energy intake, accelerated glucose uptake and maintained glucose homeostasis during high-fat feeding (Storlien *et al.*, 1997). The favourable effects of fish oil-derived PUFAs may be explained by suppression of hepatic fatty acids synthesis and increased fat oxidation. Another mechanism behind the positive effects of PUFAs on insulin sensitivity may occur through alteration in the plasma membrane composition of the cells. There is some evidence indicating that altered membrane structure may affect both insulin action and insulin binding to its receptor (Storlien *et al.*, 1996). Another possible mechanism behind the effects of PUFAs in metabolism can be attributed to changes in protein acylation. Many membrane proteins are modified by fatty acid acylation with saturated fatty acids like palmitate or myristate. Whether this has any significant effects in insulin signalling, or whether PUFAs play a role, is unknown at the present time. In summary, the metabolic effects of omega-3 PUFAs promote the reduction of triglyceride in skeletal muscle and liver, which in turn is associated with improved insulin action and glucose tolerance thereby preventing development of insulin resistance.

### 13.3.5 Islet metabolism, insulin secretion and polyunsaturated fatty acid

Besides insulin resistance defective islet function is also of importance for the development of glucose intolerance and type 2 diabetes. In fact, a normal islet function with a normal compensation in insulin secretion is a prerequisite for maintaining normal glucose homeostasis in insulin resistance (Ahren and Pacini, 2005). Therefore, to improve glucose homeostasis, effects on islet function are required. Fatty acids are known to acutely stimulate insulin secretion via several possible pathways. First, it is believed that fatty acids are taken up into the β-cell, where they are converted to long-chain acyl-CoA (LC-CoA). Through glucose metabolism the uptake and oxidation of the fatty acids are blocked through the effect of malonyl-CoA, which accumulates in the cytosol when β-cells are exposed to high glucose concentrations (Corkey *et al.*, 1989, Prentki *et al.*, 1992). Malonyl-CoA is an effective inhibitor of CPT-1, inhibiting the transport of fatty acyl-CoA into the mitochondria, resulting in increased accumulation of LC-CoA in the cytosol. LC-CoA has been found to exert effects at several levels in the β-cell to promote second-phase insulin secretion: through binding to the $K_{ATP}$ channels, affecting the exocytosis of insulin granulae, activation of protein kinases via acylation mechanism and thereby promoting insulin secretion (Corkey *et al.*, 2000, Deeney *et al.*, 2000, Yaney *et al.*, 2000). Although this seems to be a common pathway for most of the fatty acids, saturated fats are more potent in stimulating glucose-induced insulin secretion than unsaturated ones, as was recently observed in isolated human islets (Gravena *et al.*, 2002).

Another pathway for the fatty acids to stimulate insulin secretion is through the fatty acid binding protein GPR40 (Itoh *et al.*, 2003; Salehi *et al.*, 2005; Shapiro *et al.*, 2005). This is a G-protein-coupled receptor that has fatty acids as substrate. Both saturated (C12–C16) and unsaturated (C18–C22) fatty acids have the potency to induce increased intracellular $Ca^{2+}$ in Chinese hamster ovary (CHO) cells transfected with the GPR40 receptor (Itoh *et al.*, 2003; Itoh and Hinuma, 2005). A third indirect pathway for fatty acids to stimulate insulin secretion is through phospholipase $A_2$ ($PLA_2$), which is activated during glucose stimulation (Simonsson and Ahren, 2000). $PLA_2$ stimulates the formation of arachidonic acid and inhibition of $PLA_2$ results in blunted arachidonic acid formation, which was accompanied by reduced glucose-stimulated insulin secretion. Fish oil has been found to induce insulin secretion through incorporation of the omega-3 PUFAs in the plasma membrane to compete with the production of arachidonic acid.

In a recent study, inclusion of 7% omega-3 PUFAs in a high-fat diet fed to rats resulted in lower glucose-stimulated insulin secretion from isolated islets, possibly through direct effects of the fatty acids on the islets, blocking the hyper-secretion induced by saturated fatty acids (Holness *et al.*, 2003). In addition, *in vivo*, PUFA supplementation in rats fed a high-fat diet resulted in reversed insulin hyper-secretion, suggesting that PUFAs may have acute effects on islets resulting in reduced insulin secretion (Holness *et al.*, 2004). Therefore, PUFAs seems to be protective at low doses in fatty acid-induced apoptosis and may have anti-apoptotic effects in islets *in vivo*. Furthermore, the normalising effect of omega-3 PUFAs on high-fat diet-induced hyperinsulinaemia in response to glucose may have long-term beneficial effects on insulin sensitivity.

### 13.3.6 Polyunsaturated fatty acids and inflammation

It is now recognised that the adipocytes produce and actively secrete many hormones and cytokines into the circulation (Ahima and Flier, 2000). Many of these factors, collectively termed adipokines, are involved in inflammation and it has been suggested that inflammation is one important factor behind the development of obesity-related diseases (Havel, 2004; Berg and Scherer, 2005; Wellen and Hotamisligil, 2005).

The link between fatty acids and inflammation lies in the fact that the inflammatory mediators termed eicosanoids are generated from long-chain fatty acids. The role of PUFAs in inflammation has recently been thoroughly reviewed (Browning, 2003; Wu, 2004; Calder, 2005). Inflammatory cells contain high levels of the omega-6 PUFA arachidonic acid and low levels of the omega-3 PUFA EPA. The eicosanoids include prostaglandins, thromboxanes and leukotrienes, and these are typically produced from arachidonic acid. The eicosanoids in turn enhance the generation of reactive oxygen species and production of inflammatory cytokines like tumour necrosis factor-1$\alpha$ (TNF-1), interleukin-1 (IL-1) and IL-6 (Calder, 2005). Increased consumption of the omega-3 PUFAs EPA and DHA results in elevated levels of these fatty acids in the inflammatory cells, resulting in reduced production of eicosanoids with arachidonic acid as precursor. The eicosanoids produced from EPA are believed to be less potent in their inflammatory action compared with those formed from arachidonic acid. Thus, one positive effect of omega-3 PUFAs in inflammation is that less-potent eicosanoids are produced. Furthermore, EPA is precursor to a novel group of anti-inflammatory mediators (E-series resolvins) that may be of importance in the mechanism of action of PUFAs in inflammation (Serhan *et al.*, 2002).

EPA and DHA have a number of other anti-inflammatory effects downstream of the eicosanoid production. For example in cell culture systems with endothelial cells, EPA and DHA inhibited the production of IL-6 and IL-8 (De Caterina *et al.*, 1994). Dietary supplementation of fish oil in both rodents and humans has resulted in decreased production of TNF-1$\alpha$, IL-1 and IL-6 (Endres *et al.*, 1989; Yaqoob and Calder, 1995; Caughey *et al.*, 1996).

Omega-3 PUFAs may also have a direct effect on inflammatory gene expression through activation of transcription factors such as nuclear factor (NF)-κB (Novak *et al.*, 2003). Taken together, long-chain omega-3 PUFAs may function as anti-inflammatory agents in the prevention and/or treatment of obesity and its related diseases.

## 13.4 Producing omega-3 polyunsaturated fatty acids

### 13.4.1 Types and sources of polyunsaturated fatty acids

The therapeutic significance of omega-3 PUFAs has been clearly indicated in clinical trials and epidemiological studies (Bucher *et al.*, 2002; Hu *et al.*, 2002). Fatty fish or fish oils are the richest sources of long-chain omega-3 PUFAs, but as already discussed, the dietary intake of fish has decreased. However, fish stocks are also declining and there have been reports indicating the accumulation of heavy metals and pollutants in some fish (Hites *et al.*, 2004). There is thus an urgent need for alternative sources of long-chain omega-3 PUFAs and there is considerable interest in developing new techniques for this purpose. The primary producers of various omega-3 PUFAs in nature are bacteria, algae, fungi, insects and some invertebrates. Other PUFAs are extracted from oily plant seeds (Table 13.2).

### 13.4.2 Production and purification of omega-3 polyunsaturated fatty acids

The long-chain PUFAs arachidonic acid, EPA and DHA (Fig. 13.1) are of nutritional importance and also play important roles in the prevention of various diseases. Fish oil is the conventional source of EPA and DHA. However, fish oils contain a crude mixture of several different fatty acids and the omega-3 PUFAs need to be extracted and purified before they can be used for dietary supplementation in pharmacological applications. It should be noted that fish cannot produce the long-chain omega-3 PUFAs by themselves and the fatty acids that can be extracted from fish fat derive originally from marine microalgae. Many methods have been used to purify EPA and DHA from fish oil including, for example, chromatographic methods, distillation, enzymatic splitting and crystallisation. However, these processes are expensive and new methods and sources need to be identified. Microalgae produce omega-3 PUFAs and several studies have been performed to develop a commercially feasible technology to produce EPA directly from these marine plants (Wen and Chen, 2003). Even though there are a large number of EPA-containing microalgae, few have demonstrated industrial production potential. The major problems have been low growth rate, low cell density and high cost in the conventional photoautotrophic conditions. An alternative method is a heterotrophic cultivation system, where an organic carbon source such as sugar can be used as the sole energy source. This mode of culture eliminates the requirement for light and may increase productivity (Wen and Chen, 2003).

Recent progress has been made using another approach to produce long-chain PUFAs, which involves the use of transgenic plants (Napier *et al.*, 2004, Qi *et al.*, 2004). Long-chain omega-3 PUFAs such as arachidonic acid and EPA were produced and accumulated in plants that had been transfected with genes encoding enzymes participating in the omega-3/omega-6 biosynthetic pathway for formation of long-chain PUFAs. This is a new promising method for alternative production of these essential fatty acids.

## 13.5 Omega-3 and other polyunsaturated fatty acids in functional food products

Functional foods are food products that have beneficial effects on physiology and/or have the ability to reduce the risk of a disease. Functional foods may be conventional food or foods that have been enriched with functional components to provide greater health benefits, but they do not include purified substances provided in pills or capsules. Since omega-3 PUFAs have been shown to have beneficial effects in several health conditions they are considered to be a functional food. The positive effects of omega-3 PUFAs in different diseases have been established and these fatty acids have been particularly interesting in coronary heart disease but also in several other conditions such as arteriosclerosis, type 2 diabetes, cancer, depression and asthma (de Lorgeril *et al.*, 1994; Simopoulos, 1999; Ruxton *et al.*, 2004; Nettleton and Katz, 2005). The beneficial effects of omega-3 PUFAs on health have resulted in the production of dietary supplements becoming a large industry. There is also a large and growing market for producing functional foods enriched in omega-3 PUFAs, such as omega-3-enriched eggs or omega-3 PUFA-supplemented margarine. For example, in Sweden a dairy product company has produced a margarine containing 40% fat and consisting of butter, rapeseed oil and fish oil. Several companies have specialised in extracting omega-3 PUFAs from fish to provide omega-3-enriched fish oil to be used for the production of functional foods. Fish oil was earlier considered difficult to include in cooking or as a supplement in foods since it has a peculiar smell and taste. However, with today's techniques it is possible to produce fish oil extracts without this problem, making it easier to produce food products enriched with these fatty acids.

## 13.6 Future trends

### 13.6.1 Dietary recommendations and therapeutic use

As presented here, PUFAs have the potential to affect a large number of metabolic processes and, therefore, these fatty acids are beneficial in obesity and its related diseases. The most important effect of omega-3 PUFAs, and in particular EPA and DHA, is the triglyceride-lowering effect observed in humans (Connor *et al.*, 1993). Lowering circulating triglycerides has been proven to protect against coronary heart disease and the use of fish oil or increased consumption of fish after myocardial infarction reduced reinfarction and mortality (Calder, 2004). The American Heart Association have presented guidelines for dietary fish intake, proposing that patients without documented coronary heart disease should eat a variety of fish, preferably oily fish, twice a week (Kris-Etherton *et al.*, 2002). Patients with documented coronary heart disease should consume dietary supplementation of at least 1 g EPA and DHA per day. Long-chain omega-3 PUFAs derived from fish and fish oils have beneficial effects in people with pre-existing cardiovascular heart disease. One serving of fish per week may decrease the risk of mortality in heart failure by up to 40%. Patients with type 2 diabetes are often overweight or obese. To better control this disease it is important to eat healthily and to control fat intake. The American Diabetes Association recommend two to three servings of fish per week and the use of vegetable oils instead of butter in cooking (www.diabetes.org). Furthermore, the Department of Health and Human Services (HHS) and the Department of Agriculture (USDA) publish annually the *Dietary Guidelines for Americans* (www.healthierus.gov/dietaryguidelines/) providing advice on good dietary habits, which can promote health and reduce risk for major chronic diseases.

The role of PUFAs for body weight control is, however, at the present time not fully understood. Most studies indicate no change in body weight after increased intake of PUFAs. However, incorporation of a fish meal in a weight-loss programme improved the response to the diet with a tendency to increased weight loss, although this was not statistically significant (Mori *et al.*, 1999). Fasting insulin levels were significantly reduced and the lipid profile improved with decreased triglyceride levels and increased high-density lipoprotein levels. A dietary recommendation that is valid for all individuals is to consume a diet with: (1) decreased total fat content; (2) reduced saturated fat content; (3) reduced omega-6:omega-3 fatty acid ratio by increasing the intake of omega-3 PUFAs. This would be recommended to maintain body weight and whole-body glucose and lipid metabolism.

The positive effects of fish oil and omega-3 PUFAs in cardiovascular disease and mortality are apparent. However, most studies with increased fish intake or addition of dietary fish oil supplementation do not take into account that there may be other components present in fish that may be important in cardiovascular health. The recommendation by the American Heart Association is that the degree of PUFAs in the diet should be increased and that the ratio of omega-6:omega-3 PUFAs needs to be reduced. This will be achieved by increased consumption of plant-derived α-linolenic acid and marine-derived EPA and DHA (Kris-Etherton *et al.*, 2002). Another source of essential omega-3 PUFAs is walnuts, which despite being energy dense have no implications in inducing altered energy balance. Hence, incorporation of nuts into diets with low levels of saturated fats may have beneficial effects on weight reduction and maintenance (Gillen *et al.*, 2005).

In summary, different fat types have different effects on satiety. To be able to make clear recommendations regarding dietary PUFA supplementation, more studies are needed to evaluate the correct composition of fatty acids that induces satiety and maintains energy balance. Methods for prevention of metabolic abnormalities such as overweight, obesity and type 2 diabetes are urgently required and a primary long-term strategy to cure these diseases is to improve dietary habits. The use of PUFAs in the diet may, by stimulating the use of fat as an energy substrate and by reducing the accumulation of fat in the adipose tissue, significantly contribute to the maintenance or reduction of body weight.

## 13.7 Sources of further information and advice

There are many websites that can be consulted for dietary recommendations (Table 13.4). The American Dietetic Association has a site with information about food and nutrition for everyone who wants to keep a healthy lifestyle. Similar information can be found on the British Nutrition Foundation website and at the American Heart Association website.

## 13.8 Acknowledgements

This work has been supported by the Swedish Research Council (grant 6834), the European Union (grant QLK6-2002-02288, OB-AGE), the

**Table 13.4** Sources of further information and advice on dietary recommendations and PUFAs

| Organisation | Website |
|---|---|
| American Dietetic Association | www.eatright.org |
| American Diabetes Association | www.diabetes.org |
| American Heart Association | www.americanheart.org |
| British Nutrition Foundation | www.nutrition.org.uk |
| National Agricultural Library | www.nal.usda.gov/fnic |
| National Sunflower Association | www.sunflowernsa.com/oil/ |
| Pronova Biocare | www.pronovabiocare.com |
| Triomega | www.triomega.com |
| Biochemical information on lipids | www.cyberlipid.org |

Swedish Diabetes Association, Region Skåne and the Faculty of Medicine, Lund University.

## 13.9 References

AHIMA R S and FLIER J S (2000), Adipose tissue as an endocrine organ. *Trends Endocrinol Metab*, **11**, 327–332.

AHREN B and PACINI G (2005), Islet adaptation to insulin resistance: mechanisms and implications for intervention. *Diabetes Obes Metab*, **7**, 2–8.

ARNER P, POLLARE T and LITHELL H (1991), Different aetiologies of type 2 (non-insulin-dependent) diabetes mellitus in obese and non-obese subjects. *Diabetologia*, **34**, 483–487.

ASTRUP A (2001), Healthy lifestyles in Europe: prevention of obesity and type II diabetes by diet and physical activity. *Public Health Nutr*, **4**, 499–515.

AZAIN M J (2004), Role of fatty acids in adipocyte growth and development. *J Anim Sci*, **82**, 916–924.

BECKER W (1999), Dietary guidelines and patterns of food and nutrient intake in Sweden. *Br J Nutr*, **81** (Suppl 2), S113–S117.

BERG A H and SCHERER P E (2005), Adipose tissue, inflammation, and cardiovascular disease. *Circ Res*, **96**, 939–949.

BODEN G and SHULMAN G I (2002), Free fatty acids in obesity and type 2 diabetes: defining their role in the development of insulin resistance and beta-cell dysfunction. *Eur J Clin Invest*, **32** (Suppl 3), 14–23.

BORKMAN M, CHISHOLM D J, FURLER S M, STORLIEN L H, KRAEGEN E W, SIMONS L A and CHESTERMAN C N (1989), Effects of fish oil supplementation on glucose and lipid metabolism in NIDDM. *Diabetes*, **38**, 1314–1319.

BRISCOE C P, TADAYYON M, ANDREWS J L, BENSON W G, CHAMBERS J K, EILERT M M, ELLIS C, ELSHOURBAGY N A, GOETZ A S, MINNICK D T, MURDOCK P R, SAULS H R JR, SHABON U, SPINAGE L D, STRUM J C, SZEKERES P G, TAN K B, WAY J M, IGNAR D M, WILSON S and MUIR A I (2003), The orphan G protein-coupled receptor GPR40 is activated by medium and long chain fatty acids. *J Biol Chem*, **278**, 11303–11311.

BROWNING L M (2003), n-3 Polyunsaturated fatty acids, inflammation and obesity-related disease. *Proc Nutr Soc*, **62**, 447–453.

BUCHER H C, HENGSTLER P, SCHINDLER C and MEIER G (2002), N-3 polyunsaturated fatty acids in coronary heart disease: a meta-analysis of randomized controlled trials. *Am J Med*, **112**, 298–304.

CALDER P C (2004), n-3 Fatty acids and cardiovascular disease: evidence explained and mechanisms explored. *Clin Sci (Lond)*, **107**, 1–11.

CALDER P C (2005), Polyunsaturated fatty acids and inflammation. *Biochem Soc Trans*, **33**, 423–427.

CAUGHEY G E, MANTZIORIS E, GIBSON R A, CLELAND L G and JAMES M J (1996), The effect on human tumor necrosis factor alpha and interleukin 1 beta production of diets enriched in n-3 fatty acids from vegetable oil or fish oil. *Am J Clin Nutr*, **63**, 116–122.

CLARKE S D (2004), The multi-dimensional regulation of gene expression by fatty acids: polyunsaturated fats as nutrient sensors. *Curr Opin Lipidol*, **15**, 13–18.

CLARKE S D and JUMP D B (1994), Dietary polyunsaturated fatty acid regulation of gene transcription. *Annu Rev Nutr*, **14**, 83–98.

CONNOR W E, DEFRANCESCO C A and CONNOR S L (1993), N-3 fatty acids from fish oil. Effects on plasma lipoproteins and hypertriglyceridemic patients. *Ann N Y Acad Sci*, **683**, 16–34.

CORKEY B E, DEENEY J T, YANEY G C, TORNHEIM K and PRENTKI M (2000), The role of long-chain fatty acyl-CoA esters in beta-cell signal transduction. *J Nutr*, **130**, 299S–304S.

CORKEY B E, GLENNON M C, CHEN K S, DEENEY J T, MATSCHINSKY F M and PRENTKI M (1989), A role for malonyl-CoA in glucose-stimulated insulin secretion from clonal pancreatic beta-cells. *J Biol Chem*, **264**, 21608–21612.

CRAWFORD M A (1968), Fatty-acid ratios in free-living and domestic animals. Possible implications for atheroma. *Lancet*, **1**, 1329–1333.

DE CATERINA R, CYBULSKY M I, CLINTON S K, GIMBRONE M A JR and LIBBY P (1994), The omega-3 fatty acid docosahexaenoate reduces cytokine-induced expression of proatherogenic and proinflammatory proteins in human endothelial cells. *Arterioscler Thromb*, **14**, 1829–1836.

DE LORGERIL M, RENAUD S, MAMELLE N, SALEN P, MARTIN J L, MONJAUD I, GUIDOLLET J, TOUBOUL P and DELAYE J (1994), Mediterranean alpha-linolenic acid-rich diet in secondary prevention of coronary heart disease. *Lancet*, **343**, 1454–1459.

DEENEY J T, GROMADA J, HOY M, OLSEN H L, RHODES C J, PRENTKI M, BERGGREN P O and CORKEY B E (2000), Acute stimulation with long chain acyl-CoA enhances exocytosis in insulin-secreting cells (HIT T-15 and NMRI beta-cells). *J Biol Chem*, **275**, 9363–9368.

DIN J N, NEWBY D E and FLAPAN A D (2004), Omega 3 fatty acids and cardiovascular disease – fishing for a natural treatment. *Br Med J*, **328**, 30–35.

DYERBERG J, BANG H O and HJORNE N (1975), Fatty acid composition of the plasma lipids in Greenland Eskimos. *Am J Clin Nutr*, **28**, 958–966.

EATON S B, EATON S B 3rd, SINCLAIR A J, CORDAIN L and MANN N J (1998), Dietary intake of long-chain polyunsaturated fatty acids during the paleolithic. *World Rev Nutr Diet*, **83**, 12–23.

ENDRES S, GHORBANI R, KELLEY V E, GEORGILIS K, LONNEMANN G, VAN DER MEER J W, CANNON J G, ROGERS T S, KLEMPNER M S, WEBER P C, SCHAEFER E J, WOLFF S M and DINARELLO C A (1989), The effect of dietary supplementation with n-3 polyunsaturated fatty acids on the synthesis of interleukin-1 and tumor necrosis factor by mononuclear cells. *N Engl J Med*, **320**, 265–271.

FAHEY D A, SMALL D M, KODALI D R, ATKINSON D and REDGRAVE T G (1985), Structure and polymorphism of 1,2-dioleoyl-3-acyl-sn-glycerols. Three- and six-layered structures. *Biochemistry*, **24**, 3757–3764.

FELDMAN E B (2002), The scientific evidence for a beneficial health relationship between walnuts and coronary heart disease. *J Nutr*, **132**, 1062S–1101S.

FRIDAY K E, CHILDS M T, TSUNEHARA C H, FUJIMOTO W Y, BIERMAN E L and ENSINCK J W (1989), Elevated plasma glucose and lowered triglyceride levels from omega-3 fatty acid supplementation in type II diabetes. *Diabetes Care*, **12**, 276–281.

FRIEDBERG C E, JANSSEN M J, HEINE R J and GROBBEE D E (1998), Fish oil and glycemic control in diabetes. A meta-analysis. *Diabetes Care*, **21**, 494–500.

GILLEN L J, TAPSELL L C, PATCH C S, OWEN A and BATTERHAM M (2005), Structured dietary advice incorporating walnuts achieves optimal fat and energy balance in patients with type 2 diabetes mellitus. *J Am Diet Assoc*, **105**, 1087–1096.

GRAVENA C, MATHIAS P C and ASHCROFT S J (2002), Acute effects of fatty acids on insulin secretion from rat and human islets of Langerhans. *J Endocrinol*, **173**, 73–80.

GRUNDT H, NILSEN D W, HETLAND O, AARSLAND T, BAKSAAS I, GRANDE T and WOIE L (1995), Improvement of serum lipids and blood pressure during intervention with n-3 fatty acids was not associated with changes in insulin levels in subjects with combined hyperlipidaemia. *J Intern Med*, **237**, 249–259.

HAVEL P J (2004), Update on adipocyte hormones: regulation of energy balance and carbohydrate/lipid metabolism. *Diabetes*, **53** (Suppl 1), S143–S151.

HITES R A, FORAN J A, SCHWAGER S J, KNUTH B A, HAMILTON M C and CARPENTER D O (2004), Global assessment of polybrominated diphenyl ethers in farmed and wild salmon. *Environ Sci Technol*, **38**, 4945–4949.

HOLNESS M J, GREENWOOD G K, SMITH N D and SUGDEN M C (2003), Diabetogenic impact of long-chain omega-3 fatty acids on pancreatic beta-cell function and the regulation of endogenous glucose production. *Endocrinology*, **144**, 3958–3968.

HOLNESS M J, SMITH N D, GREENWOOD G K and SUGDEN M C (2004), Acute omega-3 fatty acid enrichment selectively reverses high-saturated fat feeding-induced insulin hypersecretion but does not improve peripheral insulin resistance. *Diabetes*, **53** (Suppl 1), S166–S171.

HORTON J D, GOLDSTEIN J L and BROWN M S (2002), SREBPs: activators of the complete program of cholesterol and fatty acid synthesis in the liver. *J Clin Invest*, **109**, 1125–1131.

HU F B, BRONNER L, WILLETT W C, STAMPFER M J, REXRODE K M, ALBERT C M, HUNTER D and MANSON J E (2002), Fish and omega-3 fatty acid intake and risk of coronary heart disease in women. *JAMA*, **287**, 1815–1821.

IDE T (2005), Interaction of fish oil and conjugated linoleic acid in affecting hepatic activity of lipogenic enzymes and gene expression in liver and adipose tissue. *Diabetes*, **54**, 412–423.

IKEMOTO S, TAKAHASHI M, TSUNODA N, MARUYAMA K, ITAKURA H and EZAKI O (1996), High-fat diet-induced hyperglycemia and obesity in mice: differential effects of dietary oils. *Metabolism*, **45**, 1539–1546.

ITOH Y and HINUMA S (2005), GPR40, a free fatty acid receptor on pancreatic beta cells, regulates insulin secretion. *Hepatol Res*, **33**, 171–173.

ITOH Y, KAWAMATA Y, HARADA M, KOBAYASHI M, FUJII R, FUKUSUMI S, OGI K, HOSOYA M, TANAKA Y, UEJIMA H, TANAKA H, MARUYAMA M, SATOH R, OKUBO S, KIZAWA H, KOMATSU H, MATSUMURA F, NOGUCHI Y, SHINOHARA T, HINUMA S, FUJISAWA Y and FUJINO M (2003), Free fatty acids regulate insulin secretion from pancreatic beta cells through GPR40. *Nature*, **422**, 173–176.

JUMP D B, CLARKE S D, THELEN A and LIIMATTA M (1994), Coordinate regulation of glycolytic and lipogenic gene expression by polyunsaturated fatty acids. *J Lipid Res*, **35**, 1076–1084.

KREY G, BRAISSANT O, L'HORSET F, KALKHOVEN E, PERROUD M, PARKER M G and WAHLI W (1997), Fatty acids, eicosanoids, and hypolipidemic agents identified as ligands of peroxisome proliferator-activated receptors by coactivator-dependent receptor ligand assay. *Mol Endocrinol*, **11**, 779–791.

KRIS-ETHERTON P M, HARRIS W S and APPEL L J (2002), Fish consumption, fish oil, omega-3 fatty acids, and cardiovascular disease. *Circulation*, **106**, 2747–2757.

KRIS-ETHERTON P M, TAYLOR D S, YU-POTH S, HUTH P, MORIARTY K, FISHELL V, HARGROVE R L, ZHAO G and ETHERTON T D (2000), Polyunsaturated fatty acids in the food chain in the United States. *Am J Clin Nutr*, **71**, 179S–188S.

KROMANN N and GREEN A (1980), Epidemiological studies in the Upernavik district, Greenland. Incidence of some chronic diseases 1950–1974. *Acta Med Scand*, **208**, 401–406.

LEVY J R, CLORE J N and STEVENS W (2004), Dietary n-3 polyunsaturated fatty acids decrease hepatic triglycerides in Fischer 344 rats. *Hepatology*, **39**, 608–616.

LOMBARDO Y B and CHICCO A G (2006), Effects of dietary polyunsaturated n-3 fatty acids on dyslipidemia and insulin resistance in rodents and humans. A review. *J Nutr Biochem*, **17**, 1–13.

LUO J, RIZKALLA S W, VIDAL H, OPPERT J M, COLAS C, BOUSSAIRI A, GUERRE-MILLO M, CHAPUIS A S, CHEVALIER A, DURAND G and SLAMA G (1998), Moderate intake of n-3 fatty acids for 2 months has no detrimental effect on glucose metabolism and could ameliorate the lipid profile in type 2 diabetic men. Results of a controlled study. *Diabetes Care*, **21**, 717–724.

MA D W, SEO J, SWITZER K C, FAN Y Y, MCMURRAY D N, LUPTON J R and CHAPKIN R S (2004), n-3 PUFA and membrane microdomains: a new frontier in bioactive lipid research. *J Nutr Biochem*, **15**, 700–706.

MALASANOS T H and STACPOOLE P W (1991), Biological effects of omega-3 fatty acids in diabetes mellitus. *Diabetes Care*, **14**, 1160–1179.

MANCO M, CALVANI M and MINGRONE G (2004), Effects of dietary fatty acids on insulin sensitivity and secretion. *Diabetes Obes Metab*, **6**, 402–413.

MONTORI V M, FARMER A, WOLLAN P C and DINNEEN S F (2000), Fish oil supplementation in type 2 diabetes: a quantitative systematic review. *Diabetes Care*, **23**, 1407–1415.

MORI T A, BAO D Q, BURKE V, PUDDEY I B, WATTS G F and BEILIN L J (1999), Dietary fish as a major component of a weight-loss diet: effect on serum lipids, glucose, and insulin metabolism in overweight hypertensive subjects. *Am J Clin Nutr*, **70**, 817–825.

MOURATOFF G J, CARROLL N V and SCOTT E M (1969), Diabetes mellitus in Athabaskan Indians in Alaska. *Diabetes*, **18**, 29–32.

NAKATANI T, KIM H J, KABURAGI Y, YASUDA K and EZAKI O (2003), A low fish oil inhibits SREBP-1 proteolytic cascade, while high-fish-oil feeding decreases SREBP-1 mRNA in mice liver: relationship to anti-obesity. *J Lipid Res*, **44**, 369–379.

NAPIER J A, BEAUDOIN F, MICHAELSON L V and SAYANOVA O (2004), The production of long chain polyunsaturated fatty acids in transgenic plants by reverse-engineering. *Biochimie*, **86**, 785–792.

NETTLETON J A and KATZ R (2005), n-3 long-chain polyunsaturated fatty acids in type 2 diabetes: a review. *J Am Diet Assoc*, **105**, 428–440.

NOVAK T E, BABCOCK T A, JHO D H, HELTON W S and ESPAT N J (2003), NF-kappa B inhibition by omega-3 fatty acids modulates LPS-stimulated macrophage TNF-alpha transcription. *Am J Physiol Lung Cell Mol Physiol*, **284**, L84–L89.

PRENTKI M, VISCHER S, GLENNON M C, REGAZZI R, DEENEY J T and CORKEY B E (1992), Malonyl-CoA and long chain acyl-CoA esters as metabolic coupling factors in nutrient-induced insulin secretion. *J Biol Chem*, **267**, 5802–5810.

QI B, FRASER T, MUGFORD S, DOBSON G, SAYANOVA O, BUTLER J, NAPIER J A, STOBART A K and LAZARUS C M (2004), Production of very long chain polyunsaturated omega-3 and omega-6 fatty acids in plants. *Nat Biotechnol*, **22**, 739–745.

RICCARDI G, GIACCO R and RIVELLESE A A (2004), Dietary fat, insulin sensitivity and the metabolic syndrome. *Clin Nutr*, **23**, 447–456.

RUXTON C H, REED S C, SIMPSON M J and MILLINGTON K J (2004), The health benefits of omega-3 polyunsaturated fatty acids: a review of the evidence. *J Hum Nutr Diet*, **17**, 449–459.

RUZICKOVA J, ROSSMEISL M, PRAZAK T, FLACHS P, SPONAROVA J, VECK M, TVRZICKA E, BRYHN M and KOPECKY J (2004), Omega-3 PUFA of marine origin limit diet-induced obesity in mice by reducing cellularity of adipose tissue. *Lipids*, **39**, 1177–1185.

SALEHI A, FLODGREN E, NILSSON N E, JIMENEZ-FELTSTROM J, MIYAZAKI J, OWMAN C and OLDE B (2005), Free fatty acid receptor 1 (FFA(1)R/GPR40) and its involvement in fatty-acid-stimulated insulin secretion. *Cell Tissue Res*, **322**, 207–215.

SAMPATH H and NTAMBI J M (2004), Polyunsaturated fatty acid regulation of gene expression. *Nutr Rev*, **62**, 333–339.

SANDERS T A (2000), Polyunsaturated fatty acids in the food chain in Europe. *Am J Clin Nutr*, **71**, 176S–178S.

SERHAN C N, HONG S, GRONERT K, COLGAN S P, DEVCHAND P R, MIRICK G and MOUSSIGNAC R L (2002), Resolvins: a family of bioactive products of omega-3 fatty acid transformation circuits initiated by aspirin treatment that counter proinflammation signals. *J Exp Med*, **196**, 1025–1037.

SHAPIRO H, SHACHAR S, SEKLER I, HERSHFINKEL M and WALKER M D (2005), Role of GPR40 in fatty acid action on the beta cell line INS-1E. *Biochem Biophys Res Commun*, **335**, 97–104.

SHILLABEER G and LAU D C (1994), Regulation of new fat cell formation in rats: the role of dietary fats. *J Lipid Res*, **35**, 592–600.

SHULMAN G I (2000), Cellular mechanisms of insulin resistance. *J Clin Invest*, **106**, 171–176.

SIMONSSON E and AHREN B (2000), Phospholipase A2 and its potential regulation of islet function. *Int J Pancreatol*, **27**, 1–11.

SIMOPOULOS A P (1995), Evolutionary aspects of diet: fatty acids, insulin resistance and obesity. In VanItallie, T. B., & Simopoulos, A. P., (eds.), *Obesity: New Directions in Assessment and Management.* Philadelphia: Charles Press, pp. 241–261.

SIMOPOULOS A P (1999), Essential fatty acids in health and chronic disease. *Am J Clin Nutr*, **70**, 560S–569S.

SIRTORI C R, CREPALDI G, MANZATO E, MANCINI M, RIVELLESE A, PAOLETTI R, PAZZUCCONI F, PAMPARANA F and STRAGLIOTTO E (1998), One-year treatment with ethyl esters of n-3 fatty acids in patients with hypertriglyceridemia and glucose intolerance: reduced triglyceridemia, total cholesterol and increased HDL-C without glycemic alterations. *Atherosclerosis*, **137**, 419–427.

SMALL D M (1991), The effects of glyceride structure on absorption and metabolism. *Annu Rev Nutr*, **11**, 413–434.

STORLIEN L H, BAUR L A, KRIKETOS A D, PAN D A, COONEY G J, JENKINS A B, CALVERT G D and CAMPBELL L V (1996), Dietary fats and insulin action. *Diabetologia*, **39**, 621–631.

STORLIEN L H, HIGGINS J A, THOMAS T C, BROWN M A, WANG H Q, HUANG X F and ELSE P L (2000), Diet composition and insulin action in animal models. *Br J Nutr*, **83** (Suppl 1), S85–S90.

STORLIEN L H, JENKINS A B, CHISHOLM D J, PASCOE W S, KHOURI S and KRAEGEN E W (1991), Influence of dietary fat composition on development of insulin resistance in rats. Relationship to muscle triglyceride and omega-3 fatty acids in muscle phospholipid. *Diabetes*, **40**, 280–289.

STORLIEN L H, KRIKETOS A D, CALVERT G D, BAUR L A and JENKINS A B (1997), Fatty acids, triglycerides and syndromes of insulin resistance. *Prostaglandins Leukot Essent Fatty Acids*, **57**, 379–385.

SUMMERS L K, FIELDING B A, BRADSHAW H A, ILIC V, BEYSEN C, CLARK M L, MOORE N R and FRAYN K N (2002), Substituting dietary saturated fat with polyunsaturated fat changes abdominal fat distribution and improves insulin sensitivity. *Diabetologia*, **45**, 369–377.

TANIGUCHI A, NAKAI Y, FUKUSHIMA M, KAWAMURA H, IMURA H, NAGATA I and TOKUYAMA K (1992), Pathogenic factors responsible for glucose intolerance in patients with NIDDM. *Diabetes*, **41**, 1540–1546.

TERRY P D, ROHAN T E and WOLK A (2003), Intakes of fish and marine fatty acids and the risks of cancers of the breast and prostate and of other hormone-related cancers: a review of the epidemiologic evidence. *Am J Clin Nutr*, **77**, 532–543.

TKW N (1997), Dietary fat and fibre intakes of Malaysian adults: issues and implications when 'western targets' are set as dietary goals. *Mal J Nutr*, **3**, 137–147.

TOFT I, BONAA K H, INGEBRETSEN O C, NORDOY A and JENSSEN T (1995), Effects of n-3 polyunsaturated fatty acids on glucose homeostasis and blood pressure in essential hypertension. A randomized, controlled trial. *Ann Intern Med*, **123**, 911–918.

UNGER R H (1995), Lipotoxicity in the pathogenesis of obesity-dependent NIDDM. Genetic and clinical implications. *Diabetes*, **44**, 863–870.

UNGER R H (2003), Lipid overload and overflow: metabolic trauma and the metabolic syndrome. *Trends Endocrinol Metab*, **14**, 398–403.

UNGER R H and ORCI L (2000), Lipotoxic diseases of nonadipose tissues in obesity. *Int J Obes Relat Metab Disord*, **24** (Suppl 4), S28–S32.

UNGER R H and ZHOU Y T (2001), Lipotoxicity of beta-cells in obesity and in other causes of fatty acid spillover. *Diabetes*, **50** (Suppl 1), S118–S121.

VALSTA L M (1999), Food-based dietary guidelines for Finland – a staged approach. *Br J Nutr*, **81** (Suppl 2), S49–S55.

VESSBY B (1989), n-3 fatty acids and blood glucose control in diabetes mellitus. *J Intern Med Suppl*, **731**, 207–210.

WELLEN K E and HOTAMISLIGIL G S (2005), Inflammation, stress, and diabetes. *J Clin Invest*, **115**, 1111–1119.

WEN Z Y and CHEN F (2003), Heterotrophic production of eicosapentaenoic acid by microalgae. *Biotechnol Adv*, **21**, 273–294.

WESTERVELD H T, DE GRAAF J C, VAN BREUGEL H H, AKKERMAN J W, SIXMA J J, ERKELENS D W and BANGA J D (1993), Effects of low-dose EPA-E on glycemic control, lipid profile, lipoprotein(a), platelet aggregation, viscosity, and platelet and vessel wall interaction in NIDDM. *Diabetes Care*, **16**, 683–688.

WINZELL M S and AHREN B (2004), The high-fat diet-fed mouse: a model for studying mechanisms and treatment of impaired glucose tolerance and type 2 diabetes. *Diabetes*, **53** (Suppl 3), S215–S219.

WORGALL T S, STURLEY S L, SEO T, OSBORNE T F and DECKELBAUM R J (1998), Polyunsaturated fatty acids decrease expression of promoters with sterol regulatory elements by decreasing levels of mature sterol regulatory element-binding protein. *J Biol Chem*, **273**, 25537–25540.

WU D (2004), Modulation of immune and inflammatory responses by dietary lipids. *Curr Opin Lipidol*, **15**, 43–47.

XU J, TERAN-GARCIA M, PARK J H, NAKAMURA M T and CLARKE S D (2001), Polyunsaturated fatty acids suppress hepatic sterol regulatory element-binding protein-1 expression by accelerating transcript decay. *J Biol Chem*, **276**, 9800–9807.

YANEY G C, KORCHAK H M and CORKEY B E (2000), Long-chain acyl CoA regulation of protein kinase C and fatty acid potentiation of glucose-stimulated insulin secretion in clonal beta-cells. *Endocrinology*, **141**, 1989–1998.

YAQOOB P and CALDER P (1995), Effects of dietary lipid manipulation upon inflammatory mediator production by murine macrophages. *Cell Immunol*, **163**, 120–128.

ZHOU Y T, GRAYBURN P, KARIM A, SHIMABUKURO M, HIGA M, BAETENS D, ORCI L and UNGER R H (2000), Lipotoxic heart disease in obese rats: implications for human obesity. *Proc Natl Acad Sci U S A*, **97**, 1784–1789.
ZRAIKA S, DUNLOP M, PROIETTO J and ANDRIKOPOULOS S (2002), Effects of free fatty acids on insulin secretion in obesity. *Obes Rev*, **3**, 103–112.

# 14

# Medium-chain and structured triglycerides: their role in weight control

**I. Rudkowska and P. J. H. Jones, University of Manitoba, Canada**

## 14.1 Introduction: medium-chain triglycerides and weight control

Conventional fats and oils are composed of glycerides of 12- to 18-carbon long-chain fatty acids (LCFA). These compounds are known as long-chain triglycerides (LCT) and are the predominant form of lipids in the diet. Lipids are an essential source of energy and essential fatty acids, and a vital component of body cells. Therefore, it would be beneficial to have a dietary fat with the added benefit of anti-obesity properties. Medium-chain triglycerides (MCT) have a number of unique characteristics relating to energy density, absorption and metabolism, which give them advantages over the more common LCT. Upon hydrolysis, MCT yield medium-chain fatty acids (MCFA) [caproic ($C_6$), caprylic ($C_8$), capric ($C_{10}$), lauric ($C_{12}$)] (Papamandjaris *et al.*, 1997). Naturally occurring sources of MCT are rare, but include milk fat, palm kernel oil, and coconut oil. Human consumption of MCT is currently low but intake should perhaps be greater due to the distinctive properties of MCT, which cause an increase in energy expenditure (EE) and increased satiety that may contribute to weight loss.

First, the energy density of MCFA is less than that of LCFA due to their shorter chain length. MCT provide about 10% fewer calories than LCT – 8.3 cal/g for MCT versus 9 cal/g for LCT (Bach *et al.*, 1972). Therefore, the use of MCT can decrease caloric intake and potentially decrease body weight and body fat in the long term.

Secondly, MCT demonstrate additional characteristics of evident advantage. Specifically, MCFA are readily hydrolysed from triglycerides (TGs) by lingual and gastric lipases, compared with LCFA that require intestinal lipase to cleave TGs (Babayan, 1987). MCT oils also require less bile salts and pancreatic enzymes for digestion than LCT. The intramucosal metabolism of MCFA differs from that of LCFA. MCFA have a lower affinity for esterifying and activating enzymes, and there is a minimal re-sterification of MCFA to MCT, as compared with LCFA (Babayan, 1987). In addition, the intraluminal enzymatic hydrolysis of MCT is more rapid and complete than that of LCT since the smaller molecular size of MCT allows slight amounts to enter the intestinal cell without prior hydrolysis (Babayan, 1987). These properties enable MCT to be absorbed rapidly and more completely than LCT.

Thirdly, MCT are metabolized differently from LCT as demonstrated in Fig. 14.1. MCT are disassembled and enter the bloodstream as medium-chain free fatty acids (MCFFAs). These MCFFAs are transported to the liver directly via the hepatic portal circulation, which does not require chylomicron formation. In contrast, LCT are absorbed via intestinal lymphatic ducts and transported in chylomicrons through the thoracic duct to reach the systemic circulation. MCFA are transported into hepatocytes and converted to medium-chain fatty acyl CoA esters, which are further transported into mitochondria for conversion to acetoacetate and beta-hydroxybutyrate. These substrates may be further metabolized in the liver to carbon dioxide, water, and energy. Finally, MCFA tend to be preferentially oxidized in comparison with LCFA; therefore, less ingested MCT are deposited in the body as fat.

In summary, these unique characteristics of MCT, including their caloric content, and digestive and metabolic pathways, may give them the potential to induce weight loss as well as to maintain a healthy body weight.

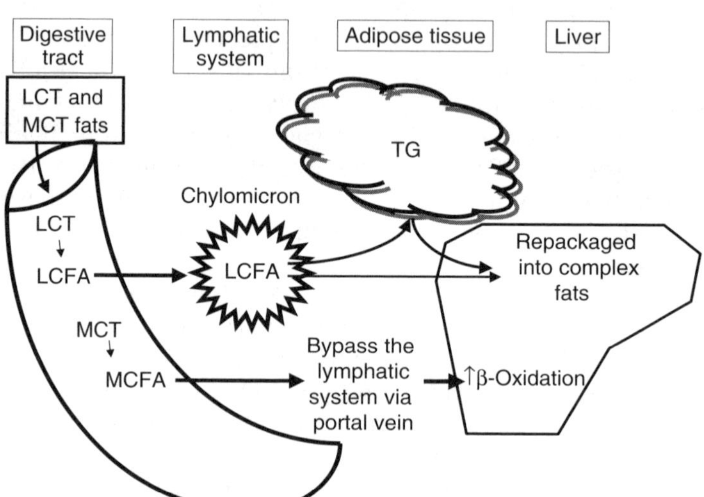


**Fig. 14.1** Mechanism of action of MCT compared with LCT.

## 14.2 Metabolic effects of medium-chain triglycerides related to weight control

### 14.2.1 Effects of medium-chain triglycerides on energy expenditure

Many animal studies have shown that diets high in MCT increase thermogenesis, leading to less fat deposition as compared with diets high in LCT (Bray *et al.*, 1980; Baba *et al.*, 1982; Geliebter *et al.*, 1983; Rothwell and Stock, 1987). An animal study by Lasekan *et al.* (1992), showed lower weight gain and 8–13% greater EE in rats fed a 3:1 mixture of MCT and LCT in emulsion compared with only LCT. Overall, animal studies suggest the possibility for MCT to increase EE in humans, thus potentially assisting in weight loss. The short-term effects of MCT on human EE are summarized in Table 14.1; long-term studies on EE are summarized in Table 14.2.

Human studies were first conducted by Flatt *et al.* (1985), who observed a greater postprandial (PP) thermogenesis and the tendency for a lower respiratory quotient, indicating a greater fat oxidation, over the first few hours following the consumption of a meal high in MCT compared with a meal high in LCT. This finding was reaffirmed by Seaton *et al.* (1986), in seven healthy men. Results demonstrated that mean PP oxygen consumption was 12% higher than basal values after the MCT meal, while it was 4% higher than the basal oxygen consumption after the LCT meal. However, these two studies examining the effect of MCT were one-meal effect and single-day experiments, which represent major limitations of these study designs.

A 1-week study assessed whether thermogenesis was affected differently in the presence of excess dietary energy as MCT in comparison to energy as LCT (Hill *et al.*, 1989). Hill *et al.* (1989) recruited ten young males who were fed 150% of estimated energy requirements in a liquid formula diet containing 40% fat as either MCT or LCT. The authors demonstrated that excess dietary energy as MCT stimulated an increase in the thermic effect of food (TEF) to a greater degree than excess energy as LCT. This increase was seen on days 1 and 7 of the study and was most probably due to enhanced hepatic lipogenesis. The group recognized that the 1-week duration of the study was a limiting factor in determining the effects of MCT on basal metabolic rate (BMR) and body weight, as changes in these parameters could not be seen over such a short study period. Hence, it is was not known whether the effects of high-MCT diets on EE in humans found in short-term studies would persist in studies of longer duration and would produce weight loss even if energy intake remained constant.

Consequently, longer studies to assess the impact of MCT on EE were undertaken. White *et al.* (1999), fed 12 non-obese, premenopausal women a diet containing 40% of energy as fat, either in the form of butter and coconut oil or beef tallow, over 14 days. On day 7, mean BMR and PP EE values were significantly greater with the MCT diet than with the LCT diet. On day 14, PP total EE was still greater with the MCT diet, but not

**Table 14.1** Human work on the acute effects (1 meal) of MCT on EE

| Study design | Study diet including amount of MCT (~g/day) | Outcomes on EE |
|---|---|---|
| **Flatt *et al.*, 1985**<br>Randomized, cross-over study<br>Controlled diet<br>7 young men | Mixed 858 kcal meal including<br>40 g MCT + 10 g LCT or<br>50 g LCT | ↑ Postprandial thermogenesis<br>↓ Respiratory quotients, ↑ fat oxidation |
| **Seaton *et al.*, 1986**<br>Randomized, cross-over study<br>Controlled diet<br>7 healthy men | Test meal containing<br>48 g MCT or<br>45 g corn oil meal | ↑ Postprandial oxygen consumption<br>NS ↓ Respiratory quotients, ↑ fat oxidation<br>↑ 3-Hydroxybutyrate concentration |
| **Scalfi *et al.*, 1991**<br>Randomized, cross-over study<br>Controlled diet<br>6 lean and 6 obese young men | Mixed meals including<br>38 g LCT or<br>30 g MCT + 8 g LCT | ↑ Postprandial thermogenesis in the lean and the obese subjects<br>↓ Respiratory quotients, ↑ fat oxidation in the lean but not obese subjects |
| **Dulloo *et al.*, 1996**<br>Randomized, cross-over study<br>Controlled diet<br>8 healthy men | Combinations of MCT and LCT in the following ratio of MCT:LCT (g/g):<br>0:30, 5:25, 15:15, and 30:0 | ↑ EE with ↑ MCT:LCT ratio<br>↑ 24-h EE with the diet providing a total of 15–30 g MCT<br>↔Respiratory quotients but trends towards ↓ |

| | | |
|---|---|---|
| **Van Wymelbeke *et al.*, 2000**<br>Randomized, cross-over study<br>Controlled diet<br>12 healthy men | 4 lunches dietary carbohydrate, fat (≈ 43 g MCT or LCT), and a basic hypoenergetic lunch | ↔ EE after the different lunches<br>↓ Carbohydrate oxidation was lower after the MCT and LCT lunches than after the Carbohydrate lunch |
| **Binnert *et al.*, 1998**<br>Randomized, cross-over study<br>Controlled diet<br>8 lean and 8 obese women | Ingested 30 g (50:50) of MCT–LCT load or 30 g LCT (olive oil) | ↓ LCT oxidation in obese versus lean<br>↑ MCT oxidation then LCT<br>↔ MCT oxidation in obese versus lean |
| **Bendixen *et al.*, 2002**<br>Randomized, cross-over study<br>Controlled diet<br>11 healthy men | 60% fat test meal, 4 different test fats: conventional fat (rapeseed oil); 3 modified fats (all 48% MCT) – lipase-structured fat, chemically structured fat, and physically mixed fat | ↔ EE between fats<br>↔ Substrate oxidation including fat oxidation<br>↔ Appetite or *ad libitum* energy intake |
| **Kasai *et al.*, 2002**<br>Randomized, cross-over study<br>Controlled diet<br>16 healthy men and women | **Study 1:** liquid meals including 10 g MCT or 5 g MCT + 5 g LCT or 10 g LCT<br>**Study 2:** margarine or mayonnaise including 5 g MCT or 5 g LCT | **Study 1:**<br>↑ TEF after 5 g MCT + 5 g LCT and 10 g MCT<br>↓ Respiratory quotients, ↑ fat oxidation<br>**Study 2:**<br>↑ TEF after 5 g MCT of both foods |

Abbreviations: MCT, medium-chain triglycerides; LCT, long-chain triglycerides; EE, energy expenditure; TEF, thermic effect of food; NS, non-significant.

**Table 14.2** Human work on the chronic effect (>1 meal) of MCT on EE

| Study design | Study diet including amount of MCT (~g/day) | Outcomes on energy expenditure |
|---|---|---|
| **Hill *et al.*, 1989**<br>Randomized, cross-over study<br>Controlled diet<br>10 non-obese men | Overfeeding period (150% of energy requirements) with 40% fat diet as ~185 g MCT or ~168 g LCT for 7 days | ↔ BW, body fat<br>↔ RMR<br>↑ TEF on day 1 and day 5<br>↑ EE on day 7<br>↓ Fat oxidation in both diets<br>↑ β-hydroxybutyrate |
| **White *et al.*, 1999**<br>Randomized, cross-over study<br>Controlled diet<br>12 healthy women | 40% fat of total energy 2540 kcal (80% from experimental oil) as ~90 g MCT for 14 days | ↔ BW, body fat<br>↑ BMR on day 7<br>↑ Postprandial total EE on day 7, but NS ↑ by day 14<br>↑ Fat oxidation on days 1 and 7 |
| **St-Onge and Jones, 2003; St-Onge *et al.*, 2003b**<br>Randomized, cross-over study<br>Controlled diet<br>24 overweight men | 40% fat of total energy (75% from experimental oil) as functional oil composed of ~64.7 g MCT* (64.7% of fat) + PS (22 mg/kg body weight) + n-3 fatty acids (5% of fat) versus ~100 g olive oil for 29 days | ↓ BW<br>↔ RMR<br>↑ Postprandial EE and TEF on days 2 and 28<br>↑ EE on day 2, NS↑ on day 28<br>↑ Fat oxidation on day 2, NS↑ on day 28 |
| **St-Onge *et al.*, 2003a**<br>Randomized, cross-over study<br>Controlled diet<br>17 overweight women | 40% fat of total energy (75% from experimental oil) as functional oil composed of ~50 g MCT* (50% of fat) + PS (22 mg/kg body weight) + n-3 fatty acids (5% of fat) versus ~100 g beef tallow for 27 days | ↓ BW to same extent as beef tallow<br>↔ RMR<br>↔ Postprandial EE and TEF<br>↑ EE on day 2 higher than day 27<br>↑ Fat oxidation on days 2 and 27 |

Abbreviations: BW, body weight; EE, energy expenditure; MCT, medium-chain triglycerides; LCT, long-chain triglycerides; NS, non-significant; PS, plant sterol; RMR, resting metabolic rate; TEF, thermic effect of food.
* Calculated based on 3000 kcal.

significantly. The authors concluded that short-term feeding of MCT-enriched diets increases total EE, but this effect may not be sustained with continued feeding. In addition, MCT were suggested to exert greater incremental increases in EE when given in a single dose than during chronic intake. In order to further explore the outcome of long-term MCT intake, a 27-day study was carried out to determine the effects of MCT versus LCT consumption in 17 obese healthy women (St-Onge *et al.*, 2003a). Long-term consumption of MCT enhanced both EE and fat oxidation on day 2, as well as on day 27, when compared with LCT consumption. A similar protocol conducted in 19 overweight men for 28 days showed comparable results, with average EE and fat oxidation being greater on day 2 and showing a tendency to increase on day 28 with MCT as compared with LCT consumption (St-Onge and Jones, 2003; St-Onge *et al.*, 2003c). These human studies demonstrated an evident increase in EE, especially in men. When data are extrapolated from trials conducted in men, the average EE is approximately 460 kJ/day greater with MCT than with LCT consumption. In contrast, data from women show differences in EE of 138 kJ/day between MCT and LCT. Using the peak difference in EE between MCT and LCT in men, it has been determined that a weight gain of 1.35 kg in 30 days could be avoided by substituting MCT for LCT. Using the lowest difference in EE between MCT and LCT, both men and women could avoid a weight gain of 0.45 kg per 30 days by consuming MCT rather than LCT.

The ingestion of MCT in low to moderate quantities may have variable effects on TEF. Dulloo *et al.* (1996), fed subjects 15–30 g of MCT in addition to a weight-maintaining diet containing 40% of energy as fat. It was reported that EE increased significantly with increasing MCT : LCT ratio. Furthermore, the difference in 24-h EE between 30 g of MCT and 30 g of LCT was 471 kJ; this increase in EE would result in about 0.45 kg of fat loss over 36 days if effects were to persist over that period. However, even smaller doses of MCT (5 and 10 g/day) have been tested (Kasai *et al.*, 2002). Results have shown that intake of small doses of MCT causes larger diet-induced thermogenesis than LCT. Therefore, both small and large doses of MCT increase EE; however, large doses may create greater TEF, which may be more beneficial for weight loss.

There may be differences in the effect of MCT on TEF between lean and obese individuals. Scalfi *et al.* (1991) first tested this possibility. Their results demonstrated that PP thermogenesis was enhanced in both lean and obese subjects when LCT were replaced with MCT, but that MCT-induced thermogenesis tended to be higher in obese than in lean individuals. Similarly to the previous study, Binnert *et al.* (1998), showed that LCT were less well oxidized in obese than in control subjects when consuming a mixed 50% LCT and 50% MCT load. The authors suggested that obesity may be associated with a defective oxidation of LCT, probably related to excessive intake of meal-derived LCT. Thus, substitution of MCT for LCT in combination with a weight-maintaining diet might prevent long-term weight gain via increased EE.

There is clear evidence that MCT create an increase in TEF in both animal and human studies within the first week of intake; however, some metabolic adaptations to MCT may occur afterwards as demonstrated in long-term feeding studies. This metabolic regulation may be due to weight loss, and techniques should be sought to avoid this metabolic adaptation. Furthermore, the effects of MCT on PP thermogenesis seem to be dose dependent, although even small doses can increase PP thermogenesis. In addition, MCT are oxidized at a faster rate than LCT which may suggest that they will lead to less fat accumulation and subsequent weight loss.

### 14.2.2 Effects of medium-chain triglycerides on appetite control

MCT may help with appetite control via their satiating properties. The satiating properties of MCT involve multiple pre-absorptive and post-absorptive mechanisms. First, MCT appear as a thin, light-yellow, clear, and odorless oil, with a nearly neutral or slightly bland taste, whereas MCFA are characterized by an odor of goat and strong bitterness (Bach *et al.*, 1996). This repulsive quality is extremely strong, as a concentration of 0.1% makes a meal unfit for human consumption (Bach *et al.*, 1996). These palatability properties are important determinants of feeding behavior of an individual, in particular satiation.

The effect of dietary MCT versus LCT on short-term food intake has been compared in rats (Maggio and Koopmans, 1982; Furuse *et al.*, 1992). The satiating effect of these two triglycerides appears to be related to their caloric content rather than to chain length (Feinle *et al.*, 2001; Westerterp-Plantenga, 2004a). In addition, the ingestion of MCT as a bolus does not stimulate contraction of the gallbladder nor raise the plasma cholecystokinin (CCK) level in the manner in which it occurs following LCT ingestion (Hopman *et al.*, 1984). This gastric relaxation by MCT is not sufficient to induce satiation; therefore, the nutrient-induced gastric relaxation occurs through other mechanisms than CCK (Furuse *et al.*, 1992; Barbera *et al.*, 2000). According to Maas *et al.* (1998), MCT inhibit gastrin-stimulated gastric acid secretion, but less so than LCT. Overall, it has been determined that the satiating effects of a fat depend on the fatty acid chain length, and moreover that the role of CCK and gastrin-stimulated gastric acid are minor.

Post-absorptive properties of MCT, including hepatic exposure to fatty acids, may lead to greater beta-oxidation by the liver than that following LCT intake. Enhanced beta-oxidation may in turn lead to increased satiety (Westerterp-Plantenga, 2004b). Thus, MCT consumption in sufficient quantities over the long term may lead to decreased caloric intake and consequently decreased body weight and fat. Van Wymelbeke *et al.* (2001), conducted a study demonstrating that ingestion of a MCT-containing lunch resulted in less food consumed at dinner in comparison with the other non-MCT-containing meals, indicating that MCT have a higher satiation power than other fats and carbohydrates. This increased satiety may also be due to greater fat oxidation after the MCT lunches. Krotkiewski (2001), demonstrated a similar decrease in hunger feelings and increase in satiety with MCT intake, related to a higher concentration of plasma ketone bodies and lower nitrogen excretion. These differences were observed during the first 2 weeks of treatment and then gradually declined during the third and fourth weeks. However, it is important to note that the increase of ketone bodies paralleled the intensity of hunger feelings, demonstrating that beta-oxidation may lead to increased satiety. These effects gradually declined, indicating subsequent metabolic adaptation, as was demonstrated in studies of MCT-related EE (Krotkiewski, 2001). Long-term effects of a diet rich in MCT or LCT on subjective appetite and *ad libitum* energy intake were compared in 24 men by St-Onge and Jones (2003) and St-Onge *et al.* (2003b). There was a trend towards decreased appetite and *ad libitum* energy intake during MCT compared with LCT consumption. Correspondingly, the average fat oxidation tended to be greater with MCT compared with LCT intake on day 2, but not on day 28. Conversely, Bendixen *et al.* (2002) observed no differences in fat oxidation, appetite, or *ad libitum* energy intake after intake of any one of three randomly provided, modified MCT-rich meals. The contradictory results between the studies may be due to different study lengths – one meal versus several days. The initial accumulation of ketone bodies may produce increased satiety, but there may be no further satiating effects when the body adapts to the higher levels of ketone bodies. Further research is required to confirm the short- and long-term appetite-suppressing effects of MCT supplementation in relation to beta-oxidation.

Although MCT have been shown to induce satiety and stimulate hormone secretion, no single hormone has been clearly associated with MCT digestion. Therefore, the exact mechanism for the satiating effects of MCT is unknown, but may possibly be explained by the distinct energy density of MCT or the increase in fat oxidation that they promote.

### 14.2.3 Effects of medium-chain triglycerides on body weight and body fat

Animal and human studies indicate enhanced EE and satiety after MCT consumption; these studies were conducted to determine if these characteristics translate into decreases in fat mass. In animals consuming MCT, body weight was lower, fat depots smaller (Lavau and Hashim, 1978; Bray *et al.*, 1980; Baba *et al.*, 1982; Geliebter *et al.*, 1983; Crozier *et al.*, 1987; Hill *et al.*, 1993), and adipose size reduced (Baba *et al.*, 1982; Crozier *et al.*, 1987) with MCT compared with LCT. These experiments suggest that the decreased deposition of fat in the MCT-fed rats may have resulted from obligatory oxidation of MCT-derived fatty acids in the liver after being transported there via the portal vein, leaving almost no MCT derivatives for incorporation into body fat. Overall, these animal studies with MCT indicate positive results relating to body weight, suggesting a potential for dietary prevention of human obesity via MCT intake.

Diets high in fat have been previously shown to induce a gain in body weight. However, substitution of a readily metabolized fat for a less well metabolized fat, within the context of a very high fat, energy-dense diet, can potentially limit excess energy intake and resultant weight gain (Stubbs and Harbron, 1996). MCT have been shown to reduce body weight effectively in numerous studies (Binnert *et al.*, 1998; Krotkiewski, 2001; Nosaka *et al.*, 2003; St-Onge and Jones, 2003; St-Onge *et al.*, 2003b). However, others have not found positive effects on body weight (Yost and Eckel, 1989; St-Onge *et al.*, 2003a). A summary of studies on the effects of MCT on body weight and composition is provided in Table 14.3.

The addition of MCT to hypocaloric diets displays variable effects. Yost and Eckel (1989) compared MCT and LCT feedings during and after 4 or 12 weeks of hypocaloric feedings in 16 obese women. It was concluded that MCT are safe, but fail to increase the rate or amount of weight loss. However, a major drawback in this study was that the authors did not measure EE or body composition. Another study tested the effects of a very low calorie diet supplemented with MCT versus a low-fat, high-carbohydrate regimen over 4 weeks (Krotkiewski, 2001). The MCT group showed a significantly greater decrease in body weight during the first 2 weeks compared with the group consuming the low-fat, high-carbohydrate diet. The contribution of body fat to the total weight loss was also higher while the contribution of fat-free mass was lower, as measured by dual-energy x-ray absorptiometry. Similarly, Nosaka *et al.* (2003) randomized 73 subjects into two groups and provided them with 2100–2400 kcal/day of energy, including 5 g/day of MCT or LCT. After 12 weeks, subjects on the MCT diet demonstrated decreases in total body fat, subcutaneous fat, and visceral fat as measured by the air-displacement method. The authors suggested that a PP increase in thermogenesis was the cause of the weight loss, but EE was not measured. Overall, the benefits of MCT supplementation in combination with a hypocaloric diet are significant; however, future studies are needed to confirm these results.

St-Onge *et al.* (2003a) recruited 17 obese women to assess body composition by magnetic resonance imaging (MRI) after long-term consumption of an MCT-supplemented diet. Changes in total and subcutaneous adipose tissue volumes were not significantly different between MCT and LCT diets. The authors hypothesized that the lack of effect on body composition in women may have been due to inadequate intake of MCT oil, and thus a smaller increase in EE. Therefore, the same investigators recruited 19 healthy, overweight men who consumed diets rich in MCT or LCT (St-Onge and Jones, 2003; St-Onge *et al.*, 2003b). This study found a greater decrease in body weight, including the upper body adipose tissue as measured by

**Table 14.3** Human work on the chronic effect of MCT and structured lipids on body weight and composition

| Study design | Study diet including amount of MCT (~g/day) | Outcomes on body weight and body composition |
|---|---|---|
| **St-Onge and Jones, 2003; St-Onge *et al.*, 2003b**<br>Randomized, cross-over study<br>Controlled diet<br>24 overweight men | 40% fat of total energy (75% from experimental oil) as functional oil composed of ~ 64.7 g MCT* (64.7% of fat) + PS (22 mg/kg body weight) + n-3 fatty acids (5% of fat) versus ~100 g olive oil for 29 days | ↓ BW and body mass<br>↓ Total adipose tissue<br>↓ Upper adipose tissue<br>NS↓ subcutaneous adipose tissue |
| **St-Onge *et al.*, 2003a**<br>Randomized, cross-over study<br>Controlled diet<br>17 overweight women | 40% fat of total energy (75% from experimental oil) as functional oil composed of ~50 g MCT* (50% of fat) + PS (22 mg/kg body weight) + n-3 fatty acids (5% of fat) versus ~100 g beef tallow for 27 days | ↓ BW to same extent as beef tallow<br>↔ Total adipose tissue<br>↔ Subcutaneous adipose tissue |
| **Beermann *et al.*, 2003**<br>Randomized, cross-over study<br>Controlled diet<br>10 healthy overweight men | 1500 kcal diet with 55.5% as fat ~53 g MCT + 16 g n-3 LCPUFA/day versus LCT (vegetable oils) for 15 days | ↓ BW<br>↓ Body fat mass |
| **Yost and Eckel, 1989**<br>Parallel arm study<br>*Ad libitum* diet<br>16 obese women | 800 kcal/day liquid diet with 30% of calories as 6% of calories as LCT (5 g) and 24% as MCT (21 g) or LCT (27 g) for 4 or 12 weeks | ↓ BW to same rate as LCT<br>↔ Serum ketones<br>↔ N balance |

**Table 14.3** *Continued*

| Study design | Study diet including amount of MCT (~g/day) | Outcomes on body weight and body composition |
|---|---|---|
| **Matsuo *et al.*, 2001**<br>Parallel arm study<br>*Ad libitum* diet<br>13 healthy male volunteers | Structured medium- and long-chain triglycerols composed of ~20 g medium- (10%) and ~180 g long-chain (90%) fatty acids versus LCT for 12 weeks | NS ↑ BW to same extent as LCT<br>↑ Body fat to same extent as LCT<br>↓ Body fat variation |
| **Tsuji *et al.*, 2001**<br>Parallel arm study<br>*Ad libitum* diet<br>78 healthy men and women | 60 g total fat including 10 g MCT or 10 g LCT for 12 weeks | ↓ BW in both groups but ↑ weight loss in MCT<br>↓ Body fat mass in both groups but ↑ in MCT in pt BMI ≥ 23<br>↓ Subcutaneous adipose tissue in pt BMI ≥ 23<br>↓ Visceral fat in pt BMI < 23 |
| **Nosaka *et al.*, 2003**<br>Randomized, crossover study<br>*Ad libitum* diet<br>73 healthy men and women | 2100–2400 kcal diet including 65–73 g/day of total fat with 5 g of MCT or 5 g of LCT (rapeseed and soybean oil) for 12 weeks | ↓ BW<br>↓ Total adipose tissue<br>↓ Subcutaneous adipose tissue<br>↓ Visceral adipose tissue |
| **Takeuchi *et al.*, 2002**<br>Randomized, cross-over study<br>*Ad libitum* diet<br>6 active young men | Structured lipids 20 g of dietary triglycerols containing (20%) medium- and (80%) long-chain fatty acids (TML) 4 g MCT versus 20 g/day of soybean oil for 3 weeks | NS ↑ BW to same extent as soybean oil<br>↓ Body fat<br>↓ Rate of variation BW |
| **Kasai *et al.*, 2003**<br>Parallel arm study<br>*Ad libitum* diet<br>82 subjects | Structured medium- and long-chain triglycerols (MLCT) diet consumed 14 g of MLCT containing 1.7 g MCFA versus LCT for 12 weeks | ↓ BW<br>↓ Body fat<br>↓ Subcutaneous and visceral fat |

Abbreviations: BW, body weight; BMI, body mass index; MCT, medium-chain triglycerides; MCFA, medium-chain fatty acids; LCT, long-chain triglycerides; LCPUFA, long-chain fatty acids; N, nitrogen; NS, non-significant; PS, plant sterol; pt, patients.
* Calculated based on 3000 kcal

MRI, with MCT compared with LCT consumption; these results were probably due to the increase in measured EE and fat oxidation observed with MCT intake (St-Onge and Jones, 2003; St-Onge *et al.*, 2003b). The authors concluded that substitution of MCT for LCT in a targeted energy-balanced diet might prevent long-term weight gain via increased EE. Furthermore, the results indicated that MCT may be a better tool in the prevention of weight gain when body weight is not yet highly elevated, since MCT consumption stimulated EE and fat oxidation to a lower extent in men of greater body weight compared with in men of lower body weight (St-Onge *et al.*, 2003b).

These studies suggest that replacing LCT with MCT oil could produce body fat loss over long periods of time, with or without reduced energy intake. However, the exact area of fat loss in the human body is still undetermined. Individual and genetic differences in the populations studied, as well as varying methods of analysis for body composition, may make generalizations more difficult.

## 14.3 Effects of structured lipids related to weight control

MCT derivatives produced by the interesterification process are referred to as structural lipids or structural TGs. Interesterification is a process by which LCFA, such as oleic acid, are introduced into the final product. In the case of MCT derivatives, the product created is a rearranged TG with both MCFA and LCFA, in the desired ratios, on the same glycerine molecule. The existence of physiological actions of structured lipids on body weight and composition is explored in this section.

Human studies have been conducted with a variety of structured lipids as demonstrated in Table 14.3. Matsuo *et al.* (2001) examined the effects of a liquid diet supplement containing structured lipid composed of 10% MCFA and 90% LCFA as compared with a liquid formula containing LCT in 13 healthy male volunteers. Although body weight increased nonsignificantly in both groups, the rates of variation in body fat percentage were lower in the structured lipid group than in the LCT group throughout the 12-week study. Despite this, in another 12-week study comparing LCT with a diet supplemented with 14 g of structured fat containing only 1.7 g MCFA, results showed decreases in body weight, including subcutaneous and visceral fat as measured by air displacement methods (Kasai *et al.*, 2003). Similarly, Takeuchi *et al.* (2002) examined the effects of 20 g of structured lipid containing MCFA and LCFA versus the same quantity of soybean oil for 3 weeks in 6 young men. The rate of variation in body fat mass as measured by bioelectrical impedance was lower with the structured lipids than with soybean oil.

Secondly, oils rich in MCT lack essential fatty acids, which makes them inappropriate to consume as the sole source of fat in the diet. For this reason, the addition of essential fatty acids such as n-6 and n-3 long-chain polyunsaturated fatty acids (n-6 and n-3 LCPUFA) to a structured lipid may be beneficial. Beermann *et al.* (2003) hypothesized that MCT combined with n-3 LCPUFA would act synergistically to stimulate fatty acid oxidation, resulting in LCFA release from adipocytes and blood lipid clearance. Ten overweight volunteers consumed a high-fat hypoenergetic diet for 15 days, including a formula containing either LCFA or a combination of MCFA and n-3 LCPUFAs (Beermann *et al.*, 2003). Both groups showed equivalent reductions in body weight and fat mass (Beermann *et al.*, 2003). However, the study measured weight loss with a scale and body fat by impedance, neither of which can give the breakdown of regional changes in body composition. Nonetheless, longer-term studies with larger sample sizes should be considered to determine the exact benefits of MCT and n-3 LCPUFA on weight loss, body composition, and blood lipid parameters.

Structured lipids have recently been tested as agents to decrease body weight and body fat accumulation and to improve lipoprotein profile in human studies. Results of these studies suggest that the daily intake of structured lipids could result in a reduction in body weight and fat accumulation. However, the exact ratio of MCT to LCT and the components of structured lipids required for optimal effects on both body composition and blood lipids need further investigation.

## 14.4 Producing oils and using medium-chain triglycerides

### 14.4.1 Producing oils containing medium-chain triglycerides

The MCT used for commercial purposes are usually derived from lauric fats, which are found primarily in palm kernel oil and coconut oil. In the process of producing MCT, lauric oils are hydrolyzed to MCFFA and glycerol. The glycerol is drawn off from the resultant mixture, and the MCFA are fractionally distilled. The MCFA fraction used commercially mainly consists of caprylic or octanoic acid (65–75% $C_8$) and capric or decanoic acid (25–35% $C_{10}$). Smaller amounts of caproic or hexanoic acid (1–2% $C_6$) and lauric acid (1–2% $C_{12}$) exist in commercial products (Babayan, 1987).

Unlike most natural oils of animal or vegetable origin, MCT are stable and resistant to oxidation, owing mainly to the saturation of the MCFA. MCT oil is also colorless, odorless, and possesses a bland flavor and low viscosity; therefore MCT oil can be used in salad dressings and cooking oils. However, MCT oil should not be heated to temperatures above 150–160 °C, because the oil oxidizes and breaks down, adversely affecting its taste. This characteristic is due to MCT oil's content of low molecular weight fatty acids, which have lower smoke, flash, and fire points than other animal or vegetable fats.

In 1991, the first product commercialized containing MCT was Caprenin, a reduced-calorie designer fat consisting of three fatty acids: caprylic, capric, and behenic acid. Behenic acid is poorly absorbed because of its very long chain length compared with other fatty acids. The combination of MCFA and behenic in Caprenin results in a fat with a total caloric density of only 5 kcal/g. Caprenin was commercialized by Procter & Gamble as a cocoa butter replacement, and was launched in two products (US Food and Drug Administration, FDA, website). Unfortunately, the products are difficult to heat due to their lower flash point and they appear to increase serum total cholesterol slightly, resulting in withdrawal from the market in September 2000. Their primary use was as flavor carriers for fat-free food products.

Since then MCT have been used in formulated liquid diets and infant formulas. They have been more recently introduced into various sports nutritional supplements, including the Cognis functional ingredient DELIOS® (Institute of Food Technologists News, 2005), Twinlab MCT Fuel, Neobee MLT-B (Stepan Co. trademark) and Smart Basics MCT Oil. In Japan, a structured lipid called Ollio – an oil containing MCFA and LCFA on the same TG molecule, is currently marketed. Other functional foods can also be mixed in with MCT, such as plant sterols in Vivola™ Oil (Forbes Medi-Tech Inc. website). This Vivola™ Oil is composed of several different oils including approximately 65% w/w of MCT, linoleic and linolenic acid, and Reducol™, which is a plant sterol mixture. Recently, Bunge Foods launched a new functional oil called Delta Oil™ which includes MCT mixed with high-oleic canola oil and added plant sterols to maintain a healthy body weight and reduce cholesterol. Future mixtures with other oils, such as diacylglycerols, should be considered for weight loss acceleration.

Fat-based fat-reduction ingredients have the same physical properties as fat, including taste, texture, and mouth feel. These products include MCT, which are highly versatile and can be used in a wide variety of foods. In addition, MCT can be mixed with other functional foods to amplify effects on weight loss or cardiovascular disease.

### 14.4.2 Optimal intake of medium-chain triglycerides

The recommended dietary allowance for healthy adults for MCT ranges from 30 to 100 g/day, which would cover up to 40% of daily energy requirements. The ingestion of too large a dose of MCT, such as 85 g, or not enough progressive incorporation into the diet may cause adverse symptoms in healthy volunteers, including nausea, vomiting, bloating, emesis, gastrointestinal discomfort, abdominal cramps, and osmotic diarrhea (Hopman *et al.*, 1984). Temporary interruption or provision of a small initial dose (i.e. half a tablespoon per day) may be necessary in order to avoid adverse effects. Tolerance improves over time in most instances (Bach *et al.*, 1996). However, some individuals who consume MCT, especially on an empty stomach, experience abdominal cramps and bloating. The general acceptance of MCT consumed in mixed meals suggests that MCT are better tolerated with other nutrients, or that tolerance simply develops over time.

Daily consumption of MCT oil by humans is safe up to levels of 1 g/kg of body weight (Traul *et al.*, 2000). Studies in animals and humans have shown MCT to be quite safe when consumed at a level of up to 50% of total dietary fat (Traul *et al.*, 2000; Nosaka *et al.*, 2002). Since ketone bodies are a product of MCT metabolism, the use of MCT oil by diabetics is not recommended unless it is part of a medically supervised treatment. Furthermore, MCT do not offer any advantages over conventional oil for glycemic control. People with liver disease should not use MCT oil because MCT are delivered rapidly to the liver and their presence would put additional stress on the liver. The maximum safe dosage of MCT in young children, pregnant or nursing women, or people with serious kidney disease has not been established; however, MCT can be consumed safely in moderation at levels of up to 10% of total fat intake. MCT supplements do not contain any essential fatty acids, nevertheless this would not present a problem unless MCT were the only source of fat in the diet. Different doses of MCT have been added to a variety of formulas and oils, with quantities of MCT ranging from 50 to 10% of structured oil.

As can be logically interpreted from the above data, MCT should be included at every meal in order to increase EE maximally. However, it has not been determined whether a large bolus of MCT has different effects on EE and overall BMR as compared with a small, frequent intake. Furthermore, the duration of intake is somewhat controversial in the literature since short-term intake increases EE, but long-term intake seems to increase EE to a less significant level.

### 14.4.3 Cost and regulation of medium-chain triglycerides in different countries

The marketplace provides a variety of MCT oils and structured lipids. Although there has been success in structured fats, these developments have come with considerable time and cost compared with simple MCT oil mixtures. The development of structured lipids will focus on cost.

Regulations regarding MCT oils and structured lipids vary between countries. Japan was the first to regulate and implement programs for functional foods. MCFA were approved as FOSHU (Foods for Specific Health Use) for health claims in the category of 'neutral fats and body fats'. In the United States, MCTs benefit from the GRAS (Generally Recognized As Safe) label provided for use by the FDA, confirming the safety of MCTs in human nutrition. In Canada, MCTs are allowed for use both as a food and as an ingredient in foods. When sold as a food, the acceptable common name is 'Medium Chain Triglycerides' and the abbreviation 'MCT' is not acceptable (Canadian Food Inspection Agency Food Safety Directorate

Bureau of Food Safety and Consumer Protection). However, claims about the function, effects, or benefits of MCT are not permitted in Canada. A variety of functional foods, including MCT, are sold in Europe. Again in the European Union, functional or health claims are the center of the problem of regulation of functional foods since they are not yet authorized. At present, Australia and New Zealand do not possess a comprehensive regulatory framework on health claims for functional foods. The competitive marketplace and demand for new functional products appears to have encouraged the food industry's interest in obtaining government approval for health claims – especially since companies have invested time and money in the development of these products. However, most health claims for MCT oils and structured lipids are still banned in many countries.

Overall, functional foods, including MCT oils and structured lipids, are readily sold in markets worldwide. However, health claims are not allowed until further proof of action on weight loss is generated.

## 14.5 Future trends

The present chapter reviewed the experimental and clinical evidence for physiological effects of MCT on weight loss. The literature provides support for the hypothesis that MCT oil increases EE and decreases body fat in the majority of studies in both animals and humans. Furthermore, MCT may have a greater effect in overweight subjects than in normal weight or obese subjects. Short-term intakes of MCT oil have shown positive results for EE; however, chronic intakes of MCT have shown diverse effects on EE, body weight, and fat mass – probably due to metabolic adaptation. Therefore, other practices should be introduced to attempt to escape metabolic adaptation to MCT oil; these practices may include exercise, dietary change, or increased dose of MCT oil. Curbing appetite may play a bigger role in weight loss than EE in long-term feedings of MCT. Satiety may be related to increases in fat oxidation during MCT feeding; no specific hormones have been identified for this mechanism. Future research should examine the precise mechanism of satiety due to MCT oil. The exact areas of the body that are affected by weight loss are still unknown and may vary in different populations.

The food industry understands that fats and oils can be distinguished from one another by the amounts and positions of fatty acids on the TG molecule. However, the optimal ratio of MCT to LCT for beneficial effects on body composition and blood lipids needs to be researched. A variety of MCT and structured oils are available on the worldwide market. However, greater proof of action on weight loss without adverse effects on lipids is required before strong claims can be made for these products. It will be especially interesting to see the results of further research using MCT blended with other functional foods such as n-3 fatty acids, plant sterols, as well as diacylglycerol oil, including the benefits of these products for cardiovascular disease and obesity.

The optimal intake of MCT remains to be determined, but they can be safely ingested as 50% of total fat intake. Consumption of low doses of MCT has beneficial effects on weight, but more research is needed to determine the exact benefits. MCT should be consumed at every meal to have the maximum PP thermogenesis; however, studies testing the effects on EE of different frequencies of MCT intake have not been completed. MCT and structured oils can be found with a variety of health claims on the markets of all major countries. Nevertheless, there are still gaps to be filled by research regarding the dosage and duration of intake of MCT in order to have optimal weight loss effects. In conclusion, there is potential for MCT and structured lipids to be incorporated in food ingredients in the diet that may help prevent the obesity epidemic.

## 14.6 Sources of further information and advice

Sources of general information on MCT and structured lipids are listed below.

- Books:

GUNSTONE F D (2001), *Structured and Modified Lipids*, Marcel Dekker, New York.

GUNSTONE F D (2004), *The Chemistry of Oils and Fats: Sources, Composition, Properties, and Uses*, CRC Press, Boca Raton, Florida.

GUNSTONE F D and PADLEY F B (1997), *Lipid Technologies and Applications*, Marcel Dekker, New York.

- Review articles:

BABAYAN V K (1987), 'Medium-chain triglycerides and structured lipids', *Lipids*, **22**, 417–420.

BACH A C and BABAYAN V K (1982), 'Medium-chain triglycerides: an update', *Am J Clin Nutr*, **36**, 950–962.

BACH A C, INGENBLEEK Y and FREY A (1996), 'The usefulness of dietary medium-chain triglycerides in body weight control: fact or fancy?', *J Lipid Res*, **37**, 708–726.

ST-ONGE M P (2005), Dietary fats, teas, dairy, and nuts: potential functional foods for weight control?, *Am J Clin Nutr*, **81**, 7–15.

ST-ONGE M P and JONES P J (2002), 'Physiological effects of medium-chain triglycerides: potential agents in the prevention of obesity', *J Nutr*, **132**, 329–332.

- Website:

DEAN W and ENGLISH J (2004), 'Beneficial Effects on Energy, Atherosclerosis and Aging Medium Chain Triglycerides (MCT)',

Nutrition Review. Last accessed September 26th, 2005. http://www.nutritionreview.org/library/mcts.html.

## 14.7 References

BABA N, BRACCO E F and HASHIM S A (1982), 'Enhanced thermogenesis and diminished deposition of fat in response to overfeeding with diet containing medium chain triglyceride', *Am J Clin Nutr*, **35**, 678–682.

BABAYAN V K (1987), 'Medium-chain triglycerides and structured lipids', *Lipids*, **22**, 417–420.

BACH A, GUISARD D, METAIS P and DEBRY G (1972), 'Metabolic effects following a short and medium chain triglycerides load in dogs. I. Infusion of an emulsion of short and medium chain triglycerides', *Arch Sci Physiol (Paris)*, **26**, 121–129.

BACH A C, INGENBLEEK Y and FREY A (1996), 'The usefulness of dietary medium-chain triglycerides in body weight control: fact or fancy?', *J Lipid Res*, **37**, 708–726.

BARBERA R, PERACCHI M, BRIGHENTI F, CESANA B, BIANCHI P A and BASILISCO G (2000), 'Sensations induced by medium and long chain triglycerides: role of gastric tone and hormones', *Gut*, **46**, 32–36.

BEERMANN C, JELINEK J, REINECKER T, HAUENSCHILD A, BOEHM G and KLÖR H-U (2003), 'Short term effects of dietary medium-chain fatty acids and n-3 long-chain polyunsaturated fatty acids on the fat metabolism of healthy volunteers', *Lipids Health Dis*, **2**, 10–20.

BENDIXEN H, FLINT A, RABEN A, HOY C E, MU H, XU X, BARTELS E M and ASTRUP A (2002), 'Effect of 3 modified fats and a conventional fat on appetite, energy intake, energy expenditure, and substrate oxidation in healthy men', *Am J Clin Nutr*, **75**, 47–56.

BINNERT C, PACHIAUDI C, BEYLOT M, HANS D, VANDERMANDER J, CHANTRE P, RIOU J P and LAVILLE M (1998), 'Influence of human obesity on the metabolic fate of dietary long- and medium-chain triacylglycerols', *Am J Clin Nutr*, **67**, 595–601.

BRAY G A, LEE M and BRAY T L (1980), 'Weight gain of rats fed medium-chain triglycerides is less than rats fed long-chain triglycerides', *Int J Obes*, **4**, 27–32.

Canadian Food Inspection Agency Food Safety Directorate Bureau of Food Safety and Consumer Protection, 'Fair Labelling Practices Program Decisions: Fats, Oils and Fatty Acids', Section: Medium Chain Triglycerides. Last Accessed: August 28th, 2005. http://www.inspection.gc.ca/english/fssa/labeti/decisions/fatgrae.shtml.

CROZIER G, BOIS-JOYEUX B, CHANEZ M, GIRARD J and PERET J (1987), 'Metabolic effects induced by long-term feeding of medium-chain triglycerides in the rat', *Metabolism*, **36**, 807–814.

DULLOO A G, FATHI M, MENSI N and GIRARDIER L (1996), 'Twenty-four-hour energy expenditure and urinary catecholamines of humans consuming low-to-moderate amounts of medium-chain triglycerides: a dose-response study in human respiratory chamber', *Eur J Clin Nutr*, **50**, 152–158.

FEINLE C, RADES T, OTTO B and FRIED M (2001), 'Fat digestion modulates gastrointestinal sensations induced by gastric distention and duodenal lipid in humans', *Gastroenterology*, **120**, 1100–1107.

FLATT J P, RAVUSSIN E, ACHESON K J and JEQUIER E (1985), 'Effects of dietary fat on postprandial substrate oxidation and on carbohydrate and fat balances', *J Clin Invest*, **76**, 1019–1024.

FURUSE M, CHOI Y H, MABAYO R T and OKUMURA J (1992), 'Feeding behavior in rats fed diets containing medium chain triglyceride', *Physiol Behav*, **52**, 815–817.

Forbes Medi-Tech Inc. Nutraceuticals, vivola oil. Last accessed: August 30th, 2005. http://www.forbesmedi.com/s/vivolaoil.asp.

GELIEBTER A, TORBAY N, BRACCO E, HASHIM S A and VAN ITALLIE T B (1983), 'Overfeeding with medium-chain triglyceride diet results in diminished deposition of fat', *Am J Clin Nutr*, **37**, 1–4.

HILL J O, PETERS J C, LIN D, YAKUBU F, GREENE H and SWIFT L (1993), 'Lipid accumulation and body fat distribution is influenced by type of dietary fat fed to rats', *Int J Obes*, **17**, 223–236.

HILL J O, PETERS J C, YANG D, SHARP T, KALER M, ABUMRAD N N and GREENE H L (1989), 'Thermogenesis in humans during overfeeding with medium-chain triglycerides', *Metabolism*, **38**, 641–648.

HOPMAN W P, JANSEN J B, ROSENBUSCH G and LAMERS C B (1984), 'Effect of equimolar amounts of long-chain triglycerides and medium-chain triglycerides on plasma cholecystokinin and gallbladder contraction', *Am J Clin Nutr*, **39**, 356–359.

Institute of Food Technologists News (2005), Cognis Tackles Two-Fold Market Need: Exclusive Ingredients Add Functionality to Foods and Drinks and Enhance Health – The Natural Way. http://www.cognis.com/framescout.html?/Press/PressReleases2005/Health_And_Functional_Ingredients_eng.html.

KASAI M, NOSAKA N, MAKI H, NEGISHI S, AOYAMA T, NAKAMURA M, SUZUKI Y, TSUJI H, UTO H, OKAZAKI M and KONDO K (2003), 'Effect of dietary medium- and long-chain triacylglycerols (MLCT) on accumulation of body fat in healthy humans', *Asia Pac J Clin Nutr*, **12**, 151–160.

KASAI M, NOSAKA N, MAKI H, SUZUKI Y, TAKEUCHI H, AOYAMA T, OHRA A, HARADA Y, OKAZAKI M and KONDO K (2002), 'Comparison of diet-induced thermogenesis of foods containing medium- versus long-chain triacylglycerols', *J Nutr Sci Vitaminol (Tokyo)*, **48**, 536–540.

KROTKIEWSKI M (2001), 'Value of VLCD supplementation with medium chain triglycerides', *Int J Obes Relat Metab Disord*, **25**, 1393–1400.

LASEKAN J B, RIVERA J, HIRVONEN M D, KEESEY R E and NEY D M (1992), 'Energy expenditure in rats maintained with intravenous or intragastric infusion of total parenteral nutrition solutions containing medium- or long-chain triglyceride emulsions', *J Nutr*, **122**, 1483–1492.

LAVAU M M and HASHIM S A (1978), 'Effect of medium chain triglyceride on lipogenesis and body fat in the rat', *J Nutr*, **108**, 613–620.

MAAS M I, HOPMAN W P, KATAN M B and JANSEN J B (1998), 'Release of peptide YY and inhibition of gastric acid secretion by long-chain and medium-chain triglycerides but not by sucrose polyester in men', *Eur J Clin Invest*, **28**, 123–130.

MAGGIO C A and KOOPMANS H S (1982), 'Food intake after intragastric meals of short-, medium, or long-chain triglyceride', *Physiol Behav*, **28**, 921–926.

MATSUO T, MATSUO M, KASAI M and TAKEUCHI H (2001), 'Effects of a liquid diet supplement containing structured medium- and long-chain triacylglycerols on body fat accumulation in healthy young subjects', *Asia Pac J Clin Nutr*, **10**, 46–50.

NOSAKA N, MAKI H, SUZUKI Y, HARUNA H, OHARA A, KASAI M, TSUJI H, AOYAMA T, OKAZAKI M, IGARASHI O and KONDO K (2003), 'Effects of margarine containing medium-chain triacylglycerols on body fat reduction in humans', *J Atheroscler Thromb*, **10**, 290–298.

PAPAMANDHARIS A A, DI BUONO M F and JONES P J (1997), 'Fatty acid chain-length designations are important to study conclusions', *Am J Clin Nutr*, **66**, 710–712.

ROTHWELL N J and STOCK M J (1987), 'Stimulation of thermogenesis and brown fat activity in rats fed medium chain triglyceride', *Metabolism*, **36**, 128–130.

SCALFI L, COLTORTI A and CONTALDO F (1991), 'Postprandial thermogenesis in lean and obese subjects after meals supplemented with medium-chain and long-chain triglycerides', *Am J Clin Nutr*, **53**, 1130–1133.

SEATON T B, WELLE S L, WARENKO M K and CAMPBELL R G (1986), 'Thermic effect of medium-chain and long-chain triglycerides in man', *Am J Clin Nutr*, **44**, 630–634.

ST-ONGE M P and JONES P J (2003), 'Greater rise in fat oxidation with medium-chain triglyceride consumption relative to long-chain triglyceride is associated with lower initial body weight and greater loss of subcutaneous adipose tissue', *Int J Obes Relat Metab Disord*, **27**, 1565–1571.

ST-ONGE M P, BOURQUE C, JONES P J, ROSS R and PARSONS W E (2003a), 'Medium- versus long-chain triglycerides for 27 days increases fat oxidation and energy expenditure without resulting in changes in body composition in overweight women', *Int J Obes Relat Metab Disord*, **27**, 95–102.

ST-ONGE M P, ROSS R, PARSONS W D and JONES P J (2003b), 'Medium-chain triglycerides increase energy expenditure and decrease adiposity in overweight men', *Obes Res*, **11**, 395–402.

STUBBS R J and HARBRON C G (1996), 'Covert manipulation of the ratio of medium- to long-chain triglycerides in isoenergetically dense diets: effect on food intake in ad libitum feeding men', *Int J Obes Relat Metab Disord*, **20**, 435–444.

TAKEUCHI H, KASAI M, TAGUCHI N, TSUJI H and SUZUKI M (2002), 'Effect of triacylglycerols containing medium- and long-chain fatty acids on serum triacylglycerol levels and body fat in college athletes', *J Nutr Sci Vitaminol (Tokyo)*, **2**, 109–114.

TRAUL K A, DRIEDGER A, INGLE D L and NAKHASI D (2000), 'Review of the toxicologic properties of medium-chain triglycerides', *Food Chem Toxicol*, **38**, 79–98.

TSUJI H, KASAI M, TAKEUCHI H, NAKAMURA M, OKAZAKI M and KONDO K (2001), 'Dietary medium-chain triacylglycerols suppress accumulation of body fat in a double-blind, controlled trial in healthy men and women', *J Nutr*, **131**, 2853–2859.

VAN WYMELBEKE V, LOUIS-SYLVESTRE J and FANTINO M (2001), 'Substrate oxidation and control of food intake in men after a fat-substitute meal compared with meals supplemented with an isoenergetic load of carbohydrate, long-chain triacylglycerols, or medium-chain triacylglycerols', *Am J Clin Nutr*, **74**, 620–630.

WESTERTERP-PLANTENGA M S (2004a), 'Modulatory factors in the effect of energy density on energy intake', *Br J Nutr*, **92**, S35–39.

WESTERTERP-PLANTENGA M S (2004b), 'Fat intake and energy-balance effects', *Physiol Behav*, **83**, 579–585.

WHITE M D, PAPAMANDJARIS A A and JONES P J H (1999), 'Enhanced postprandial energy expenditure with medium-chain fatty acid feeding is attenuated after 14 d in premenopausal women', *Am J Clin Nutr*, **69**, 883–889.

YOST T J and ECKEL R H (1989), 'Hypocaloric feeding in obese women: metabolic effects of medium-chain triglyceride substitution', *Am J Clin Nutr*, **49**, 326–330.

# 15

# *Trans*-free oils and fats

**E. Flöter and G. van Duijn, Unilever Research and Development Vlaardingen, The Netherlands**

## 15.1 Introduction

The functionality of fats and oils in food products is twofold. These two main, unfortunately contradicting, aspects are nutrition and physical structure – related to oils and fats (solids) respectively. The term oil implies compositions essentially free of solid material at ambient temperature. Fats in contrast are at least semi-solid lipid materials. The physical functionality of fats is strongly related to the presence of saturated and *trans* fatty acids (TFA). These types of fatty acids do not, except for the delivery of energy, contribute much to the nutritional value of a food product. An often cited paper in 1993 (Willet *et al.*, 1993) is the starting point for the significant attention that the negative health effects of dietary TFA have received over the last decade. As a result of subsequent studies and publications it is widely agreed that a limitation of the intake of TFA is desirable. Fats high in saturated and/or *trans* fatty acids are used to give structure to semi-solid food emulsions like margarines, spreads and shortenings. In these emulsions the other main components are oil and water. A reduction of the energy content of such emulsions, for weight control, can be obtained by reducing the total oil and fat content. In such an exercise, the remaining oils and fats mixture should still be balanced for nutritional value (fatty acid composition) and should have sufficient structure to maintain the physical properties of the product. This chapter discusses the structuring functionality of different fat compositions with special attention to the role of TFA and their possible elimination.

### 15.1.1 The meaning of *trans*-free

In industrial practice there is practically no such thing as fat that is completely free of TFA. This is because fat compositions, except for in laboratory conditions, will almost always contain small amounts of TFA. They evolve either from natural processes or are due to configurational changes of the unsaturated bonds in fatty acids on exposure to elevated temperatures. However, these TFA are typically found at low levels, so their nutritional contribution can be neglected. This is not strictly true for ruminant fat with TFA levels of several per cent. Consequently the term 'virtually *trans* free' (VTF), implying levels of TFA of less than 1% in the fat phase seems an appropriate description for products that contain no deliberately generated or added TFA. The translation of the desire to restrict the consumption of TFA by legislators has so far resulted in quite divergent approaches. On the one hand, the Danish Veterinary and Food Administration issued an order (Stender and Dyerberg, 2003) that limits the concentration of TFA in fat phases of food products to a level below 2 weight per cent. Naturally occurring TFA in animal fats and conjugated linoleic acid are excluded from this restriction. On the other hand, the labeling of '0g *Trans*' in the United States as per 1 January 2006, according to the Food and Drug Administration (Food and Drug Administration, 2003), is related to an uptake of TFA of less than 0.5g per serving of the food product. Here the official definition of TFA reads 'all unsaturated fatty acids that contain one or more isolated double bonds in a *trans* configuration'. The FDA also excludes conjugated fatty acids from this definition. These quite divergent definitions and regulations allow for different technical solutions to compliance requirements.

### 15.1.2 Functional benefits of *trans* fatty acids

In the early 1990s partially hydrogenated fats could be found in essentially all fat applications that involved some kind of challenge to the fat composition. Partially hydrogenated fats were the most important and versatile ingredient for fat technologists. In simple terms, this role was based on three distinct properties: (1) the high chemical stability against oxidation of the partially hydrogenated fats, corresponding to the significantly reduced levels of polyunsaturated fatty acids (PUFA) compared with native oils; (2) the possibility of manipulating the melting profile of fat compositions as a function of the degree of hydrogenation; (3) partially hydrogenated fats have favorable crystallization properties as they crystallize quickly and effectively deliver structure to fat phases. An additional benefit of the application of partially hydrogenated fats is the fact that the final fat functionality is more dependent on the hydrogenation process than on the actual native starting fat. This feature creates a fair amount of raw material flexibility with its known benefits – a phenomenon described as 'interchangeability'.

Mildly hydrogenated oils are preferred in frying applications because their semi-liquid nature permits convenient handling while their chemical composition, in particular the absence of linolenic acid (18:3), ensures longevity of the frying medium. The extremely steep melting behavior related to high levels of TFA qualifies partially hydrogenated fats as good cocoa butter substitutes and coating fats. Compared with alternative fats with a similar melting range, TFA-containing fats show a solidification behavior that is clearly superior in manufacturing processes under quiescent conditions (the term 'quiescent' indicates the absence of shear during crystallization). A number of other applications require long-term storage at ambient temperatures. Examples are bouillon cubes, cookies and the like. In these applications aspects such as chemical stability, crystallization behavior for manufacturing and melting profile are of key importance. While the first two aspects are self-evident, the melting profile in these applications is related to a compromise between the absence of solid fatty residue or waxy mouthfeel when consumed and the integrity of the product over its shelf life. For this type of commodity the storage conditions are in essence not controlled and robust designs are necessary. Last but not least, the application of partially hydrogenated fats in spread products such as margarine is highly favored by the ease of manufacturing and the good structuring and melting behavior. In this product area the substitution of TFA has been widely achieved in Europe as the elimination process started in the mid 1990s. Before starting a detailed product-specific discussion of the conversion from partially hydrogenated fats to VTF fats it is necessary to consider aspects such as crystallization behavior, product integrity or stability, and melting behavior explicitly. Detailed discussions on the different aspects of chemical stability can be found elsewhere (Allen and Hamilton, 1994; Chan, 1987).

### 15.1.3 Crystallization behavior

To what extent a fat composition is suited to supply the necessary structure in a certain product application depends on a combination of the structuring potential of the formulation and the manufacturing process. Without reiterating the discussion of fat structures elsewhere (e.g. Marangoni *et al.*, 2006), a few basic comments on the structuring of fat phases must be made here. In a first rough approximation the structure or hardness of a semi-solid fat mixture is proportional to the amount of solid fat present (de Bruijne and Bot, 1999; Kloek, 1998). Taking a more refined view without going into any details, the number of continuous connections through the bulk of the mass and the strength of these connections drive the bulk rheological properties. The first aspect can be directly linked to the size and shape of the crystals present in the system. The rule of thumb supports the line of thought that smaller crystals are favorable. To get a comprehensive view of crystal–crystal interaction is far more complicated. In cases where only secondary bonds are considered, one might assume that the van de Waals adhesive forces between the various crystals are similar. They will, however, be very different if primary bonds come into play. Primary bonds are related to the so-called 'sintering'. As the term suggests this is the formation of solid bridges between the crystals of the primary network due to additional material crystallizing on the original fat crystal scaffolding (Johansson and Bergenstahl, 1995a). The presence of primary bonds delivers much harder structures but is accompanied by a dramatic increase in the brittleness of the semi-solid material. For products that are meant to be plastic, these primary bonds have to be avoided (Haighton, 1965). This is easily understood by appreciating that the slow relaxation of the sintered bonds involves re-crystallization of the bridging material.

The solid state of fats is characterized by monotropic polymorphism; polymorphism is the ability to appear in different forms. The different crystal structures – α, β′ and β – relate to different molecular packing arrangements. Each structure has its specific set of physical properties. The term 'monotropic' indicates that for a given composition only one of the three basic polymorphic forms is thermodynamically stable. More detailed descriptions of the polymorphism of fats can be found elsewhere (e.g. Sato, 1999, 2001). According to the basic principles of thermodynamics the molecular composition of a fat defines how much solid material can at best exist at any given temperature. If one ignores the fact that fats are complex multi-component mixtures, composed of numerous triacylglycerols (TAGs), knowledge of the physical properties for a given composition makes it possible to calculate the equilibrium solubility of each polymorph (Wesdorp, 1990). The solubility is straightforwardly – as usual this expression relates to a cumbersome exercise – converted into the so-called 'solid fat content' (SFC) at any given temperature. Typically, fat compositions are characterized according to their SFC. A few typical SFC lines are shown in Fig. 15.1. Owing to overriding kinetic influences, these are not a reflection of equilibrium states. The basic nature of the multi-component systems with possibly multiple solid phases in combination with a complicated crystallization behavior make the equilibration of these systems highly unlikely. The various TAGs that are supersaturated with respect to the system's temperature form multiple mixed crystals. How this process evolves is strongly dependent on the actual crystallization conditions. The main parameters by which to classify the process are: the supersaturation, the speed at which the supersaturation is generated and the shear the system is exposed to during the crystallization process. These parameters influence the essential processes of crystallization, i.e. nucleation and growth. The final size of the resulting crystals is strongly related to the management of these two processes. In instances of abundant nucleation, a large number of small crystals will evolve from the crystallization process. Nucleation increases with increasing supersaturation, as does crystal growth. However, the polymorphism of fats complicates this picture. When substantial supersaturation is

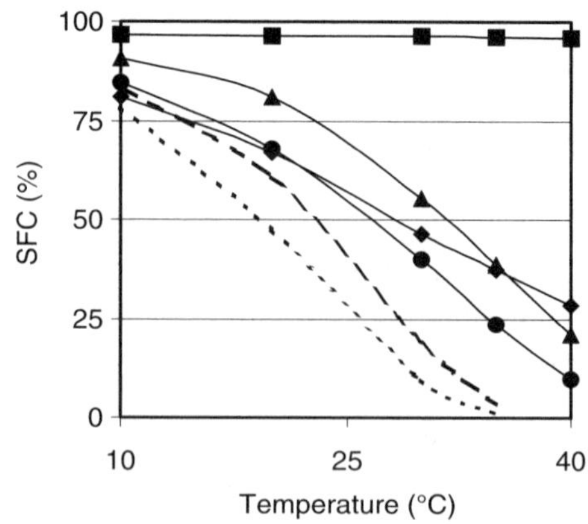


**Fig. 15.1** Solid fat content versus temperature lines for selected fats: - - - -, partially hydrogenated rapeseed oil (slip melting point, 32 °C); — — —, partially hydrogenated rapeseed oil (slip melting point, 36 °C); ●, interesterified fat based on palm oil and palm kernel fat; ◆, dry fractionated stearin of palm oil; ▲, partially hydrogenated palm oil (slip melting point, 44 °C); ■, fully hydrogenated palm oil (slip melting point, 58 °C).

applied the crystallizing material behaves according to Ostwald's famous rule of stages (Ostwald, 1897). This rule implies that a less-stable polymorph appears as an intermediate state in the crystallization process. Obviously this is subject to the necessary condition that this less-stable polymorph is also supersaturated. Consequently, a high supersaturation crystallization process takes place in the following order: supersaturated liquid → crystall ization α → transition into β′ or β.

In light of the fact that cocoa butter has a fairly simple structure – only three main TAGs account for 80% of the composition – and yet has six polymorphic forms, the above scheme is only a first approximation. The initial crystallization of the α polymorph can be controlled by the cooling process and occurs almost instantaneously once the solution is supersaturated with respect to the α form. In contrast to this, the solid-to-solid transition processes towards more stable polymorphic forms primarily depend on the fat composition. In the process description above, it is referred to as the β′ structure, as this more commonly persists over time in typical fat mixtures. In pure TAGs the β structure is considered the most stable polymorph due to the better crystal packing, but the β′ form is often energetically more favorable for crystals containing many different TAGs. Even though the crystallization process outlined above is more complicated than a single-step process, it is preferably applied in industrial practice. This is because this detour via the metastable crystal form is the fastest – and sometimes the only – way to create solid fat in the preferred final polymorph. The main complication resulting from this process is the adjustment of the manufacturing processes to the kinetics of the polymorphic transition, which is primarily a function of fat composition. Depending on the molecular composition of TAGs and also other minor components such as partial glycerides, the time scale of the polymorphic transition can vary between tens and thousands of seconds. To avoid the development of primary bonds it is advisable to manufacture in such a way that the polymorphic transition is largely achieved before packaging of the product (Bot *et al.*, 2003).

### 15.1.4 Product stability

The stability or integrity of products always has to be seen in the light of the challenge the product is potentially exposed to. For the fat-based products discussed here, the main challenge is typically the fluctuation of the storage temperature. Other minor challenges are of a mechanical nature due to handling and transportation. Another driver for product disintegration is obviously gravity. As discussed above the products also have the potential to change because they are not found in their true equilibrium state. This is particularly true as fat crystal structures tend to change over time even in the most controlled storage conditions. These changes are mainly due to relaxation processes in the network and Ostwald ripening (Bot and Pelan, 2000). Ostwald ripening describes the phenomenon where large crystals actually grow larger at the expense of small crystals. This process is driven by a difference in chemical potential that results from the higher surface energy contribution in the small crystals. Additionally, a typical industrial crystallization process, with high driving forces, results mostly in kinetically frozen non-equilibrium states (Bot *et al.*, 2003). This is possible because the speed at which the mixed solid system approaches its equilibrium state is extremely low.

At a macroscopic level there are principally five types of instabilities. These are: changes in the product hardness; product clumping for powders; oil exudation (meaning the separation of liquid oil out of the semi-solid mass); coalescence of droplets or change of the even distribution of the dispersed particles for emulsions and suspensions; and product inhomogeneity.

The hardness of a product might increase or decrease through a temperature challenge but change also occurs under well-controlled storage conditions. The reduction in hardness is accounted for by the coarsening of crystals. This is stimulated by temperature fluctuations since they involve a change in solubility. At higher temperatures some of the original solid material dissolves into the liquid oil and is re-deposited onto the solid material once the temperature is reduced again. Depending on whether the re-deposited solid forms solid bridges on the original scaffolding or just induces growth of the existing crystals, this process results in increased or reduced hardness respectively. Furthermore, either parts of or the whole crystal structure can undergo a polymorphic transition. This is either accompanied by a steep loss of product hardness or, in cases of a distinct segregation of specific TAGs into a certain conformation, by the occurrence of large crystals or distinct crystal agglomerates. A well-known example of this is the development of tropical graininess related to the separate crystallization of TAGs of the palmitic–oleic–palmitic type (Watanabe, 1992) derived from palm oil or its fractions in spherulitic crystals. The diameter of these particles can be as big as 2 mm. Another problem is the so-called 'sandiness' caused by large needle-like crystals that evolve from re-crystallization of TAGs made up from stearic and elaidic acid. The resulting particles are truly a product defect because their sizes are clearly above the threshold of oral perception, approximately 30 microns.

The process of clumping together of particles of a free-flowing powder is clearly related to temperature fluctuations. Adjacent particles partially melt and become greasy at elevated temperatures, forming a joint liquid layer. On cooling, this joint layer reverts to a solid or semi-solid structure gluing the particles together. Through this process a free-flowing powder can be easily converted into a solid brick.

The three other defects are strongly related to the coarsening of the crystalline network. The capacity of the fat crystal network to hold oil is based on capillary forces and adhesion similar to the function of a sponge. Smaller crystals generate much more surface and thus a finer sponge. On coarsening, it is less capable of holding oil. In most fat-based water-in-oil emulsion products, the main mechanism to stabilize the oil–water interface is Pickering stabilization (Pickering, 1907). This means that solid particles, in our case fat crystals, wet and cover the oil–water interface and thus prevent the coalescence of the water droplets (Johansson and Bergenstahl, 1995b; Johansson *et al.*, 1995a, 1995b; Rousseau *et al.*, 2003). Upon either crystal coarsening or depletion of the crystals due to higher temperatures the protective coverage of the interface might become incomplete or crystals start bridging the individual droplets and thus permit coalescence. This becomes a macroscopical problem only when excessive coalescence changes the product appearance. However, relatively limited progression of coalescence might also have detrimental effects on product quality. This is so because small droplets of diameters below 7 µm suppress microbiological growth through confinement (Verrips and Zaalberg, 1980; Verrips *et al.*, 1980). At larger droplet sizes, microbiological stability can usually only be ensured by use of preservatives such as potassium sorbate. Consequently, the microbiological stability of emulsion products free of preservatives relies on the maintenance of the small droplets.

Lastly, inhomogeneous distribution of solid material is most likely to occur in systems that are best described as viscous liquids. Here also the coarsening or partial dissolution of the fat crystal network is the main cause of the defective distribution of the particles. In such cases the fat scaffolding turns out not to be strong enough to immobilize the dispersed phase. This can yield either sedimentation or creaming of the dispersed phase.

### 15.1.5 Mouthfeel

The mouthfeel of a product is a multidimensional oral sensation. The main aspects of the mouthfeel are the structure breakdown on mastication, the release of flavor as a function of emulsion break-up, the cooling effect due to melting and, preferentially, the absence of waxy aftertaste due to high melting material. The fat crystals present directly influence these properties to a great extent. On mastication and heating the fat crystals start to melt and to dissolve. Intense mixing with saliva helps the heat transfer and also the dissolution. Additionally, kneading further improves heat transfer and softens the product, as fat crystal networks are sensitive to shear. The effects that the fat crystals have on the oral sensation are consequently mainly linked to SFC and crystal size. The cooling effect of a disintegrating product depends on how much solid material is actually melting in the mouth. This correlates to the steepness of the SFC curve in the temperature range from 20 to 34°C. This sensation is modulated by the speed of product disintegration, which depends on the heat transfer and shear, and also on the crystal size. Smaller crystals melt or dissolve much more quickly than bigger ones. The liberation of flavors from an emulsified water phase happens upon product inversion (Bot and Pelan, 2000; de Bruijn and Bot, 1999, de Bruijn *et al.*, 1993); this means during the emulsion breakdown induced by insufficient stabilization of the droplets by fat crystals (see Section 15.1.4). Finally if the amount of fatty material that remains solid in the mouth is too high, a few per cent, there is a risk that instead of the desirable lubrication, combined with beneficial flavor perception enhancement, a waxy sensation persists. TAGs melting above 50°C are typically associated with this phenomenon.

## 15.2 Requirements for *trans*-free fat compositions

There are two main requirements with respect to *trans*-free fat compositions: on the one hand the functional specification relating to the actual product application; on the other hand even though the TFA are eliminated, the formulation should not compromise the overall nutritional value of the composition. Furthermore one has to take into account that, for the successful elimination of TFA, time is also an important parameter. Immediate solutions can not afford to be registered as novel foods or suffer from long clearance procedures. Lastly, it is not very likely that the consumer will be willing to pay a premium for TFA-free products because the elimination of TFA is not an additional benefit but more a correction of the status quo driven by general consensus.

### 15.2.1 Functional requirements for successful *trans* fatty acid elimination

Every approach to substitute another fat for *trans*-containing partially hydrogenated fats in product applications is doomed to fail if one tries only to match the properties of the fat. With such a substitution only a limited set of the physical properties can be matched. Consequently the substitution process has to be based on a deep understanding of the application at hand. Consideration should also be given to how far it is acceptable that the change in fat composition is accompanied by a perceivable change of the product.

Starting from the simple end, chemical stability is based mainly on the absence of PUFA. Therefore alternative high stability oils, as used in frying applications, should also have a limited amount of PUFA. Another condition related to chemical deterioration is related to products containing enzymes, such as those present in herb preparations. Products containing herbs and significant amounts of medium-chain fatty acids such as lauric or myristic acid tend to develop a soapy taste over time through lipolysis.

In applications that rely on partially hydrogenated fats for structure, three aspects of the TFA are key to their success. These are the excellent crystallization behavior, the steep melting profile and the reliable formation of small crystals with the consequent high structuring effectiveness of the solid material. Consequently, successful substitutes will in the first place need to form small crystals to maintain product structure and stability. For manufacturing processes under more or less quiescent conditions with relatively low supersaturation, as for example found for bouillon cubes, it is necessary that the crystallization from a slurry to a solid mass proceeds in a comparable timeframe to the TFA-containing reference. Crispness and form stability of the product and the absence of stickiness are important attributes in the further manufacturing or packing of products.

Manufacturing processes with high supersaturation and high shear are related to high throughput and intrinsically to polymorphic transitions. These applications, such as spreads, necessitate that the substituting fat undergoes the polymorphic transition quickly. TFA containing fats undergo the polymorphic transition very quickly, often in less than 100 s. As the throughput of the manufacturing process scales inversely with the transition time, unless the hardware configuration of the manufacturing equipment is changed, dramatic increases of the transition time are prohibitive. As the final consumer remains king, obviously no substitution scenarios should yield a deterioration of properties perceived by the consumer, such as mouthfeel.

### 15.2.2 Nutritional constraints

Next to the functional and cost restrictions in the substitution of partially hydrogenated fats, a few other aspects have to be taken into account. TFA are considered to have more adverse effects on health than saturated fats (SFA). However, it is not desirable that the elimination of TFA results in final fat compositions with levels of saturated fats that are substantially higher than the original combined levels of TFA and SFA. It should also be mentioned that consumer understanding about TFA is limited and that therefore the discrimination between partially hydrogenated fats, high-*trans* and fully hydrogenated fats, and virtually zero *trans*, is blurred. An illustration of this is readily available via an Internet search on '*trans* fatty acids' status in spring 2005.

## 15.3 Production of *trans*-free fats and their application

The main tools that we find at our disposal for the fabrication of suitable fats for the substitution of partially hydrogenated fats are: hydrogenation, preferentially executed to iodine values close to zero; chemical or enzymatic interesterification; fractionation; and the search for new raw materials, possibly executed via modern plant breeding (e.g. Bockisch, 1993).

### 15.3.1 Full hydrogenation

A very low maximum TFA level can only be achieved by either no hydrogenation or by full hydrogenation. Full hydrogenation delivers fats with very high SFC levels. Tropical oils and fats are in their natural state already relatively saturated and therefore high in solids. They might be subjected to fractionation, see Section 15.3.3, in order to further increase their level of SFA. These two sources of concentrated SFA, hydrogenated fats or tropical fats, form the starting point for the manufacture of hardstocks, the structuring fats in a fat composition, by interesterification. Liquid oils contain hardly any solids. Therefore use of interesterification and/or fractionation alone as a means of reducing TFA in food compositions based on liquid oils used for hardstock production is not an option. Use of full hydrogenation is an option to generate a starting fat that is rich in SFA. As fully hydrogenated fats are, for reasons discussed above (melting profile and mouthfeel), only suited to a limited number of applications they are normally subject to further oil modification.

Factory-scale hydrogenation processes under normal conditions do not achieve complete saturation of all double bonds. Thus, the residual iodine value (IV) of a fully hydrogenated product is normally around 1–2. The IV is a measure of the degree of unsaturation of an oil or a fat, it gives the amount of iodine (in grams) that reacts with 100 g of oil or fat. A residual IV of 1 corresponds to 1.15% remaining monounsaturated fatty acids in the fat composition. For 'fully hydrogenated' fats (IV = 1–2), the thermodynamic equilibrium ratio between the *cis* and *trans* configuration of unsaturated fatty acids is reached (28/72). Combining these two pieces of evidence one finds that each IV point of the fully hydrogenated fat corresponds to 0.85% TFA. To obtain a product with a *trans* level below 1.25%, the hydrogenation should be continued until an IV below 1.5 is reached (the 'practical' specification of a fully hydrogenated product).

### 15.3.2 Interesterification

Interesterification permits a rearrangement or redistribution of the fatty acids on the glycerol backbone of the TAG molecules. Interesterification is promoted by an alkaline catalyst or by lipase. The most commonly used alkaline catalysts are sodium methylate and sodium ethylate. The mechanism of interesterification is described in detail in the literature (Rozendaal and Macrae, 1997). Alkaline-catalysed reactions produce a mixture of TAGs where the fatty acids are distributed randomly over all three positions of all TAG molecules.

In contrast to chemical interesterification, lipase catalysed reactions are more gentle. They proceed slowly and at lower temperatures. Temperature limitations are, for example, dictated by the thermal stability of the enzyme used. When applied to high-melting fats, for example, this can be a source of viscosity-related problems. For most enzymes used in fat technology, less than a handful beyond academic applications, only the two terminal positions of the glycerol backbone are randomized. The selectivity of the enzymes in many cases is not only limited to the configuration of the TAG but also to certain fatty acids. These are thus converted at specific reaction rates. Key parameters in the operation of enzyme-catalyzed rearrangement, an industrial application still in an infant state, are water activity, raw material pre-treatment and enzyme utilization. Since the process proceeds at a much lower rate than the chemical interesterification, it allows an abundance of different fat phases to be created from a given starting mixture. This is so because the process can, through variation of contact time, be managed such that only partial randomization is achieved.

The alkaline (sodium (m)ethylate)-catalysed reaction takes place in prerefined oil (low in water and in free fatty acids) at elevated temperatures (100–110 °C). The reaction is very fast; full randomization is reached within a few minutes even in factory-scale vessels (10–40 tons oil content). After the reaction, the catalyst is deactivated by water addition; sodium hydroxide and (m)ethyl esters will be formed. Sodium hydroxide will react with fatty acids and oil to form soap, which is subsequently removed by water washing and decanting. (M)ethyl esters are more volatile than TAG molecules and are removed during standard downstream processing, i.e. high-temperature deodorization.

The modification of the fatty acid distribution of the TAG molecules by interesterification will in general lead to a modification of the solid phase line, resulting in a change in the crystallization behavior. This is particularly true because typically a mixture of fats and/or oils with different SFC profiles is subjected to this process.

### 15.3.3 Fractionation

Fractionation is a process that separates a fat phase into two phases according to the crystallization behavior of its molecular species. This slow, well controlled crystallization process aims at the manufacture of preferentially large crystals to be separated from the surrounding mother liquor. The resulting high-melting fraction, solid crystals plus liquid entrapment after filtration, is referred to as stearin. The remaining liquid fraction, with the same composition as the entrapment, is called olein. It is easily appreciated that unless additional solvent is added to the system (solvent fractionation) only a limited amount of solid material, typically less than 25%, can be separated out of a fat composition.

By far the most important oil fractionated worldwide is palm oil; the main reason being the demand for clear liquid oil (palm olein). More recently there has been a growing interest in the solid product of palm oil fractionation (palm stearin), for production of cocoa butter equivalents, cocoa butter replacers and margarine hardstocks. Besides palm oil, palm kernel oil, partly hydrogenated liquid oils, cottonseed oil and milk fat are also fractionated.

The fractionation process consists of the following steps:

1 Crystal nucleation.
2 Crystal growth.
3 Crystal slurry filtration.
4 Filter cake squeezing/pressing.

There are two defined forms of nucleation: primary and secondary. Primary nuclei are formed when oil is supersaturated or under-cooled; this is the driving force of the fractionation process. Secondary nucleation is the result of 'mechanical' attrition of existing crystals. The presence or addition of secondary crystals shortens the induction time necessary for primary nucleation and can initiate a better-controlled crystal growth regime. The aim for fractionation is to grow large, dense crystal agglomerates that can easily be separated from the liquid oil. The level of supersaturation and the presence of growth nuclei essentially drive crystal growth. Crystal slurry is made up of potentially fragile crystal agglomerates. This slurry must not experience high shear stresses during the transfer to the filter and inside the filter. The filtration characteristics of the slurry depend on size of the crystal agglomerates, the separation efficiency of the slurry and the solid phase content. Most modern fractionation plants use membrane filter presses. These enable the filter cake, produced by simple filtration, to be squeezed to both increase the yield of olein and produce a harder stearin.

The combination of process conditions influencing these fractionation steps determines the characteristics and yield of both the olein and stearin. The most important parameters for solid fat production are:

- the type and quality of the feedstock;
- the crystallization temperature;
- the type and size of the crystals;
- the efficiency of the separation process.

### 15.3.4 *Trans*-free fat production

Full hydrogenation offers a simple answer to the search for chemically stable fatty materials, as required for example in frying applications. However, replacing a *trans*-containing viscous liquid with a solid block of fully hydrogenated fat for frying applications might not be agreeable; particularly because fully hydrogenated oils have slip melting points above 65 °C and would quickly generate a solid fat layer around fried goods. In the recent past there has been a lot of activity from oil suppliers associated with the launch of new *trans*-free oils. In 2004, Dow AgroSciences, Bunge and DuPont all launched their various brands of zero- or low-*trans* oils, with Cargill and Bayer CropScience joining in 2005. Most of these oils are supposed to be an answer to the limited chemical stability of conventional oils as these new oils are high-oleic (low-linoleic) fatty acid variants of soybean, canola or other seed oils. The new traits have been developed by conventional breeding or by genetic modification techniques. Alternatively, one could attempt the procurement of more stable oils through fractionation of, for example, palm oil. In doing so, however, it has to be noted that even a double-fractionated palm olein is relatively rich in SFA, approximately 30%, as this is just the nature of the TAGs present in palm oil; it contains a large fraction of palmitic–oleic–oleic acid-based TAGs.

For applications that rely on the structuring function of TFA-containing TAGs, the substitution can be much more difficult. While in the applications focusing on chemical stability the absence of PUFA is the key objective, here specific TAGs that truly functionally substitute for the TFA-containing TAGs have to be identified. This means that, depending on the specific application, tailor-made solutions have to be sought. Applications of fats where high temperature stability and manufacturability are key can be served by fat compositions rich in fully saturated TAGs. These are most easily generated by full hydrogenation, producing a fat composition rich in stearic acid. If, for reasons of consumer preference, hydrogenation has to be avoided then stearin fractions of palm oil also offer the starting point for compositions rich in fully saturated TAGs. Either wet (solvent-supported) fractionation or multiple-step dry fractionation deliver palm stearins with levels of SFA of more than 80%. Both routes outlined above create fat compositions rich in only a single TAG, typically tristearin in fully hydrogenated seed oils and tripalmitin in palm stearin. This may not deliver the functionality of mixed crystals, which tend to be small. To this end, one could either just mix these fats or subject them conjointly to an interesterification process. If the melting behavior of a fat composition is important not only for the stability and integrity of a product, but also for the mouthfeel or deposition behavior, then the fat has to satisfy a much narrower specification. Fully saturated TAGs based solely on palmitic or stearic acid have to be used in very limited amounts on such occasions. The steep melting of partially hydrogenated fats and their good mouthfeel are based on the physical properties of TAGs containing both stearic acid and elaidic acid. These yield a range of individual TAG melting points well above body temperature but below 60 °C. Nature delivers TAGs with melting points in this range very sparingly. These glycerol esters are composed of two saturated and one unsaturated fatty acid with the fatty acids typically arranged in a symmetric fashion (SUS: saturated–unsaturated–saturated). They can be found in, for example, cocoa butter, well appreciated for its melting behavior, and a range of other exotic fats, such as sal fat, kokum fat, shea nut oil, mango kernel oil and obviously also palm oil. A significantly increased use of palm oil and palm oil fractions is already anticipated by oil suppliers as they currently enlarge their production capacities. An alternative way to manufacture a fat composition rich in SUS- and SSU-TAGs is currently promoted by ADM and Novozymes. One of their enzymatically interesterified hardstocks is based on fully hydrogenated soybean oil and native soybean oil. This is particularly interesting for the United States because of the relatively low acceptance of palm oil. Besides this approach there have been numerous attempts to develop seed oils with elevated levels of stearic acid, rich in SUS-TAGs, none of which has yet generated a fat that is available on an industrial scale.

The SUS-TAGs unfortunately have a melting point very close to body temperature and typically show a complicated and slow crystallization behavior. The relatively low melting point of SUS-TAGs necessitates that, for elevated temperature structuring, high levels of these TAG are present. The two features mentioned, in combination with their price and limited availability, make these TAG less suited for robust commodity applications.

Alternatively, TAGs composed of saturated medium-chain and long-chain fatty acids also melt in the desired intermediate temperature range (see also Garti and Sato, 1988). Unfortunately these do not exist naturally. They can be fabricated by esterification of a mixture of fats containing adequate amounts of long-chain SFA, derived from palm oil from full hydrogenation, and medium-chain fatty acids present in palm kernel or coconut fat. Since interesterification always delivers a statistical mix of triglycerides in accordance with the starting fatty acid mixture, the concentration of the targeted, high-melting (HM) TAGs, of di-long-chain, mono-medium-chain fatty acids is always limited.

Alternatively, similar high melting fats with good crystallization properties can be fabricated by full hydrogenation of palm kernel fat. To further optimize the characteristics of this fat, highly suitable for coating and other cocoa-butter-like applications, it is often subsequently interesterified to randomize the distribution of its fatty acids. In spite of the suggestion that interesterified fully hydrogenated palm kernel fat is a good alternative for partially hydrogenated fats, its application in other products remains limited due its price and its interaction with enzymes.

For the replacement of partially hydrogenated fats in spreads and similar applications other constraints apply. In the first place, modern spreads, soft tub products, are typically designed to deliver high amounts of healthy liquid oils. This implies that the structuring fat, in general referred to as hardstock, is used in limited quantities. Similar fats as discussed above qualify for use in spreads. As already outlined, for manufacturing processes under high supersaturation, the kinetics of the polymorphic transition is of prime importance. It turns out that fat rich in TAGs composed of medium- and long-chain SFA (HM-TAG) actually have short transition times. Furthermore, this type of TAG, possibly driven by the fairly complex packing at the molecular level into the crystal lattice, produce smaller crystals than for example fully saturated long-chain fatty acid-based TAGs. This makes the mixed saturated TAGs particularly suitable candidates for the substitution of partially hydrogenated fats. It has to be noted here that, in this substitution, the melting profile of the products will also change according to the illustration in Fig. 15.1. Interesterified fats yield relatively straight SFC versus temperature lines that can be manipulated by the composition of the interesterification mixture. With straightforward application of interesterified fats, the limits of a high SFC at 20 °C in combination with very low SFC levels at 35 °C are quickly reached. In order to create significantly steeper SFC lines, either TAGs of the SUS type or HM-TAG levels have to be optimized in the formulation. This can be achieved by combination of different hardstocks. However, in mixing, for example, an HM-TAG hardstock with cocoa butter fat, economically not very attractive for spreads, one can find that instead of a synergistic benefit quite the opposite occurs. At certain mixing ratios, immiscibility of the TAG in the solid phase occurs and both SFC and structuring potential actually drop. This illustrates that the mixing behavior of the TAGs, which can be influenced by the processing conditions, is a key element in the design of functional fat compositions. In the attempt to fabricate highly functional hardstocks, fractionation plays an important role. There are two possible applications of fractionation: it can be applied either pre- or post-interesterification. The economics of the application of fractionation depend heavily on the value and usage of the secondary fraction evolving from the separation process. For example, to increase the concentration of HM-TAG in a fat, one could improve the yield of the interesterification with respect to the HM-TAG concentration by optimizing the fatty acid composition of the starting materials towards two-thirds of stearic plus palmitic acid mixed with one-third of lauric acid. The elimination of unsaturated fatty acids from the interesterification mixture can be achieved by utilization of fully hydrogenated starting materials. However, for non-hydrogenated fat compositions, fractionation of the starting materials is the only tool available to move in this direction. The abundant use of palm stearin in interesterifications, which due to the good market value of palm olein is economically attractive, is the most prominent example of this process. Again this supports the installation of increased palm oil manufacturing capacities as mentioned before. Higher yields of functional TAGs in the hardstock fats can be achieved by fractionation applied after interesterification. However, there are two downsides to this manufacturing approach. First, the TAGs one wants to concentrate are characterized by mixed crystal formation with relatively small crystal sizes. This feature obviously has adverse effects on the smooth execution of the fractionation process, as the separation of the stearin and the olein fractions will be negatively affected. Remedies to this drawback can either be the use of solvent fractionation, with significant cost implications, or redesign of the process. Secondly, the by-product from post-fractionation processes is less likely to be of high value, hence possibly creating prohibitive cost for the overall application. In general it is fair to conclude that post-fractionation of hardstock fats is considered a last resort in the substitution of partially hydrogenated fats as it will add substantial cost. However, for other high-value applications, the process discussed might very well be suitable.

## 15.4 Implementation of *trans*-free fats in manufacturing and the supply chain

The nature of the successful replacement of partially hydrogenated fats, as outlined above, yields a number of specific solutions to specific product applications. The identification of the respective best set of solutions for a manufacturer is more complicated. On implementing a technical solution, the balance between utilization of a special fat composition, re-design of the manufacturing process and complexity of the supply chain – more raw materials on-site – has to be found. All three factors are related to additional costs. Consequently, they should all be subject to optimization after initial *trans*-free solutions are established. The complexity of a new *trans*-free raw material portfolio could be a 'show stopper' in cases where layout and tank capacity of a manufacturing site do not allow implementation. Either investment in hardware or preferentially harmonization of raw materials can overcome this impasse. This harmonization of *trans*-free raw materials needs to involve process optimization and the re-evaluation of product specifications. In retrospective consideration of the elimination of *trans*-fatty acids in practically all European spreads, one finds that actually the industry as a whole has undergone such a process of harmonization towards an optimal raw material base. Subsequent to the original elimination of TFA in the mid 1990s, initial solutions have been further optimized.

Products have slowly changed and it turns out that finally a wide range of products use a limited set of structuring fats. This industry-wide optimization process has obviously also been helped by the consolidation of the oil and fat suppliers.

## 15.5 Future trends

Future developments with respect to the elimination of TFA will depend to a great extent on non-technical issues. The choice of the legal framework can drive the evolution of technology. The Danish legislation practically bans partially hydrogenated fats from food. In contrast to this, the FDA endorsed the limitation of uptake of TFA per serving, which can in some instances be met with lower fat products still based on partially hydrogenated fats. Finally, consumer preference will decide what product technology will prevail, for example whether consumers accept full hydrogenation or not. The power of consumer preference is documented in the fact that canola oil is well appreciated as a very healthy oil in Scandinavia but is practically unsaleable in Spain because of its unhealthy image, due to a malpractice involving canola oil in 1981. Similarly, Europeans use a vast amount of products based on palm oil, which is only sparingly found in US products.

The main future technology developments relevant to TFA elimination, beyond those already mentioned, are the increased use of non-TAG structuring. This is already advocated by ingredient suppliers and is the subject of numerous research projects. However, these mainly emulsifier-based structuring techniques have not yet found widespread application. This is because, among other reasons, the known systems such as those based on monoglycerides or combinations of fatty acids and fatty alcohols are not suited for emulsion systems.

## 15.6 Conclusions

The replacement of partially hydrogenated fats – with their role in aerating, emulsifying, lubricating and providing texture, structure and flavor characteristics to food products – is a challenge for food developers. Due to the versatility and robustness of partially hydrogenated fats their substitution is strongly application specific. An understanding of the specific application of partially hydrogenated fats and the resulting functional specifications of alternative fats is a necessary pre-requisite for a successful substitution. This process eliminates some historical specifications and could result in a change in technological paradigms. Local consumer preference and legal frameworks have a strong influence on technology evolution with respect to the *trans*-free challenge. Finally, in the short term, technological solutions are likely to be based on the smart combination of conventional oil modification techniques.

## 15.7 References

ALLEN J C and HAMILTON R J (1994), *Rancidity in Foods*, 3rd edition, Glasgow, Blackie Academic & Professional.

BOCKISCH M (1993), *Nahrungsfette und Öle, Handbuch der Lebensmitteltechnologie*, Stuttgart, Ulmer Verlag.

BOT A and PELAN E (2000), 'Food emulsions inside and outside the mouth', *Food Ingredients and Analysis International*, **22** (6), 53–58.

BOT A, FLÖTER E, LAMMERS J G and PELAN E (2003), 'Controlling the texture of spreads', in McKenna B M (Ed.), *Texture in Foods*, volume 1: *Semi-solid Foods*, Cambridge, Woodhead Publishing, pp. 350–372.

CHAN H W-S (1987), *Autoxidation of Unsaturated Lipids*, London, Academic Press.

DE BRUIJNE D W and BOT A (1999), 'Fabricated fat-based foods', in Rosenthal A J (Ed.), *Food Texture: Measurement and Perception*, Gaithersburg, Aspen, pp. 185–227.

DE BRUIJNE D W, HENDRICKX H C A M, ALDERLIESTEN L and DE LOOFF J (1993), 'Mouthfeel of foods', in Dickinson E and Walstra P (Eds), *Food Colloids and Polymers: Stability and Mechanical Properties*, Cambridge, Royal Society of Chemistry, pp. 204–213.

Food and Drug Adminstration (2003), *Food Labeling: Trans Fatty Acids in Nutrition Labeling, Nutrient Content Claims, and Health Claims*, Federal Register – 68 FR 41433 July 11, 2003.

GARTI N and SATO K (1988), *Crystallization and Polymorphism of Fats and Fatty Acids*, New York, Marcel Dekker.

HAIGHTON A J (1965), 'Worksoftening of margarine and shortening', *Journal of American Oil Chemists' Society*, **42**, 27–30.

JOHANSSON D and BERGENSTAHL B (1995a), 'Sintering of fat crystal networks in oil during post-crystallisation processes', *Journal of the American Oil Chemists' Society*, **72**, 911–920.

JOHANSSON D and BERGENSTAHL B (1995b), 'Wetting of fat crystals by triglyceride oil and water II. Adhesion to the oil/water interface', *Journal of the American Oil Chemists' Society*, 72, 933–938.

JOHANSSON D, BERGENSTAHL B and LUNDGREN E (1995a), 'Wetting of fat crystals by triglyceride oil and water I. The effect of additives', *Journal of the American Oil Chemists' Society*, **72**, 921–931.

JOHANSSON D, BERGENSTAHL B and LUNDGREN E (1995b), 'Water-in-triglyceride emulsions. Effect of fat crystals on stability', *Journal of the American Oil Chemists' Society*, **72**, 939–950.

KLOEK W (1998), Mechanical properties of fats in relation to their crystallization, PhD Thesis, University of Wageningen, The Netherlands.

MARTINI S, AWAD T and MARANGONI A G (2006), 'Structure and properties of fat crystal networks', in Gunstone F (Ed.), *Modifying Lipids for Use in Food*, Chapter 8, Cambridge, Woodhead Publishing Limited, pp. 142–169.

OSTWALD W (1897), 'Studien uber die Bildung und Umwandlung Fester Korper', *Zeitschrift der Physikalischen Chemie*, **22**, 289–293.

PICKERING S U (1907), 'Emulsions', *Journal of the Chemical Society*, **91**, 2001–2021.

ROUSSEAU D, ZILNIK L, KHAN R and HODGE S M (2003), 'Dispersed phase destabilisation in table spreads', *Journal of the American Oil Chemists' Society*, **80**, 957–961.

ROZENDAAL A and MACRAE A R (1997), 'Interesterification of oils and fats', in Gunstone F D and Padley F B (Eds), *Lipid Technologies and Applications*, New York, Marcel Dekker, pp. 223–263.

SATO K (1999), 'Solidification and phase transformation behaviour of food fats – a review', *Fett/Lipid*, **101**, 467–474.

SATO K (2001), 'Crystallization behaviour of fats and lipids – a review', *Chemical Engineering Science*, **56**, 2255–2265.

STENDER S and DYERBERG J (2003), *The Influence of Trans Fatty Acids on Health*, 4th edition, Danish Nutritional Council.

VERRIPS C T and ZAALBERG J (1980), 'The intrinsic stability of water-in-oil emulsions. 1. Theory', *European Journal of Applied Microbiology and Biotechnology*, **10**, 187–196.

VERRIPS C T, SMID D and KERKHOF A (1980), 'The intrinsic stability of water-in-oil emulsions. 2. Experimental', *European Journal of Applied Microbiology and Biotechnology*, **10**, 73–85.

WATANABE A, TASHIMA I, MATSUZAKI N, KURASHIGE J and SATO K (1992), 'On the formation of granular crystals in fat blends containing palm oil', *Journal of the American Oil Chemists' Society*, **69**, 1077–1080.

WESDORP L H (1990), Liquid-multiple solid phase equilibria in fats, theory and experiments, PhD Thesis, TU Delft, The Netherlands.

WILLETT W C, STAMPFER M J, MANSON J E, COLDITZ G A, SPEIZER F E, ROSNER B A, SAMPSON L A and HENNEKENS C H (1993), 'Intake of TFA and risk of coronary heart disease among women', *Lancet*, **341** (8845), 581–585.

# Index